The 10-Minute Diagn

Symptoms and Signs in the

D1586526

Editor

Robert B. Taylor, M.D.
Professor of Family Medicine
Oregon Health Sciences University School of Medicine
Portland, Oregon

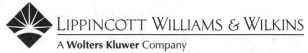

LIPPINCOTT WILLIAMS & WILKINS
A **Wolters Kluwer** Company
Philadelphia · Baltimore · New York · London
Buenos Aires · Hong Kong · Sydney · Tokyo

Acquisitions Editor: Richard Winters
Developmental Editor: Michelle LaPlante
Production Editor: Emily Lerman
Manufacturing Manager: Kevin Watt
Cover Designer: Patricia Gast
Compositor: Circle Graphics
Printer: R. R. Donnelley, Crawfordsville

© 2000 by **LIPPINCOTT WILLIAMS & WILKINS**
530 Walnut Street
Philadelphia, PA 19106 USA
LWW.com

All rights reserved. This book is protected by copyright. No part of this book may be reproduced in any form or by any means, including photocopying, or utilized by any information storage and retrieval system without written permission from the copyright owner, except for brief quotations embodied in critical articles and reviews. Materials appearing in this book prepared by individuals as part of their official duties as U.S. government employees are not covered by the above-mentioned copyright.

Printed in the USA

Library of Congress Cataloging-in-Publication Data

Manual of 10-minute diagnosis : how to evaluate symptoms and signs in the time-limited encounter / [edited by] Robert B. Taylor.
        p. ; cm.
    Includes bibliographical references and index.
    ISBN 0-7817-2732-4 (alk. paper)
        1. Symptoms—Handbooks, manuals, etc. 2. Diagnosis—Handbooks, manuals, etc. I. Title: Manual of ten minute diagnosis. II. Taylor, Robert B.
        [DNLM: 1. Diagnosis—Handbooks. WB 39 M2949 2000]
    RC69 .M364 2000
    616.07´5—dc21

                                                                        00-020705

Care has been taken to confirm the accuracy of the information presented and to describe generally accepted practices. However, the authors, editor, section editors, and publisher are not responsible for errors or omissions or for any consequences from application of the information in this book and make no warranty, expressed or implied, with respect to the currency, completeness, or accuracy of the contents of the publication. Application of this information in a particular situation remains the professional responsibility of the practitioner.

The authors, editor, section editors, and publisher have exerted every effort to ensure that drug selection and dosage set forth in this text are in accordance with current recommendations and practice at the time of publication. However, in view of ongoing research, changes in government regulations, and the constant flow of information relating to drug therapy and drug reactions, the reader is urged to check the package insert for each drug for any change in indications and dosage and for added warnings and precautions. This is particularly important when the recommended agent is a new or infrequently employed drug.

Some drugs and medical devices presented in this publication have Food and Drug Administration (FDA) clearance for limited use in restricted research settings. It is the responsibility of the health care provider to ascertain the FDA status of each drug or device planned for use in their clinical practice.

10 9 8 7 6 5 4 3 2

CONTENTS

1. PRINCIPLES OF THE 10-MINUTE DIAGNOSIS
Robert B. Taylor

2. UNDIFFERENTIATED PROBLEMS
Eric M. Walsh, Section Editor

3. MENTAL HEALTH PROBLEMS
Thomas L. Campbell, Section Editor

4. PROBLEMS RELATED TO THE NERVOUS SYSTEM
Anne Cather Cutlip, Section Editor

5. EYE PROBLEMS
John E. Sutherland, Section Editor

6. EAR, NOSE, AND THROAT PROBLEMS
Frank S. Celestino, Section Editor

7. CARDIOVASCULAR PROBLEMS
Jim Nuovo, Section Editor

8. RESPIRATORY PROBLEMS
Joseph E. Scherger, Section Editor

9. GASTROINTESTINAL PROBLEMS
Michael R. Spieker, Section Editor

10. RENAL AND UROLOGIC PROBLEMS
R. Whitney Curry, Jr., Section Editor

11. PROBLEMS RELATED TO THE FEMALE REPRODUCTIVE SYSTEM
Kathryn M. Andolsek, Section Editor

12. MUSCULOSKELETAL PROBLEMS
Elise M. Coletta, Section Editor

13. DERMATOLOGIC PROBLEMS
Michael L. O'Dell, Section Editor

14. ENDOCRINE AND METABOLIC PROBLEMS
Richard D. Blondell, Section Editor

15. VASCULAR AND LYMPHATIC SYSTEM PROBLEMS
Paul M. Paulman, Section Editor

16. LABORATORY ABNORMALITIES:
HEMATOLOGY AND URINE DETERMINATIONS
Lars C. Larsen, Section Editor

17. LABORATORY ABNORMALITIES:
BLOOD CHEMISTRY AND IMMUNOLOGY
Judith A. Fisher, Section Editor

18. DIAGNOSTIC IMAGING ABNORMALITIES
Enrique S. Fernandez, Section Editor

CONTRIBUTING AUTHORS

Samuel B. Adkins, III, M.D.
Assistant Professor of Family Medicine, East Carolina University School of Medicine, Greenville, North Carolina
16.2 Eosinophilia

Gowri Anandarajah, M.D.
Clinical Assistant Professor of Family Medicine, Brown University School of Medicine, Providence, Rhode Island
12.9 Shoulder Pain

Kathryn M. Andolsek, M.D., M.P.H.
Clinical Professor of Community and Family Medicine, Duke University School of Medicine, Durham, North Carolina
11.7 Pap Smear Abnormality

Mark Douglas Andrews, M.D.
Assistant Professor of Family and Community Medicine, Wake Forest University School of Medicine, Winston-Salem, North Carolina
6.1 Halitosis

David E. Anisman, M.D.
Assistant Clinical Professor of Family and Community Medicine, University of California, Davis, School of Medicine, Sacramento, California; Department of Family Practice, David Grant Medical Center, Travis Air Force Base, California
7.6 Heart Murmur, Diastolic

Mark Bajorek, M.D.
Assistant Professor of Family Medicine, Oregon Health Sciences University School of Medicine, Portland, Oregon
2.11 Night Sweats

Cindy Barter, M.D.
Faculty Physician, Mercy Family Medicine, St. John's Mercy Medical Center, St. Louis, Missouri
9.6 Epigastric Distress

Thomas C. Bent, M.D.
Associate Clinical Professor of Family Medicine, University of California, Irvine, College of Medicine, Irvine, California
8.9 Wheezing

Dale Bishop, M.D.
Clinical Professor of Family Medicine, University of California, Davis, School of Medicine, Sacramento, California
7.7 Heart Murmur, Systolic

Melissa B. Black, M.D.
Assistant Professor of Family and Community Medicine, University of Alabama School of Medicine, Birmingham, Alabama
13.2 Erythema Multiforme

Shawn H. Blanchard, M.D.
Assistant Professor of Family Medicine, Oregon Health Sciences University School of Medicine, Portland, Oregon
2.1 Anorexia

Duane Bland, M.D.
Assistant Clinical Professor of Family and Community Medicine, University of
California, Davis, School of Medicine, Sacramento, California; Shasta-Cascade
Family Practice Residency Program, Redding, California
7.8 Hypertension

Carol Blenning, M.D.
Assistant Professor of Family Medicine, Oregon Health Sciences University
School of Medicine, Portland, Oregon
2.8 Hypersomnia

Richard D. Blondell, M.D.
Professor of Family and Community Medicine, University of Louisville
School of Medicine, Louisville, Kentucky
14.3 Hirsutism

Kent D. W. Bream, M.D.
Clinical Instructor, Department of Family Practice and Community Medicine,
University of Pennsylvania School of Medicine, Philadelphia, Pennsylvania
17.5 Hyperkalemia
17.6 Hypokalemia

James M. Brian, M.D.
Staff Family Physician, Occupational and Community Health, National Naval
Medical Center, Bethesda, Maryland
9.10 Jaundice

Douglas G. Browning, M.D., A.T.C.
Assistant Professor of Family Medicine, Wake Forest University School of Medicine,
Winston-Salem, North Carolina
6.4 Nosebleed

Charles L. Bryner, Jr., M.D.
Director of Clinical Services, U.S. Naval Hospital, Rota, Spain
9.12 Steatorrhea

David E. Bybee, M.D.
Assistant Clinical Professor of Medicine, University of Louisville School of Medicine,
Louisville, Kentucky
14.4 Hypothyroidism
14.6 Thyroid Enlargement/Goiter
14.7 Thyroid Nodule
14.8 Thyrotoxicosis/Hyperthyroidism

Thomas L. Campbell, M.D.
Professor of Family Medicine and Psychiatry, University of Rochester
School of Medicine and Dentistry, Rochester, New York
3.1 Anxiety

Rosemarie Cannarella, M.D.
Associate Professor of Family Medicine, West Virginia University School of Medicine,
Harpers Ferry, West Virginia
4.6 Parathesia and Dysesthesia

Rachelle L. Cassity, M.D.
Assistant Professor of Family Medicine, University of Alabama School of Medicine
at Huntsville, Huntsville, Alabama
13.7 Urticaria

Frank S. Celestino, M.D.
Associate Professor of Family and Community Medicine, Wake Forest University School of Medicine, Winston-Salem, North Carolina
6.5 Pharyngitis
6.9 Vertigo

S. Shekar Chakravarthi, M.B., B.S.
Associate Clinical Professor of Family Medicine, East Carolina University School of Medicine, Greenville, North Carolina
16.1 Anemia

Ku-Lang Chang, M.B., B.Ch.
Clinical Assistant Professor of Family Medicine, University of Florida College of Medicine, Gainesville, Florida
10.2 Hematuria

Marcia J. Chesebro, M.D.
Associate Professor of Family Medicine, University of Alabama School of Medicine at Huntsville, Huntsville, Alabama
13.8 Vesicular and Bullous Eruptions

James C. Chesnutt, M.D.
Assistant Professor of Family Medicine, Oregon Health Sciences University School of Medicine, Portland, Oregon
2.12 Syncope

C. Randall Clinch, D.O.
Assistant Professor of Family Medicine, Uniformed Services University of the Health Sciences; Director, Division of Predoctoral Programs, Department of Family Medicine, National Naval Medical Center, Bethesda, Maryland
9.2 Ascites

John Coe, M.D.
Assistant Professor of Family and Community Medicine, University of California, Davis, School of Medicine, Sacramento, California; Shasta-Cascade Family Practice Residency Program, Redding, California
7.4 Cardiomegaly

Elise M. Coletta, M.D.
Assistant Professor of Family Medicine, Brown University School of Medicine, Providence, Rhode Island
12.3 Hip Pain
12.7 Neck Pain

Joyce A. Copeland, M.D.
Clinical Associate Professor of Family Medicine, Duke University School of Medicine, Durham, North Carolina
11.2 Breast Mass
11.6 Nipple Discharge

Susan C. Cullom, D.O.
Assistant Professor of Family Medicine, Uniformed Services University of the Health Sciences, Bethesda, Maryland
9.8 Hepatitis

Alicia J. Curtin, R.N., M.S.N.
Senior Clinical Teaching Associate of Family Medicine, Brown University School of Medicine, Providence, Rhode Island
12.2 Calf Pain

L. Gail Curtis, B.A., P.A.-C.
Assistant Professor of Family and Community Medicine, Wake Forest University School of Medicine, Winston-Salem, North Carolina
6.3 Hoarseness

Anne Cather Cutlip, M.D.
Associate Professor of Family Medicine, West Virginia University School of Medicine, Morgantown, West Virginia
4.2 Coma
4.4 Dementia

Mark D. Darrow, M.D.
Associate Professor of Family Medicine, East Carolina University School of Medicine, Greenville, North Carolina
16.7 Thrombocytopenia

Stephen Davis, M.D.
Clinical Associate Professor of Family Medicine, Brown University School of Medicine, Providence, Rhode Island
12.5 Low Back Pain

Gehan Devendra, M.D.
Clinical Instructor of Internal Medicine, University of California, Davis, Medical Center, Sacramento, California
7.12 Tachycardia

L. Allen Dobson, Jr., M.D.
Cabarrus Family Medicine Residency Program, Concord, North Carolina; Assistant Clinical Professor of Community and Family Medicine, Duke University School of Medicine, Durham, North Carolina
11.1 Amenorrhea

Michael J. Dodard, M.D.
Associate Professor of Clinical Family Medicine and Community Health, University of Miami, School of Medicine, Miami, Florida
18.4 Solitary Pulmonary Nodule

Gregory A. Doyle, M.D.
Associate Professor of Family Medicine, West Virginia University School of Medicine, Morgantown, West Virginia
4.8 Stroke

Alexandra Duke, D.O.
Assistant Clinical Professor of Family Medicine, University of California, Irvine, College of Medicine, Irvine, California
8.8 Stridor

Charles B. Eaton, M.D.
Associate Professor of Family Medicine, Brown University School of Medicine, Providence, Rhode Island
12.4 Knee Pain

Richard W. Emerine, M.D., M.P.H.
Faculty of Family Medicine, Family Practice Residency, Naval Hospital, Camp Pendleton, California; Assistant Clinical Professor of Family Medicine, University of California, San Diego, School of Medicine, La Jolla, California; Clinical Assistant Professor of Family Practice, Uniformed Services University of the Health Sciences, Bethesda, Maryland
9.1 Abdominal Pain

Ted Epperly, M.D.
Chairman, Department of Family and Community Medicine, Eisenhower Army Medical Center, Fort Gordon, Georgia
9.11 Rectal Bleeding

Paul Evans, D.O.
Associate Professor of Family Medicine, Associate Dean for Curricular Affairs, Oklahoma State University College of Osteopathic Medicine, Tulsa, Oklahoma
2.3 Edema

Lyle J. Fagnan, M.D.
Associate Professor of Family Medicine, Oregon Health Sciences University School of Medicine, Portland, Oregon
2.6 Fever

Gerald F. Farnell, M.D.
Staff Physician, David Grant Medical Center, Department of Family Practice, Travis Air Force Base, California
7.6 Heart Murmur, Diastolic

David B. Feller, M.D.
Assistant Professor of Family Medicine, University of Florida College of Medicine, Gainesville, Florida
10.6 Priapism

Scott A. Fields, M.D.
Associate Professor of Family Medicine, Oregon Health Sciences University School of Medicine, Portland, Oregon
2.1 Anorexia

Judith A. Fisher, M.D.
Assistant Professor of Family Practice and Community Medicine, University of Pennsylvania School of Medicine, Philadelphia, Pennsylvania
17.1 Alkaline Phosphatase, Elevated
17.2 Aminotransferase Levels, Elevated
17.3 Antinuclear Antibody Titer, Elevated
17.4 Hypercalcemia
17.5 Hyperkalemia
17.6 Hypokalemia

Michael B. Foster, M.D.
Associate Professor of Pediatrics, University of Louisville School of Medicine, Louisville, Kentucky
14.1 Diabetes Mellitus

Cara K. Fox, B.S., P.A.S.
Department of Occupational and Community Health, National Naval Medical Center, Bethesda, Maryland
9.10 Jaundice

Marcia W. Funderburk, M.D.
Clinical Associate Professor of Family Medicine, University of Florida College of Medicine, Jacksonville, Florida
10.5 Oliguria and Anuria

Kathleen E. Gallagher, M.D.
Assistant Clinical Professor of Family Medicine, University of California, Irvine, College of Medicine, Irvine, California
8.6 Pneumothorax

Joseph P. Garry, M.D.
Assistant Professor of Family Medicine, East Carolina University School of Medicine, Greenville, North Carolina
16.3 Erythrocyte Sedimentation Rate, Elevated

Barbara A. Gawinski, Ph.D.
Associate Professor of Family Medicine, University of Rochester School of Medicine and Dentistry, Rochester, New York
3.4 Suicidal Risk

Mark F. Giglio, M.D.
Associate Clinical Professor of Family Medicine, University of California, Irvine, College of Medicine, Irvine, California
8.4 Pleural Effusion

M. Gina Glazier, M.B., B.Ch.
Clinical Instructor of Family Practice and Community Medicine, University of Pennsylvania School of Medicine, Philadelphia, Pennsylvania
17.1 Alkaline Phosphatase, Elevated
17.4 Hypercalcemia

Arnold Goldberg, M.D.
Clinical Assistant Professor of Family Medicine, Brown University School of Medicine, Providence, Rhode Island
12.8 Polymyalgia

Meredith A. Goodwin, M.D.
Assistant Professor of Family Medicine, Brown University School of Medicine, Providence, Rhode Island
12.1 Arthralgia
12.3 Hip Pain
12.7 Neck Pain

David B. Graham, M.D.
Clinical Assistant Professor of Family Medicine, Oregon Health Sciences University School of Medicine, Portland, Oregon; Private Practice, Strawberry Wilderness Family Clinic, John Day, Oregon
2.13 Weight Loss

Pepi Granat, M.D.
Professor of Family Medicine, University of Miami School of Medicine, Miami, Florida
18.1 Bone Cyst
18.2 Mediastinal Mass
18.3 Osteopenia

Tahany Maurice-Habashy, M.D.
Assistant Clinical Professor of Family Medicine, University of California, Irvine, College of Medicine, Irvine, California
8.8 Stridor

Irene M. Hamrick, M.D.
Assistant Clinical Professor of Family Medicine, East Carolina University School of Medicine, Greenville, North Carolina
16.6 Proteinuria

Richard W. Harper, M.D.
Assistant Clinical Professor of Family Medicine, University of California, Davis, School of Medicine, Sacramento, California
7.3 Bradycardia

Jeffrey D. Harrison, M.D.
Assistant Professor of Family Medicine, University of Nebraska College of Medicine, Omaha, Nebraska
15.1 Lymphadenopathy, Generalized

Robert L. Hatch, M.D., M.P.H.
Associate Professor of Family Medicine, University of Florida College of Medicine, Gainesville, Florida
10.7 Scrotal Mass

Meg Hayes, M.D.
Assistant Professor of Family Medicine, Oregon Health Sciences University School of Medicine, Portland, Oregon
2.5 Fatigue

Charles E. Henley, D.O., M.P.H.
Professor and Chair of Family Medicine, Oklahoma State University College of Osteopathic Medicine, Tulsa, Oklahoma
2.9 Insomnia

Douglas I. Ivins, M.D.
Clinical Instructor of Family Practice and Community Medicine, University of Pennsylvania School of Medicine, Philadelphia, Pennsylvania
17.2 Aminotransferase Levels, Elevated
17.3 Antinuclear Antibody Titer, Elevated

Anthony F. Jerant, M.D.
Assistant Professor of Family and Community Medicine, University of California, Davis, School of Medicine, Sacramento, California
7.5 Congestive Heart Failure

Victoria S. Kaprielian, M.D.
Associate Clinical Professor of Family Medicine, Duke University School of Medicine, Durham, North Carolina
11.8 Postmenopausal Bleeding

Stephen H. Keiser, M.D.
Assistant in Family Medicine and Sports Medicine, Wake Forest University School of Medicine, Winston-Salem, North Carolina
6.4 Nosebleed

W. Robert Kiser, M.D., M.A.
Assistant Professor of Family Medicine, Uniformed Services University of the Health Sciences, Naval Hospital, Jacksonville, Florida
9.3 Constipation

Mark Knudson, M.D.
Associate Professor of Family Medicine, Wake Forest University School of Medicine, Winston-Salem, North Carolina
6.2 Hearing Loss

Mary Knudtson, M.S.N., N.P.
Assistant Clinical Professor of Family Medicine, University of California, Irvine, College of Medicine, Irvine, California
8.3 Hemoptysis

Charles M. Kodner, M.D.
Assistant Professor of Family Medicine, University of Louisville School of Medicine, Louisville, Kentucky
14.2 Gynecomastia

Louis Kuritzky, M.D.
Courtesy Clinical Assistant Professor, University of Florida College of Medicine, Gainesville, Florida
10.3 Impotence

Kathryn M. Larsen, M.D.
Clinical Professor of Family Medicine, University of California, Irvine, College of Medicine, Irvine, California
8.3 Hemoptysis

Bruce A. Leibert, M.D.
Assistant Clinical Professor of Family Medicine, University of Texas Health Sciences Center, San Antonio, Texas; Director, Family Practice Residency Program, Valley Baptist Medical Center, Harlingen, Texas
9.9 Hepatomegaly

Gary I. Levine, M.D.
Associate Professor of Family Medicine, East Carolina University School of Medicine, Greenville, North Carolina
16.5 Polycythemia

Désirée A. Lie, M.D., M.S.Ed.
Associate Clinical Professor of Family Medicine, University of California, Irvine, College of Medicine, Irvine, California
8.1 Cough

Jeffrey M. Lyness, M.D.
Associate Professor of Psychiatry, University of Rochester School of Medicine and Dentistry, Rochester, New York
3.3 Depression

Mark A. Marinella, M.D.
Assistant Clinical Professor of Internal Medicine, Wright State University School of Medicine, Dayton, Ohio
7.10 Pericardial Friction Rub

Gail S. Marion, P.A.C., Ph.D.
Associate Professor of Family and Community Medicine, Wake Forest University School of Medicine, Winston-Salem, North Carolina
6.6 Rhinitis

Richard C. Mauer, M.D.
Department of Ophthalmology, Allen Memorial Hospital and Covenant Medical Center, Waterloo, Iowa; University of Iowa School of Medicine, Iowa City, Iowa
5.2 Diplopia
5.4 Papilledema

Albert A. Meyer, M.D.
Associate Clinical Professor of Community and Family Medicine, Duke University School of Medicine, Durham, North Carolina
11.3 Chronic Pelvic Pain
11.4 Dysmenorrhea
11.5 Menorrhagia
11.9 Vaginal Discharge

Cynthia M. Moore-Sledge, M.D.
Assistant Professor of Family Medicine, University of Alabama at Birmingham, Birmingham, Alabama
13.1 Alopecia

John Muench, M.D.
Assistant Professor of Family Medicine, Oregon Health Sciences University
School of Medicine, Portland, Oregon
2.2 Dizziness

Laeth S. Nasir, M.D.
Associate Professor of Family Medicine, University of Nebraska College of Medicine,
Omaha, Nebraska
15.2 Lymphadenopathy, Localized

Soraya Nasraty, M.D.
Assistant Professor of Family and Community Medicine, University of Louisville
School of Medicine, Louisville, Kentucky
14.5 Polydipsia

Konrad C. Nau, M.D.
Associate Professor of Family Medicine, West Virginia University School of Medicine,
Harpers Ferry, West Virginia; Director, Rural Family Medicine Residency Program,
Jefferson Memorial Hospital, Ranson, West Virginia
4.5 Memory Impairment

Sara Lynn Neal, M.D.
Assistant Director of Residency Training, Department of Family and Community
Medicine, Wake Forest University School of Medicine, Winston-Salem, North Carolina
6.8 Tinnitus

Janis F. Neuman, M.D.
Assistant Clinical Professor of Family Medicine, University of California, Riverside,
School of Medicine, Riverside, California; Residency Director, Kaiser Permanente
Fontana, Fontana, California
8.2 Cyanosis

Mark W. Nickels, M.D.
Clinical Assistant Professor of Psychiatry, University of Rochester School of Medicine
and Dentistry, Rochester, New York
3.2 Confusion

Jim Nuovo, M.D.
Associate Professor of Family and Community Medicine, University of California,
Davis, School of Medicine, Sacramento, California
7.1 Chest Pain, Atypical

Vincent H. Ober, M.D.
Assistant Clinical Professor of Community Health and Family Medicine,
University of Florida College of Medicine, Jacksonville, Florida
10.4 Nocturia

Francis G. O'Connor, M.D.
Assistant Professor of Family Medicine, Uniformed Services University of the Health
Sciences, Bethesda, Maryland
9.4 Diarrhea

Michael L. O'Dell, M.D.
Associate Professor of Family Medicine, University of Alabama School of Medicine
at Huntsville, Huntsville, Alabama
13.3 Maculopapular Rash
13.4 Pigmentation Disorders
13.6 Rash Accompanied by Fever

Michael Ostapchuk, M.D.
Assistant Professor of Family Medicine, University of Louisville School of Medicine, Louisville, Kentucky
14.1 Diabetes Mellitus

Audrey Paulman, M.D.
Assistant Clinical Professor of Family Medicine, University of Nebraska College of Medicine, Omaha, Nebraska
15.4 Splenomegaly

Gary K. Phelps, M.D.
Department of Ophthalmology, Covenant Medical Center, Waterloo, Iowa
5.1 Blurred Vision
5.5 Pupillary Inequality

Michael J. Puk, M.D.
Department of Ophthalmology, Covenant Medical Center, Allen Memorial Hospital, Waterloo, Iowa
5.3 Nystagmus
5.7 Scotoma

David M. Quillen, M.D.
Assistant Professor of Community Health and Family Medicine, University of Florida College of Medicine, Gainesville, Florida
10.1 Dysuria

Richard Rathe, M.D.
Associate Professor of Family Medicine, University of Florida College of Medicine, Gainesville, Florida
10.10 Urinary Incontinence

Brian V. Reamy, M.D., Lt. Col., U.S.A.F.
Residency Director, Department of Family Practice, David Grant Medical Center, Travis Air Force Base, California; Clinical Associate Professor of Family Practice, University of California, Davis, School of Medicine, Sacramento, California
7.11 Raynaud's Phenomenon

Julie A. Reeves, M.D.
Clinical Instructor of Family Medicine, East Carolina University School of Medicine, Greenville, North Carolina
16.4 Neutropenia

Paul C. Riggle, M.D.
Assistant Clinical Professor of Family Medicine, University of California, Davis, School of Medicine, Sacramento, California
7.3 Bradycardia

Omart Robaina, M.D.
Assistant Professor of Clinical Family Medicine and Community Health, University of Miami School of Medicine, Miami, Florida
18.1 Bone Cyst

Jay S. Roitman, D.O.
Assistant Clinical Professor of Family and Community Medicine, University of California, Davis, School of Medicine, Sacramento, California; Shasta-Cascade Family Practice Residency Program, Redding, California
7.8 Hypertension

Joseph E. Ross, M.D.
Clinical Assistant Professor of Family Medicine, University of Illinois College of Medicine at Rockford, Rockford, Illinois
2.4 Falls

Michael P. Rowane, D.O., M.S.
Assistant Professor of Family Medicine, Case Western Reserve University School of Medicine, Cleveland, Ohio
2.3 Edema

Robert B. Sammel, M.D.
Assistant Professor of Family Medicine, West Virginia University School of Medicine, Harpers Ferry, West Virginia
4.1 Ataxia

George P. N. Samraj, M.D., M.R.C.O.G.
Assistant Professor of Family Medicine, University of Florida College of Medicine, Gainesville, Florida
10.9 Urethral Discharge

Ron Sand, M.D.
Shasta-Cascade Family Practice Residency Program, Redding, California; Assistant Professor of Family and Community Medicine, University of California, Davis, School of Medicine, Sacramento, California
7.4 Cardiomegaly

Linda M. Savory, M.D.
Professor of Family Practice, Marshall University School of Medicine, Huntington, West Virginia
4.7 Seizures

Siegfried Schmidt, M.D., Ph.D.
Clinical Assistant Professor of Community Health and Family Medicine, University of Florida College of Medicine, Gainesville, Florida
10.2 Hematuria

Stephen Schmidt, M.D.
Assistant Clinical Professor, Dwight D. Eisenhower Army Medical Center, Fort Gordon, Georgia
11.7 Pap Smear Abnormality

David M. Schneider, M.D.
Faculty Physician, Mercy Healthcare Sacramento Family Practice Residency Program; Assistant Clinical Professor of Family and Community Medicine, University of California, Davis, School of Medicine, Sacramento, California
7.9 Palpitations

Linda P. Shields, M.D.
Assistant Professor of Family Medicine, West Virginia University School of Medicine, Harpers Ferry, West Virginia
4.3 Delirium

Hal S. Shimazu, M.D.
Assistant Clinical Professor of Family Medicine, University of California, Irvine, College of Medicine, Irvine, California
8.5 Pleuritic Pain

John L. Smith, M.D.
Assistant Professor of Family Medicine, University of Nebraska College of Medicine, Omaha, Nebraska
15.3 Petechiae and Purpura

John G. Spangler, M.D., M.P.H.
Assistant Professor of Family and Community Medicine, Wake Forest University School of Medicine, Winston-Salem, North Carolina
6.7 Stomatitis

Michael R. Spieker, M.D.
Assistant Professor of Family Medicine, Uniformed Services University of the Health Sciences, Naval Hospital, Jacksonville, Florida
9.5 Dysphagia

Mark B. Stephens, M.D.
Assistant Professor of Family Medicine, Uniformed Services University of the Health Sciences, Bethesda, Maryland
9.7 Gastrointestinal Bleeding

John E. Sutherland, M.D.
Clinical Professor of Family Medicine, University of Iowa College of Medicine, Iowa City, Iowa; Program Director, Northeast Iowa Family Practice Residency, Waterloo, Iowa
5.6 Red Eye

Robert B. Taylor, M.D.
Professor of Family Medicine, Oregon Health Sciences University School of Medicine, Portland, Oregon
2.7 Headache

Peter G. Teichman, M.D., M.P.A.
Assistant Professor of Family Medicine, West Virginia University School of Medicine, Harpers Ferry, West Virginia
4.9 Tremor

Robert M. Theal, M.D.
Family Practice Residency Program, Kaiser Permanente Fontana, Fontana, California
8.7 Shortness of Breath

Margaret A. Tryforos, M.D.
Clinical Assistant Professor of Family Medicine, Brown University School of Medicine, Providence, Rhode Island
12.6 Monarticular Joint Pain

Beverly A. VonderPool, M.D.
Associate Professor of Family and Community Medicine, University of Alabama School of Medicine at Birmingham, Birmingham, Alabama
13.5 Pruritis

Eric M. Walsh, M.D.
Assistant Professor of Family Medicine, Oregon Health Sciences University School of Medicine, Portland, Oregon
2.10 Nausea and Vomiting

Douglas C. Warren, M.D., Lt. Col., U.S.A.F.
Associate Residency Director, Department of Family Practice, David Grant Medical Center, Travis Air Force Base, California; Clinical Assistant Professor of Family and Community Medicine, University of California, Davis, School of Medicine, Sacramento, California
7.11 Raynaud's Phenomenon

Stephen F. Wheeler, M.Ch.E., M.D.
Assistant Professor of Family Medicine, University of Louisville School of Medicine, Louisville, Kentucky
14.4 Hypothyroidism
14.6 Thyroid Enlargement/Goiter
14.7 Thyroid Nodule
14.8 Thyrotoxicosis/Hyperthyroidism

Darryl G. White, M.D.
Assistant Clinical Professor of Family Practice, University of Texas Health Science Center, San Antonio, Texas; Faculty, Valley Baptist Family Practice Residency Practice, Harlingen, Texas
9.9 Hepatomegaly

George R. Wilson, M.D.
Associate Professor of Community Health and Family Medicine, University of Florida College of Medicine, Jacksonville, Florida
10.8 Scrotal Pain

Anna M. Wright, M.D.
Clinical Assistant Professor of Community Health and Family Medicine, University of Florida College of Medicine, Jacksonville, Florida
10.4 Nocturia

Marie K. Yamamotoya, M.D.
Academic and Clinical Fellow of Family and Community Medicine, University of California, Davis, School of Medicine, Sacramento, California
7.2 Chest Pain, Substernal

SECTION EDITORS

Kathryn M. Andolsek, M.D., M.P.H.
Clinical Professor of Community and Family Medicine, Duke University School of Medicine, Durham, North Carolina
11. Problems Related to the Female Reproductive System

Richard D. Blondell, M.D.
Professor of Family and Community Medicine, University of Louisville School of Medicine, Louisville, Kentucky
14. Endocrine and Metabolic Problems

Thomas L. Campbell, M.D.
Professor of Family Medicine and Psychiatry, University of Rochester School of Medicine and Dentistry, Rochester, New York
3. Mental Health Problems

Frank S. Celestino, M.D.
Associate Professor of Family and Community Medicine, Wake Forest University School of Medicine, Winston-Salem, North Carolina
6. Ear, Nose, and Throat Problems

Elise M. Coletta, M.D.
Assistant Professor of Family Medicine, Brown University School of Medicine, Providence, Rhode Island
12. Musculoskeletal Problems

R. Whitney Curry, Jr., M.D.
Professor and Chairman, Department of Community Health and Family Medicine, University of Florida College of Medicine, Gainesville, Florida
10. Renal and Urologic Problems

Anne Cather Cutlip, M.D.
Associate Professor of Family Medicine, West Virginia University School of Medicine, Morgantown, West Virginia
4. Problems Related to the Nervous System

Enrique S. Fernandez, M.D., M.S.Ed.
Associate Professor of Clinical Family Medicine and Community Health, University of Miami School of Medicine, Miami, Florida
18. Diagnostic Imaging Abnormalities

Judith A. Fisher, M.D.
Assistant Professor of Family Practice and Community Medicine, University of Pennsylvania School of Medicine, Philadelphia, Pennsylvania
17. Laboratory Abnormalities: Blood Chemistry and Immunology

Lars C. Larsen, M.D.
Assistant Dean for Generalist Programs, East Carolina University School of Medicine, Greenville, North Carolina
16. Laboratory Abnormalities: Hematology and Urine Determinations

Jim Nuovo, M.D.
Associate Professor of Family and Community Medicine, University of California, Davis, School of Medicine, Sacramento, California
7. Cardiovascular Problems

Michael L. O'Dell, M.D.
Associate Professor of Family Medicine, University of Alabama School of Medicine at Huntsville, Huntsville, Alabama
13. Dermatologic Problems

Paul M. Paulman, M.D.
Professor of Family Medicine, University of Nebraska Medical Center, Omaha, Nebraska
15. Vascular and Lymphatic System Problems

Joseph E. Scherger, M.D.
Professor and Chair, Department of Family Medicine and Associate Dean for Clinical Affairs, University of California, Irvine, School of Medicine, Irvine, California
8. Respiratory Problems

Michael R. Spieker, M.D.
Assistant Professor of Family Medicine, Uniformed Services University of the Health Sciences, Naval Hospital, Jacksonville, Florida; Residency Program Director, Puget Sound Family Medicine Residency Program, Bremerton, Washington
9. Gastrointestinal Problems

John E. Sutherland, M.D.
Clinical Professor of Family Medicine, University of Iowa College of Medicine, Iowa City, Iowa; Program Director, Northeast Iowa Family Practice Residency, Waterloo, Iowa
5. Eye Problems

Robert B. Taylor, M.D.
Professor of Family Medicine, Oregon Health Sciences University School of Medicine, Portland, Oregon
1. Principles of the 10-Minute Diagnosis

Eric M. Walsh, M.D.
Assistant Professor of Family Medicine, Oregon Health Sciences University School of Medicine, Portland, Oregon
2. Undifferentiated Problems

PREFACE

The 10-Minute Diagnosis Manual is intended to be a quick-reference source for the primary care clinician faced with a diagnostic problem such as headache, fatigue, anemia, or jaundice. The book is structured in the same way in which we arrive at a diagnosis, starting not with a disease label, but with a chief complaint or, perhaps, an unexpected clinical finding. Chapter topics were selected because they occur commonly in the primary care setting or because they are likely to be first encountered by the primary care clinician. These topics include symptoms (e.g., dizziness), physical abnormalities (e.g., splenomegaly), and laboratory determinations (e.g., proteinuria). The chapters in the book are about diagnosis, and therapy is mentioned only if it might be relevant to diagnosis, such as the response of an inflamed joint to colchicine.

The "10-minute" premise of the book is based on studies showing that 10-minute office visits are the norm in primary care today.[1] Even with longer duration visits, the time devoted to diagnosis—and not to therapy, procedures, patient education, and so forth—is likely to be about ten minutes. Also, to the degree possible in a quick-reference guide, authors have presented information using an evidence-based approach.[2] For more on the book's premise and approach, see Chapter One.

Chapters are of a uniform length that is convenient for rapid reading during a patient care session, and each chapter is organized according to six major headings: Approach, History, Physical Examination, Testing, Diagnostic Assessment, and References.

I am grateful to the 18 section editors and to the 139 contributing authors. I also thank the following individuals who assisted with the development and production of this book: Coelleda O'Neil and Victoria Brown of the Department of Family Medicine of the Oregon Health Sciences University, Executive Editor Richard Winters and Developmental Editor Michelle LaPlante of Lippincott Williams & Wilkins, and Production Editor Emily Lerman.

I hope that you will find this book a useful guide to commonly encountered symptoms and signs, and that you will reach for this book first when you need help with diagnosis during a busy practice day.

Robert B. Taylor, M.D.
Portland, Oregon

---

[1] Stange KC, Zyzanski SJ, Jaen CR. Illuminating the "black box": a description of 4454 patient visits to 138 family physicians. *J. Fam Pract* 1998;46:377–389.
[2] Rosser WW. Application of evidence from randomized controlled trials to general practice. *Lancet* 1999;353:661–664.

1. PRINCIPLES OF THE 10-MINUTE DIAGNOSIS

ROBERT B. TAYLOR

1. Principles of the 10-Minute Diagnosis

Robert B. Taylor

Ten minutes for diagnosis? Really?

Yes, really!

If only we had 90 minutes to perform a diagnostic evaluation, as we did as third-year medical students on hospital rotations. Or, if we even had 30 minutes for diagnosis, as I recall from internship. But those days are gone. Today—as clinicians practicing in the age of evidence-based, cost-effective healthcare—office visits are of much shorter duration than in years past. For example, in a recent study of 4,454 patients seeing 138 physicians in 84 practices, the mean visit duration was 10 minutes (1). Another study of 19,192 visits to 686 primary care physicians estimated the visit duration to be 16.3 minutes (2). Even when the total visit duration exceeds 10 minutes, the time actually devoted to diagnosis—and not to greeting the patient, explaining treatment, doing managed care paperwork, or even the patient's dressing and undressing—is seldom more that 10 minutes.

So, if you and I generally have only 10 minutes per office visit for diagnosis, we need to be focused, while remaining medically thorough and prudent. Actually such an approach is possible, and is how experienced clinicians tend to practice. The following are some practice guidelines to the 10-minute diagnosis (*Dx10*). And, to illustrate, let us consider a patient: *Joan S., a 49-year-old married woman in your office for a first visit whose chief complaint is severe, one-sided headaches that have become worse over the past year.* (For a more complete approach to the diagnosis of headache, see Chapter 2.7.)

Search for Diagnostic Cues Throughout the Clinical Encounter

Note how the patient relates to the staff, takes off a jacket, and sits in the examination room. How does the patient begin to describe the problem and what does he or she seem to want from the visit? Who accompanies the patient to the office and who seems to do the talking?

Be sure to use "tell me about" open-ended questions. The inexperienced clinician moves early to closed-ended "Yes" or "No" questions, but the veteran *Dx10* clinician has learned that using narrow questions too early can lead to misleading conclusions, which, at least in the long run, are wasteful of time and, at worst, dangerous. An example would be inappropriately attributing chest pain to gastroesophageal reflux disease because the patient has a past history of esophageal reflux and responds affirmatively to questions about current heartburn and intolerance to spicy foods.

Watch the facial reaction to issues discussed. Tune in to hesitation and evasive answers, and be willing to follow these diagnostic paths, which may lead to the otherwise hidden problems such as drug abuse or domestic violence. *In the case of Joan S., does she answer questions readily, or does she seem evasive when addressing some topics, such as family concerns or her home life?*

Think "Most Common" First

I remind medical students of the time-honored aphorism that "the most common problems occur most commonly." When working with a patient, the physician develops diagnostic hypotheses early in the encounter. When faced with a patient with headache, we should initially consider tension headache and migraine rather than temporal arteritis. Of course, the *Dx10* clinician thinks of special concerns, such as the possibility that the headache patient might possibly have a brain tumor. The initial history seeks the characteristics and chronology of the symptoms. Then the clinician uses selected questions that help to rule in or out the diagnostic hypotheses: "What seems to precede the headache pain?" "Has the nature or the severity of your pain changed in any way?" The clinician also seeks important past medical, social, and family history: "What stress are you experiencing that may be influencing your symptoms?" "Does anyone else in your family have a headache problem?"

The physical examination should be limited to the body areas likely to contribute to the diagnosis, and a "full physical examination" is actually seldom needed. *Thus, for our patient with recurrent headaches, Joan S., the* Dx10 *examination is likely to be limited to the vital signs, head, and neck, with a screening of coordination, deep tendon reflexes, and cranial nerve function. Examination of the chest, heart, and abdomen is unlikely to contribute to the diagnosis.*

Tests should be limited to those that will help confirm or rule out a diagnostic hypothesis or, later, those that would help make a therapeutic decision. For most patients with headache as a presenting complaint, no laboratory test or diagnostic imaging is needed.

Of course, the uncommon problem occurs *sometimes.* Occasionally, you will encounter the unexpected finding: the headache patient with unanticipated unilateral deafness or the fatigued person with an enlarged spleen. Stop and think when you note a cluster of similar unexpected findings; such alertness helped clinicians identify the Muerto Canyon virus as the cause of the 1993 outbreak of the hantavirus pulmonary syndrome in the southwestern United States and also the occurrence of primary pulmonary hypertension in patients using dexfenfluramine for weight control. A few times in your career you will have the opportunity to experience a diagnostic epiphany; the *Dx10* clinician will seize this opportunity by staying alert for the unexpected diagnostic clue.

Use All Available Assistance

In addition to your professional knowledge, experience, and time, your diagnostic resources include your staff, the patient and family, and the vast array of medical reference sources available.

Your office and hospital staff can be valuable allies in determining the diagnosis. Important clues may be offered when the patient calls for an appointment or when being escorted to the examination room. If a patient remarks to the receptionist or nurse that his chest pain is "just like my father had before his heart attack" or if another wonders if her heartburn could be related to her 15-year-old daughter's misbehavior, the staff member should ask the patient's permission and then share the information with the physician.

The patient and the family generally have some insight into the cause of symptoms such as fatigue, diarrhea, or loss of appetite. In a study of the patient's differential diagnosis of cough, Bergh found that while physicians considered a mean of 7.6 diagnostic possibilities, patients reported a mean of 6.5 possibilities, with only 2.8 possibilities common to both (3). *Joan S. and perhaps her family may offer diagnostic suggestions that you have not strongly considered; also, these other hypotheses represent concerns that should eventually be addressed in order to provide reassurance. For example, might Joan be in the office today chiefly because an old friend has recently been diagnosed with brain cancer and she has become concerned about the significance of her own headaches?*

Consider the Psychosocial Aspects of the Problem

To continue the case of the patient with headache, a migraine diagnosis is incomplete if it fails to include the contribution of marital or job stress to the symptoms as well as the impact on others of family event cancellations, trips to the emergency room, and large pharmacy bills for sumatriptan injections. No diagnosis of cancer or diabetes is complete without considering the impact on the patient's life and the lives of family members (4).

The *Dx10* clinician will be especially wary of ICD-9 (*International Classification of Diseases*, 9th ed.) diagnostic categories, which facilitate statistical analysis and managed care payments, but which lack the richness of narrative and also the personal and family context. For example, compare "diabetes mellitus, uncomplicated, ICD-9 code 250.00" with "type 2 diabetes mellitus in an elderly patient with poor diet, marginal retirement income, and isolation from the family."

Failure to consider the psychosocial aspects of disease invites an incompletely understood or even a missed diagnosis: How many instances of child abuse have been overlooked as busy emergency room physicians care for childhood fractures without also exploring the cause of the injury and the home environment?

In eliciting a medical history from Joan S., it will be important to learn the current stresses at work and at home, and how she thinks her life would be different if the headaches were gone.

Seek Help When Needed

Today, healthcare, including diagnosis, must be "evidence-based" and not grounded in anecdote or even in your "years of clinical experience." The evidence is, of course, the vast body of medical knowledge, including research reports and metaanalyses found in clinical journals (5), on the worldwide web (6), and in reference books such as *The 10-Minute Diagnosis Manual. In thinking about Joan S., you might search the literature for recent articles on the approach to migraine headaches.*

Help is also available from colleagues. Consider a consultation when you have a diagnosis that is somehow not "satisfying." A personal physician in a long-term relationship with a patient can develop a blind spot and the diagnosis may be apparent only to someone taking a fresh look. What is needed at such a time may be a rethinking of the problem—almost the antithesis of continuity.

Help can be available from the same-specialty colleague down the hall or from a subspecialist.

Think in Terms of a Continually Evolving Diagnosis

You do not always need to make the definitive diagnosis on the first visit; in fact, such an approach tends to foster prolonged visits, excessive testing, overly biomedical diagnoses, and high cost medicine without adding quality. When faced with an elusive diagnosis, the best test is often the passage of time and a follow-up visit. For example, we all know that headaches often are influenced by stressful life events. Yet, a new patient may not be ready to share his or her personal, often embarrassing, burdens, and it is only when a trustful relationship has been established that the clinician learns about the abusive spouse, the pregnant teenager, or the impending financial disaster.

Often it is useful to use the descriptive, categorical diagnosis, and seek the definitive diagnosis over time. Examples include the teenage girl with chronic pelvic pain, the young adult with cough for 3 months, the middle-aged person with loss of appetite, and the older person with fatigue or insomnia. Sometimes, on an initial visit, this approach is the only reasonable option.

The *Dx10* clinician will be careful not to "fall in love" with the initial diagnosis, and realizes that the depressed patient losing weight might also have cancer and that it is too easy to attribute all new symptoms to a known diagnosis of menopause or diabetes mellitus. *If Joan S.'s headaches fail to respond as expected over time, you may wish to reconsider your original diagnosis and perhaps seek further testing that would have seemed excessive on the initial visit. For example, might the "1 year" duration of increased severity merit imaging if a favorable response to initial therapy does not occur?*

In your daily practice, use the time saved in the steps described here to consider and reconsider your diagnoses—as you review chart notes, read medical journals, search medical web sites, and see the patient in follow-up visits. The *Dx10* clinician will remain open to rethinking the patient's diagnostic problem list. In the end, patience and perseverance—often measured in 10-minute aliquots over time—will yield an insightful, biopsychosocially inclusive, and clinically useful diagnosis.

References

1. Stange KC, Zyzanski SJ, Jaen CR. Illuminating the black box: a description of 4454 patient visits to 138 family physicians. *J Fam Pract* 1998;46:377–389.
2. Blumenthal D, Causino N, Chang YC. The duration of ambulatory visits to physicians. *J Fam Pract* 1999;48:264–271.
3. Bergh KD. The patient's differential diagnosis: unpredictable concerns in visits for cough. *J Fam Pract* 1998;46:153–158.
4. Taylor RB. Family practice and the advancement of medical understanding: the first 50 years. *J Fam Pract* 1999;48:53–57.
5. Richardson WS, Wilson MC, Guyatt GH, Cook DJ, Nishikawa J. User's guide to the medical literature: how to use an article about disease probability for differential diagnosis. *JAMA* 1999; 281:1214–1219.
6. Hersh W. A world of knowledge at your fingertips: the promise, reality, and future directions of on-line information retrieval. *Acad Med* 1999;74:240–243.

2. UNDIFFERENTIATED PROBLEMS

ERIC M. WALSH

2.1 Anorexia

Shawn H. Blanchard and Scott A. Fields

Anorexia is defined as the lack or loss of appetite, which can lead to unintentional weight loss. Interestingly, only 50% of people complaining of anorexia actually have documentable weight loss (Chapter 2.13).

I. **Approach.** Two objectives for the patient encounter are (a) to ascertain the cause of this complaint and (b) to understand the effect that the patient's loss of appetite has had on his or her well-being. Patient age and gender play a role in the evidence-based approach to anorexia as well. If the patient is a young woman, the clinician may suspect anorexia nervosa (5% prevalence in the population), whereas depression is a predominant factor in elderly persons with anorexia (1). Possible causes of anorexia are listed in Table 2.1. The diagnostic pathways are divided into four categories: pathologic, pharmaceutic, psychiatric, and psychosocial.

   A. **Pathologic.** Acute loss of appetite can be as significant as a surgical emergency. Existing chronic disease can substantially reduce the appetite and should not be overlooked. Processes that negatively reward consumption and digestion can also lead to a change in eating behavior. Infectious diseases to consider include human immunodeficiency virus (HIV), tuberculosis, viral hepatitis, parasites, and intestinal protozoa (2). Pathologic or medical causes rarely present without related complaints or constitutional symptoms.

   B. **Pharmaceutic.** Recreational drugs, prescription medications, or the discontinuation of either, are far more likely to be responsible for loss of appetite than are medical causes. Tobacco, alcohol, and amphetamines can cause varying degrees of anorexia. Withdrawal from narcotics, marijuana, and stimulants can cause loss of appetite. Use of prescription anorectic medications and over-the-counter products, including dietary supplements, can lead to anorexia.

   C. **Psychiatric.** Time spent eliciting the history is likely to lead to a diagnosis. This includes time interviewing family members and significant others. Psychiatric diagnoses, including anorexia nervosa, depression, personality disorders, conversion disorder, schizophrenia, and obsessive-compulsive disorder, can affect appetite and, thus, cause loss of weight (3). It is important to remember that depressive illnesses are the most common cause for loss of appetite in the elderly and are often comorbidly associated with chronic progressive disease (4) (Chapter 3.3).

   D. **Psychosocial.** Current social history may identify factors responsible for a change in the desire to eat. Loneliness or loss of a loved one, for example, can cause a patient to lose interest in meal preparation (4). Changes in social situation—a recent move away from a support group; a brief stress reaction; and even a sudden increase in positively perceived events such as preparation for a wedding, a recent graduation, or a job promotion—can affect one's appetite.

II. **History**

   A. **History of present illness.** The patient must provide a careful explanation of the problem: How is it affecting daily life? What does the patient think is responsible for the problem? Is the patient describing early satiety, dysphagia, or social dissatisfaction associated with eating? Do symptoms fluctuate? How are symptoms associated with meals? What has been tried to increase appetite and what does the patient think is responsible for the problem? Is there weight loss, or other associated symptoms?

   B. **Past medical history.** Is there any history of eating disorders, chronic medical conditions, or history of psychiatric diagnosis?

   C. **Medications.** Prescription and nonprescription medications as well as recreational drugs, herbal medications, and dietary supplements need to be

Table 2.1 Potential causes of anorexia

Pathologic	Pharmaceutical	Psychiatric
NEOPLASM	Narcotics	Depression
Lymphoma	Tobacco	Anxiety
Colon cancer	Alcohol	Personality disorder
Lung cancer	Amphetamines	Schizophrenia
ENDOCRINE	Serotonin reuptake	Eating disorders
Diabetes mellitus	inhibitors	
Addison's syndrome	Xanthines	
Hyponatremia	Antihistamines	
Hypercalcemia	Anticonvulsants	
Hypothyroidism	Caffeine	
INFECTIOUS	Ephedrine	
Viral hepatitis	Chromium	
Human immunodeficiency	Marijuana	
virus		
Tuberculosis		
Intestinal protozoa		
CHRONIC DISEASE		
Anemia		
Obstructive pulmonary		
disease		
Chronic renal failure		
Congestive heart failure		
Parkinson's disease		
Alzheimer's dementia		
Multiple sclerosis		
INFLAMMATORY		
Pancreatitis		
Inflammatory bowel		
disease		
Peptic ulcer		
Duodenal ulcer		
Cholelithiasis		
Appendicitis		
OTHER		
Poor dentition		
Dysphagia		
Irritable bowel syndrome		

listed. Over-the-counter medications are often overlooked by physicians, as well as by patients. Ask if any medications have recently been discontinued and why. Antidepressants, for example, can have anorexia as a withdrawal symptom.

   D. **Social history**. The major focus is on recent life stressors that may play a pertinent role. Stressors can be positively perceived and still be constitutionally disabling. Take a brief life satisfaction survey of the patient. Anniversary dates of lost loved ones or marked changes in lifestyle can also be important.

   E. **Review of systems**. A careful review of systems beginning with weight loss is necessary. An accurate diet history, either retrospective or prospective (with a dietary log), can prove helpful. Include signs and symptoms of depression and a brief psychiatric inventory. Consider a mental status examination. Are there any negative rewards for eating or any pain or difficulty swallowing? The patient may have painful dentition, nausea, vomiting, bloating, diarrhea, constipation, or bleeding associated with food ingestion. Finally, ask about recent head injury, or general neurologic changes suggestive of postconcussion syndrome, a central lesion, or cerebral vascular accident (5).

III. **Physical examination**
  A. **General appearance**. Any level of anxiety behavior consistent with a personality disorder should be noted. Signs of systemic disease should be evaluated with vital signs, orthostatic blood pressure assessment, and temperature. Accurate weight documentation is critical in the evaluation for loss of appetite complaints. Serial measurements over time are required.
  B. **Head, eyes, ears, nose, and throat (HEENT)**. Dentition and neck examination, including observation of swallowing and thyroid examination, are important.
  C. **Cardiovascular and respiratory systems**. Examine for cardiac arrhythmia and heart failure, including jugular venous distention, rales, peripheral edema, and hepatic congestion. Lungs should be examined for chronic obstructive pulmonary disease.
  D. **Gastrointestinal**. Pain or rigidity of an acute abdomen, absent or hyperactive bowel sounds, ascites, and hepatomegaly should be evaluated. Rectal examination and stool guaiac testing should be done.
  E. **Skin**. Look for the possible presence of skin tracks, cyanosis, or lanugo (fine, white, downy hairs sometimes seen in patients with anorexia nervosa). Jaundice or hyperpigmentation should be noted. Changes in hair pattern may be a clue to peripheral vascular disease.
  F. **Neurologic examination**. Cranial nerve examination, including olfactory sensation and taste, should be performed. Deficits in these basic sensations can affect appetite significantly. Motor weakness, focal or asymmetric proprioception, and gait disturbance may show evidence of cerebral pathology. Most chronic neurologic disease and acute cerebral vascular events will include loss of appetite. Mental status needs to be assessed, if indicated. Organic brain syndrome, dementia, delirium, and psychosis can all play a role in loss of appetite.

IV. **Testing**
  A. **History and physical examination** should guide clinical laboratory testing. A general evaluation should include a complete blood count and a metabolic panel to assess electrolyte balance and hepatorenal function. Other specific laboratory studies to consider include HIV serology, viral hepatitis panel, calcium, thyroid-stimulating hormone, and albumin levels. Also, low levels of prealbumin can indicate malnutrition or impaired protein metabolism. Suspicion may direct the physician toward a urine drug screen, in addition to a urine dipstick test to screen for glucose, protein, and pH.
  B. **Special studies** may include a chest radiograph, esophagoduodenoscopy (EGD), abdominal ultrasound, abdominal angiogram, or computed tomography (CT) scan. A tuberculosis skin test may be useful.
  C. **Psychological testing** can include a formal depression scale, psychiatric consultation, or pharmaceutical trial with an (orexigenic) antidepressant, such as tricyclics.

V. **Diagnostic assessment**. Loss of appetite as a chief complaint rarely stands alone as the only problem when an effective history and physical examination are performed. The acuity of onset and the physical well-being of the patient may direct the urgency of the evaluation. The spectrum of additional constitutional symptoms in a complete review of systems will assist the examiner. The plan of action should be predicated by the assessment. Focus is then on treating the underlying condition: consider a trial of orexigenic therapy and nutritional supplementation to alleviate both the cause and the symptom of loss of appetite.

References
1. Morton KI, Sox HC, Krupp JR. Involuntary weight loss: diagnostic and prognostic significance. *Ann Intern Med* 1981;95(5):568–567.
2. Summerbell CD, Perrett JP, Gazzard BG. Causes of weight loss in human immuno-deficiency virus infection. *Int J STD AIDS* 1993;4:234–236.
3. Garfinkel PE, Garner DM, Kaplan AS, Rodin G, Kennedy S. Differential diagnosis of emotional disorders that cause weight loss. *CMAJ* 1983;129(9):939–945.
4. Morley JE. Anorexia in older persons: epidemiology and optimal treatment. *Drugs Aging* 1996;8(2):134–135.
5. Evans RW. The post concussion syndrome and the sequelae of mild head injury. *Neurol Clin* 1992;10(4):815–847.

2.2 Dizziness

John Muench

Dizziness is a disturbance in a patient's subjective sensation of relationship to space. It can be the clinical presentation for many different diagnoses. It is the 15th most common reason for all visits to primary care physicians, and is especially common in the elderly (1).

I. **Approach.** Dizzy patients are best categorized as having primarily vertigo, presyncope, disequilibrium, or a more vague lightheadedness. Temporal factors, related symptoms, and the physical examination can then be used to narrow the diagnosis. Screening for a psychogenic component should be part of the workup of all dizzy patients. It is important to eliminate the rare occurrence when dizziness represents a true life-threatening emergency, but once having done so, watchful waiting can be a useful primary care strategy.

A. **Dizziness types and typical causes**
   1. Lightheaded or giddiness (various studies indicate this group comprises between 9% and 24% of all dizzy patients) (2). Psychological presentations of dizziness are usually described more as a nonspecific lightheadedness, which may be associated with other somatic symptoms of anxiousness including perioral and extremity tingling, chest pressure, and difficulty breathing or hyperventilation. Anxiety, depression, panic disorder, and somatization can cause these symptoms.
   2. Presyncope (3% to 16% of all dizzy patients) reflects cerebral hypoperfusion that impairs consciousness. Typical causes are cardiac arrhythmias, ischemic or valvular heart disease, hypertrophic cardiomyopathy, vasovagal, orthostatic hypotension, or anemia.
   3. Disequilibrium (1% to 17%): Elderly patients may complain of dizziness when degenerative changes in the vestibular apparatus, vision, or proprioception make it difficult to maintain balance. This occurs when standing or walking, but generally not when sitting (a diagnostic clue). Disequilibrium can also be caused by cerebellar disease, Parkinsonism and peripheral neuropathies (e.g., from diabetes mellitus or vitamin B_{12} deficiency).
   4. Vertigo is described by patients as a spinning or whirling sensation. It is caused by pathology of the vestibular system. Peripheral vertigo is to be differentiated from central vertigo.

B. **Common causes of peripheral vertigo** (38% to 46%)
   1. Benign paroxysmal positional vertigo (BPPV) (12% to 23%) has very specific characteristics. A latency (2 to 20 seconds) is seen between assuming the position and the vertigo. The episode lasts less than 1 minute. Attempting several times in a row to induce the vertigo with repeated

head positioning will result in less severe episodes each time (fatigability). These episodes usually self-resolve within a period of months, but can recur later. Diagnosis is confirmed with the Dix-Hallpike maneuver: With the patient supine and head and shoulders extending off the examination table, the examiner supports the head and rotates it to the one side to observe for nystagmus; then the maneuver is repeated on the other side.

2. **Vestibular neuronitis (viral labyrinthitis) (3% to 9%).** This condition often follows a viral upper respiratory infection (URI) in the days prior to onset. Vertigo gradually develops over minutes to hours, usually peaks within 24 hours, and then slowly resolves over several days to weeks. Head movement aggravates the symptoms. Spontaneous nystagmus is present in the acute phase. Residual unsteadiness can last for several weeks but complete recovery usually occurs within 3 months.

3. **Ménière's disease (3% to 8%)** is a syndrome characterized by spontaneous recurrent episodes of vertigo that begin with a sense of ear fullness and pressure, a roaring tinnitus, and a characteristic fluctuating low-frequency hearing loss. Vertigo rapidly follows; it peaks within minutes and subsides over several hours. Patients can have as many as thirty attacks in a year in the active phase. Initially, the hearing loss is completely reversible, but later on, a hearing deficit will remain and worsen.

C. **Typical central vestibular causes of vertigo** (7% to 23%). Brainstem or cerebellar ischemia; acoustic neuroma or other central nervous system (CNS) tumors; multiple sclerosis; and basilar artery migraine can all have a component that is perceived as dizziness by patients.

D. **Differentiating serious acute central vertigo from other causes.** Dizziness rarely presents a life-threatening problem unless accompanied by other focal neurologic symptoms. Be more alert with elderly patients or those with risk factors for CNS hemorrhage or ischemia. A patient with vascular risk factors who presents with severe spontaneous vertigo, profound imbalance, and especially with other neurologic symptoms, should proceed with immediate magnetic resonance imaging (MRI) to rule out a cerebellar hemorrhage or infarct (3).

II. **History.** The patient should be allowed, in his or her own words, to describe what is meant by dizziness. A description of the first attack can be helpful. What is the time course of subsequent attacks? How long do the episodes last? How frequent are they? Do any particular positions or movements bring on episodes? Is there any associated nausea, headache, fever, hearing loss, ear pain, or tinnitus? Are there other neurologic symptoms? What medications is the patient taking?

III. **Physical examination.** A focused physical examination usually confirms rather than makes the diagnosis. An otoscopic examination should be done looking for impacted cerumen or signs of infection. A focused neurologic examination should be done. The patient's eyes should be observed for spontaneous, gaze-evoked or positional nystagmus. A Dix-Hallpike maneuver should be done when BPPV is suspected. The patient should be observed walking to assess cerebellar function and disequilibrium.

IV. **Testing.** A screening audiogram can sometimes be helpful to detect slight asymmetrical hearing loss the patient may not have noted. To rule out cerebellar infarct or hemorrhage, an MRI—the study of choice—should be done if the diagnosis does not become clear after a period of watchful waiting. MRI is also warranted for a persistent, unilateral hearing loss to rule out acoustic neuroma. Other ancillary tests are usually not helpful unless targeted at specific symptoms (e.g., complete blood count if anemia is suspected).

V. **Diagnostic assessment.** Because dizziness can be a somatic presentation for many diagnoses, it is important to be methodical in the workup. First, attempt to classify the dizzy patient primarily in one of the four general categories noted above. A description of near-syncope allows one to pursue causes of cerebral hypoperfusion (e.g., heart disease, dehydration, anemia). Elderly patients who have noticed a gradual inability to maintain balance while walking or standing should be evaluated for treatable causes of disequilibrium, including peripheral neuropathies, vision problems, and medication side effects. Most patients, but especially the young patient who describes a vague "swimming" lightheadedness or symptoms of panic or anxiety (e.g., shortness of breath, chest pain, or numbness in arms or legs) should be primarily questioned about feelings of depression and abnormal stressors. Finally, if a patient presents with the whirling symptoms of vertigo, assess for risk of CNS ischemia or hemorrhage by taking into account the patient's cardiovascular risks and presence of associated neurologic symptoms. Temporal factors and physical examination maneuvers can help differentiate between the primary causes of peripheral vestibular disease—BPPV, Ménière's disease, and vestibular neuronitis.

References

1. Sloan PD. Dizziness in primary care: results from the National Ambulatory Medical Care Survey. *J Fam Pract* 1989;29:33–38.
2. McGee SR. Dizzy patients: diagnosis and treatment. *West J Med* 1995;162:37–42.
3. Baloh RW. Dizziness: neurological emergencies. *Neurol Clin* 1998;16(2):305–321.

2.3 Edema

Paul Evans and Michael P. Rowane

Edema is defined as a clinically apparent increase in interstitial fluid volume (1–3). A number of possible factors cause edema.

I. **Approach**. The diagnostic process begins by determining if edema is *localized* or *generalized*.
- A. **Localized edema.** This can present as hydrothorax (excess fluid in the thoracic cavity) or ascites (excess fluid in the peritoneal cavity).
- B. **Generalized edema.** The patient may or may not have hypoalbuminemia:
  1. Normal serum albumin level. Consider congestive heart failure (CHF) and renal causes (oliguria or anuria).
  2. Hypoalbuminemia (<2.5 g/dl). Initial considerations should include cirrhosis, severe malnutrition, protein-losing gastroenteropathy, and nephrotic syndrome.

II. **History**
- A. **Onset**. When the onset of edema is sudden, consider the following possible causes: cellulitis, deep venous thrombosis (DVT), compartment syndrome, trauma, and exacerbation of chronic problems (systemic disease, medications, venous insufficiency, lymphedema).
  When the onset is *gradual*, consider the causes listed below.
- B. **Clinical course.** Is the edema intermittent or recurrent, or is it chronic?
- C. **Painful edema** most likely results from (3):
  1. Cellulitis
  2. Trauma
  3. Ruptured Baker's cyst
  4. Compartment syndrome
  5. DVT
- D. **Painless edema** or bilateral edema usually results from a systemic cause.
- E. **Associated systemic symptoms**
  1. Fever and chills can be caused by cellulitis, lymphangitis, or venous thrombosis.
  2. Dyspnea and orthopnea suggest that the edema is of cardiac origin.
  3. Either a history of streptococcal throat infection or recurrent urinary tract infection (UTI) points to renal causes.

F. **Medications** that can be associated with edema include the following: diazoxide, minoxidil, hydralazine, calcium channel blockers, alpha- and beta-blockers, reserpine, guanethidine, nonsteroidal antiinflammatory drugs (NSAIDs), carbenicillin, amantadine, lithium, phenothiazines, thioridazine, monoamine oxidase (MAO) inhibitors, corticosteroids, testosterone, estrogen, progesterone, or interleukin-2 (2, 3).

G. **Endocrine diseases**
   1. Hypothyroidism can present with pretibial myxedema (Chapter 14.4).
   2. Cushing's syndrome can cause edema.

H. **Miscellaneous causes of edema.** These include:
   1. Pregnancy
   2. Sodium overload
   3. Malnutrition
   4. Stopping laxatives
   5. Prolonged dependent position
   6. Cyclic edema in women
   7. Lymphatic obstruction (neoplastic, parasitic, iatrogenic)
   8. Idiopathic

III. **Physical examination**
   A. **Generalized edema** manifests in the most dependent area (e.g., pedal edema in ambulatory patients, presacral edema in bedbound patients).
   B. **Peripheral edema** (3)
      1. Sparing of the feet suggests lipedema.
      2. Pitting edema present for more than 3 months usually indicates a low serum protein level. Chronic edema can have fibrosis as well.
      3. Assessment of color
         a. Redness suggests infection or phlebitis.
         b. A red-blue color suggests DVT.
         c. A slightly cyanotic color bilaterally suggests CHF (Chapter 7.5).
         d. The presence of ecchymosis suggests trauma.

IV. **Testing**. Routine studies can include complete blood count (CBC), urinalysis, chest films, electrocardiogram (ECG), and biochemical screening to include albumin, total protein, total cholesterol, liver function tests, and thyroid function tests (4). Specific tests or imaging studies are indicated in clinical situations listed below.

V. **Diagnostic assessment**
   A. **Edema affecting the arms only**
      1. Edema exclusively of the upper extremities, caused by increased venous pressure, points to superior vena cava syndrome. A venogram will be useful.
      2. If venous obstruction is suspected, obtain a venogram and Doppler or ultrasound studies.
      3. If a thoracic outlet syndrome is suggested, computed tomography (CT), magnetic resonance imaging (MRI), or plain films may be helpful.
   B. **Edema of the arms and legs**
      1. Cardiac causes include CHF and constrictive pericarditis (Chapter 7.5). Diagnostic studies include a chest x-ray (CXR) study and ECG.
      2. A leading hepatic cause is cirrhosis. Liver function tests are indicated.
      3. Renal causes
         a. Nephrotic syndrome: order 24-hour urine protein and lipids.
         b. Glomerulonephritis or acute tubular necrosis: obtain urinalysis with sediment evaluation.
         c. Preeclampsia: laboratory tests include urine protein, urate, blood urea nitrogen (BUN), creatinine, and serum bilirubin (5).
      4. Other causes of generalized edema and tests that may be useful include hypothyroidism [thyroid-stimulating hormone, (TSH)], aldosteronism (serum potassium), Cushing's disease (cortisol or dexamethasone test), malnutrition (prealbumin), beriberi (thiamine), malabsorption (total

protein), angioedema, inflammatory bowel disease (sigmoidoscopy), serum sickness, malignancies (CT or MRI), and idiopathic edema (6).
- C. **Unilateral edema of the legs only** points to a local peripheral cause such as trauma, venous obstruction, mass, or inflammation.
- D. **Bilateral chronic edema of the legs only**
    1. If tenderness is present, consider lipedema if no foot involvement, or varicose veins if the foot is involved.
    2. Consider the possibility of a medication-related cause: see above.
    3. An elevated TSH may point to a diagnosis of hypothyroidism or Grave's disease.
    4. Unilateral left-sided edema could be caused by iliac compression or pelvic mass obstructing venous outflow. A venogram, CT, or MRI may be helpful.

References

1. Braunwald E. Edema. In: Fauci AS, ed. *Harrison's principles of internal medicine*, 14th ed. New York: McGraw Hill, 1998:210–214.
2. Powel AA, Armstrong MA. Peripheral edema. *Am Fam Physician* 1997;55:1721–1726.
3. Weber R. Leg edema. In: Rakel RE, ed. *Saunders manual of medical practice*. Philadelphia: WB Saunders, 1996:207–209.
4. Friedman HH. Edema. In: Friedman HH, ed. *Problem oriented medical diagnosis*, 6th ed. Boston: Little, Brown and Company, 1996:1–4.
5. Taylor RB. *Manual of family practice*. Boston: Little, Brown and Company, 1997: 497–499.
6. MacGregor GA, deWardner HE. Idiopathic edema. In: Schrier RW, Gottschalk CW, eds. *Diseases of the kidney*, 5th ed. Boston: Little, Brown and Company, 1993: 2493–2501.

2.4 Falls

Joseph E. Ross

Falls are most common at age extremes. In children aged more than 1 year, injuries are the number one cause of death. Falls account for 25% of these deaths. Bike injuries account for 68% of falls for children aged 5 to 14 years (1). The incidence of falls in patients aged more than 65 years is 30%; in those more than age 80 years, it is above 50%. Accidents are the fifth leading cause of death in the age group 65 years and older. Falls account for two-thirds of these deaths. Of elderly patients hospitalized for falls, only half are alive 1 year later (2).

- I. **Approach**. Factors contributing to falls need to be identified and evaluated for preventive measures to be taken. Children fall from heights; elderly fall from level surfaces.
    - A. **Children and adolescents**. Falls from heights over 3 feet and falls of infants aged less than 1 year old result in greater risk for skull fracture and intracranial bleeding. Emergent evaluation is needed in cases of loss of consciousness, behavioral changes, seizures, or ongoing vomiting.
    - B. **Falls in the elderly**. One-half of falls are secondary to accidents, including factors affecting stability. The other half are secondary to medical disorders (Table 2.2). If syncope occurred with a fall, it must be determined whether the cause is cardiac or noncardiac (Table 2.3) (Chapter 2.12). Cardiac mortality in falls related to syncope at 1 year is 20% to 30%, whereas noncardiac mortality is less than 5% (3).
- II. **History**
    - A. **History of the fall.** An interview of a witness to the fall is essential. This may identify any seizure activity, loss of consciousness, and method of fall. Ask what the patient was doing prior to the fall, including occurrence with

Table 2.2 Factors affecting falls

Factors affecting stability	Medical problems contributing to falls
Decreased muscle tone/strength	Arthritis
Changes in gait	Previous stroke
Changes in postural control	Hip fracture
Decreased depth perception	Dementia
Decreased hearing	Osteoporosis
Decreased proprioception	Parkinsonism
Decreased vision	Foot disorders
Slower reflexes	Peripheral neuropathies
Hazardous living arrangements	Hypothyroidism
(e.g., poor lighting, slick floors,	Alcoholism
loose rugs, stairways, unstable	Medications
furniture)	Hypertension
	Hypotension
	Myocardial infarction
	Arrhythmias
	Congestive heart failure
	Acute stroke
	Internal bleeding
	Infections
	Valvular heart disease
	Seizures

positional changes or after voiding, eating, or constipation. Are there associated palpitations implying arrhythmia? Did the patient have a fall or syncope during exercise, which may indicate a cardiac cause? Is there any confusion that is new or changed from the past that suggests central nervous system trauma or seizure? Was urine or bowel incontinence present? Are any musculoskeletal injuries present? Questions concerning home and risk factors should be raised (Table 2.2).

B. Past history. Explore coexisting illness that may have contributed to the fall (Table 2.2). A family history of sudden death can imply arrhythmias. Also inquire about any history of prior falls.

Table 2.3 Causes of syncope

Cardiac	Non-cardiac
OSBTRUCTIVE	VASOVAGAL
Valvular disease	Pain
Hypertrophic cardiomyopathy	Voiding
Pulmonary hypertension	Increased stress
Pulmonary emboli	Cough
Myxomas	Simple faint
ARRHYTHMIA	Carotid sinus disease
Sick sinus syndrome	ORTHOSTATIC
Atrial fibrillation	Medication
Arrhythmias	Volume depletion
	Diabetes
	Parkinsonism
	NEUROLOGIC
	Stroke
	Seizure
	Migraine

III. **Physical examination should include:**
   A. Assessment of vital signs, including heart rate and rhythm, orthostatic blood pressure changes, temperature, and respiratory rate.
   B. A general body survey for any evidence of trauma.
   C. Examination of the eye (funduscopic, visual acuity and fields), mouth (tongue lacerations), neck (bruits), lung (congestive heart failure or infection), and cardiovascular (murmurs and rhythm).
   D. A detailed musculoskeletal examination to evaluate strength, focal weakness, range of motion, foot abnormality, and possible fractures.
   E. A neurologic examination that includes mental status, evaluation of balance, gait, mobility, and tests for peripheral neuropathy.
IV. **Testing**
   A. **Clinical laboratory tests**. Most blood tests are of low yield and should be done to confirm clinical suspicion. An electrocardiogram is useful in the elderly to rule out arrhythmia, atrioventricular block, prolonged QT syndrome, or ischemia. Diagnosis of the cause of the fall can be obtained in 50% to 60% of cases based on history, physical, and electrocardiographic study (4).
   B. **Diagnostic imaging**. Skull x-ray (fracture) and computed tomography studies to detect intracranial bleeding are recommended in all infants aged less than 1 year or if the fall was from over 3 feet. Also consider imaging with any loss of consciousness, evidence of head trauma, behavioral changes, seizure disorder, ongoing vomiting, or focal neurologic deficits.
   C. **Other testing** to consider includes echocardiogram (valvular heart disease), electroencephalogram (seizure), carotid ultrasound (bruits), carotid sinus massage (if suggested by history), and tilt table testing (if a vasovagal cause of fall is considered).
V. **Diagnostic assessment**. A fall by an elderly person frequently requires a home visit to evaluate factors contributing to falls and correct unsafe conditions (Table 2.2). Symptoms of cardiac disease can occur with exertion or straining. Cardiac arrhythmias tend to be sudden without warning, although at times patients can complain of palpitations. Noncardiac causes include the vasovagal reaction in which the patient generally complains of dizziness or lightheadedness prior to a fall, often with changes in position or when upright. These can be associated with sweating and nausea. Orthostatic noncardiac causes have gradual onset and resolution. These are most often associated with medications, including antihypertensives, sedatives, anxiolytics, antidepressants, hypoglycemics, psychotropics, histamine-2 (H_2) blockers, alcohol, over-the-counter cold medicines, and medications with extended half-lives. Neurologic noncardiac events can usually be diagnosed by history and physical examination. A psychiatric cause for falls is less likely, but one should be suspicious in cases of frequent symptoms with no injury.

References
1. Gruskin KD, Schutzman SA. Head trauma in children younger than 2 years: are there predictors for complications? *Arch Pediatr Adolesc Med* 1999:153:15–20.
2. Steinweg KK. The changing approach to falls in the elderly. *Am Fam Physician* 1997:56:1815–1824.
3. Wiley TM. A diagnostic approach to syncope. *Resid Staff Physician* 1998:44:29–41.
4. Hupert N, Kapoor WN. Syncope: a systemic approach for the cause. *Patient Care* 1997:31:136–147.

2.5 Fatigue

Meg Hayes

Fatigue is both a normal human response as well as a symptom of physical or psychological disease. It is a subjective sensation that is multicausal and nonspecific for which no one definition is universally accepted, nor can it be quantified or diagnosed with laboratory or imaging studies. Fatigue is the seventh most common symptom in primary care, accounting for more than 10 million office visits every year (1). Women present for medical care with fatigue more often than men, although it is not clear that a gender prevalence exists in the population. Among the large number of patients who seek primary medical care for the symptom of chronic fatigue, only 2% to 5% are found to have an organic disorder, and a similar number meets the criteria for chronic fatigue syndrome (CFS). The most common underlying cause of fatigue is an affective disorder, either depression or somatic anxiety (Chapters 3.1 and 3.3). In many cases, no medical diagnosis can be made and demands of work and social responsibilities seem to be the cause of fatigue (2).

I. **Approach**
   A. **Onset and chronicity**. The complaint of fatigue should first be approached in terms of onset and chronicity as a means of further differentiating the cause from among physical (e.g., hypothyroidism), psychogenic (e.g., depression), physiologic (e.g., overwork), or a combination of those factors. The recent onset of fatigue, less than 1 month in duration and becoming worse, is more likely to be caused by physical illness. Chronic fatigue, greater than 6 months duration, is more likely to have a psychogenic or multifactorial cause. In a case of chronic fatigue for which diagnosis is elusive, the criteria for chronic fatigue syndrome should be considered.
   B. **Patient–physician communication**. Communication between the physician and patient is key to successful management. Establishing rapport, demonstrating a flexible approach and personal concern with the aim of cultivating a respectful and therapeutic relationship, can lead to an appropriate and mutually satisfactory set of expectations for the pace of evaluation and treatment. It is important to elicit the patient's diagnostic beliefs, as many attribute the fatigue to an organic medical disorder, and, therefore, resist psychiatric diagnosis or even questions that probe into that realm (3).
II. **History**. A thorough medical, social, and family history must be conducted to identify comorbid or contributing conditions that require treatment or suggest lifestyle modification.
   A. **The fatigue should be assessed in terms of duration, onset, level of impairment, and character**. Specifically, fatigue should be distinguished from weakness and hypersomnolence.
   B. **A complete review of systems** may point to a cardiovascular, neurologic, psychiatric, infectious, autoimmune, hematologic, pulmonary, endocrine, or malignant cause to pursue.
   C. **Attention should also be given to medication**—both prescription and over-the-counter—and to diet, exercise, substance abuse, and sleep disturbance.
   D. **Lifestyle issues** to explore include caretaking for young children, an elderly or ill relative, and the number of hours worked outside the home. Life stresses or major family transitions such as relocation, death, divorce, financial difficulties and past or current abuse or trauma should also be assessed.
III. **Physical examination**. A thorough physical examination should be done to investigate findings of underlying disease. This is also an important prerequisite to satisfy the patient's concern regarding the possibility of an organic cause if a psychiatric diagnosis is made. Particular attention should be given to the presence of pallor, cardiac arrhythmia, dyspnea, fever or other indication of infection; weight loss; lymphadenopathy; evidence of inflammatory arthritis, occult blood loss, organomegaly, or abdominal masses; neurologic signs of impaired coordination; hypertension; edema; generalized pruritus; obesity; peripheral neuropathy; goiter; dry hair or skin; hemoptysis; or pregnancy. Conduct a mental status examination to identify abnormalities in mood, intellectual function, memory, and personality. Pay special attention to assessment of symptoms of depression or anxiety, suicidal ideation, and psychomotor retardation.
IV. **Testing.** If diagnostic or patient concerns remain following the history and physical examination, a minimum battery of laboratory screening tests should be performed in the evaluation of fatigue. This should include a complete blood count

with leukocyte differential, serum levels of alanine aminotransferase, total protein, albumin, globulin, alkaline phosphatase, calcium, phosphorus, glucose, blood urea nitrogen, creatinine, electrolytes, thyroid-stimulating hormone, erythrocyte sedimentation rate, and urinalysis. The choice of any further investigations should be guided by clinical assessment of the patient to confirm or exclude other causative possibilities; for example, obtain a chest x-ray study in the case of exposure to tuberculosis or a magnetic resonance imaging study of the brain if multiple sclerosis is suspected. In such cases, further investigation should be conducted according to accepted clinical standards. In particular, the use of other screening tests to diagnose CFS is not recommended in the clinical setting, but should be reserved for investigation in the setting of protocol-based research (4).

V. **Diagnostic assessment**

  A. **Organic and psychogenic causes**. If the evaluation through history, physical examination, and laboratory studies reveals an organic or psychogenic cause, the diagnosis of "fatigue" should be replaced with a more precise etiologic diagnosis. The most common biomedical causes of fatigue are psychogenic (57%), usually depression or anxiety, and organic causes (37%) with infection representing the largest subgroup followed by cardiovascular and endocrine abnormalities. Cases of cancer and connective tissue disease first presenting as fatigue are rare at 1% each (5). In the case that environmental factors are identified that contribute to fatigue, a trial of behavior modification may eliminate the complaint. Prolonged fatigue is defined as self-reported, persistent fatigue lasting 1 month or longer.

  B. **Chronic fatigue syndrome**. A diagnosis of CFS is made by two criteria: (a) severe chronic fatigue of 6 months or longer duration with other known medical conditions excluded by clinical diagnosis; and (b) concurrent presence of four or more of the following symptoms: substantial impairment in short-term memory or concentration; sore throat; tender lymph nodes; muscle pain, multiple joint pain without swelling or redness; headaches of a new type, pattern, or severity; unrefreshing sleep and postexertional malaise lasting more than 24 hours. The conditions must have persisted or recurred during 6 or more consecutive months of illness and must not have predated the fatigue (4). For fatigue of undetermined cause present for 6 or more months that does not meet criteria for CFS, a diagnosis of idiopathic chronic fatigue is made.

References

1. Kroenke K, Wood DR, Mangelsdorff AD, Meier NJ, Powell JB. Chronic fatigue in primary care: prevalence, patient characteristics, and outcome. *JAMA* 1988; 260(7):929–934.
2. Komaroff AL, Buchwal DS. Chronic fatigue syndrome: an update. *Annu Rev Med* 1998;49:1–13.
3. Godwin M, Delva D, Miller K, et al. Investigating fatigue of less than six month's duration. Guidelines for family physicians. *Can Fam Physician* 1999;45:373–379.
4. Fukuda K, Strauss S, Hickie I, Sharpe MC, Dobbins JG, Komaroff AL, and the International Chronic Fatigue Syndrome Study Group. The chronic fatigue syndrome: a comprehensive approach to its definition and study. *Ann Intern Med* 1994; 121:953–959.
5. Valdini AF. Fatigue of unknown etiology—a review. *Fam Pract* 1985;2(1):48–53.

2.6 Fever

Lyle J. Fagnan

Fever is a physiologic state in which the body temperature is elevated above the individual's normal temperature. Patients and clinicians consider fever an important sign of illness.

I. **Approach to the febrile patient.** The presence or absence of fever is frequently addressed in the patient interview and a measurement of temperature is one of the vital signs recorded as a part of the physical examination.

   A. **The mean oral temperature for healthy adults** is 36.8°C ± 0.4°C (98.2°F ± 0.7°F) with a maximal high of 37.2°C (98.9°F) at 6 AM and a maximal high of 37.7°C (99.9°F) at 4 PM. Rectal temperatures are 0.6°C (1.0°F) higher. Axillary temperatures are 0.55°C (1.0°F) less than oral readings. Helpful centigrade–Fahrenheit conversions are 40.0°C = 104.0°F; 37.0°C = 98.6°F; and 35.0°C = 95.0°F.

   B. **Hyperpyrexia** is when the oral temperature exceeds 41.1°C (106.0°F). This is a medical emergency.

   C. **A number of factors affect baseline values,** including race, postprandial state, pregnancy, ovulation, physical activity, clothing, ambient temperature, and endocrine states.

II. **History**

   A. **Taking a detailed patient history** is critical; include questions relating to travel, animal exposure, occupation, injuries or operations, household members or contacts who are ill, medications, past illnesses, and a complete review of systems.

   B. **Chills, malaise, myalgia, headache, and fever** are common with infectious diseases.

   C. **The febrile pattern** may be helpful in making a diagnosis. Antipyretics, antibiotics, and glucocorticoids affect the fever pattern. Specific patterns of fever are shown in Table 2.4.

III. **Physical examination**

   A. The examination should include the skin, lymph nodes, eyes, nail beds, heart, lungs, abdomen, joints, nervous system, and genitourinary system, including rectal and bimanual pelvic examinations.

   B. Infections will increase the pulse rate approximately 10 beats per minute for each 0.5°C (1.0°F) temperature increase.

Table 2.4 Fever patterns

1. **Continuous (sustained)** fever is one with persistent temperature elevations and remissions with variations not exceeding 1°F. Diseases include lobar pneumonia, rickettsial disease, central nervous system disorders, tularemia, and falciparum malaria.

2. **Intermittent** fever exaggerates the normal circadian rhythm with normal or low temperatures in the morning and a peak at 4 to 6 PM. **Hectic** or **septic** fever indicates extreme exaggerations of this pattern. Disease causes include localized pyogenic infections, bacterial endocarditis, malignancy, and drug fevers.

3. With **quotidian fever,** a temperature spike occurs daily.

4. **Tertian** and **quartan** fevers spike every third and fourth day, respectively. This pattern can occur with malaria.

5. A **biphasic** or **saddle back** fever refers to several days of fever and a gap of a day followed by several more days of fever. Disease causes include dengue fever, yellow fever, rat-bite fever, influenza, poliomyelitis, Colorado tick fever, and Rift Valley fever.

6. **Pel–Ebstein fever** is defined as elevated temperatures lasting 3 to 10 days, followed by afebrile periods of 3 to 10 days. Disease causes include Hodgkin's disease, other lymphomas, and brucellosis.

7. **With reversal of the diurnal pattern of fever,** the highest temperature occurs in the early morning hours. Disease causes include typhoid fever and disseminated tuberculosis.

8. **The Jarish–Herxheimer** febrile pattern occurs when the temperature is markedly increased following the initiation of antibiotics. Disease causes include syphilis, leptospirosis, and brucellosis.

    C. When fever is present, the respiratory rate will frequently increase above the usual 12 to 14 breaths per minute.

    D. Infections with *Mycoplasma pneumonia*, psittacosis, and typhoid fever are often associated with a relative bradycardia.

IV. Testing. In cases of a fever in which the cause is unclear, a number of diagnostic tests may be useful, depending on history and physical examination. These include:

    A. Urinalysis with microscopic examination

    B. Blood cultures, both aerobic and anaerobic

    C. Blood tests: human immunodeficiency virus (HIV), rapid plasma reagent (RPR), antistreptolysin-O (ASO) titer, rheumatoid arthritis (RA) factor, antinuclear antibody (ANA), sedimentation rate, and serum enzymes and chemistries

    D. Tuberculosis (TB) skin test

    E. Spinal fluid examination

    F. Diagnostic imaging: chest film, abdominal ultrasound, abdominal computed tomography (CT), bone scan

    G. Biopsies: liver, bone marrow, lymph node, skin, muscle, temporal artery

V. Diagnostic assessment. The approach to the febrile patient involves a number of considerations, including the patient's age, clinical history, risk factors, community illness pattern, and physical presentation. In the family physician's office, most febrile illnesses are the result of self-limited viral illnesses (e.g., upper respiratory infections). A number of cases of fever will be caused by bacterial infections (e.g., streptococcal pharyngitis or urinary tract infections). The challenge is to select those studies with the highest sensitivity and specificity to increase the probability of a correct diagnosis. When the diagnosis continues to be elusive, repeat the history and the physical examination. Special considerations in specific populations and certain types of fever include:

    A. The elderly: 10% of elderly patients will fail to generate a febrile response with pneumonia (1). Fever in the elderly is more likely to indicate a bacterial infection than a fever in younger adults (2).

    B. Fever of unknown origin (FUO). An FUO is characterized by the first three criteria listed below:

        1. A temperature greater than 38.3°C (101.0°F) on several occasions

        2. A duration of 3 weeks

        3. Unclear cause after a full physical examination, routine blood tests, cultures, and chest x-ray studies

        4. The cause of FUOs will be determined 90% of the time; it will often be a common illness that presents in an unusual manner.

        5. Two leading causes of FUO are tuberculosis and infective endocarditis.

        6. Other causes include hepatic or subphrenic abscess, neoplasm, and lymphomas such as Hodgkin's disease.

    C. Factitious fever. Factitious fever is a consideration in a patient with a complex emotional disorder. The absence of a normal diurnal pattern, pulse elevation, and diaphoresis may suggest a diagnosis of factitious fever.

    D. Drug fever. Drugs are an important cause of noninfectious fever (3).

        1. This is a diagnosis of exclusion and requires the fever to coincide with the prescribing of the drug and the resolution of the fever on discontinuing the medication.

        2. Drug-associated fevers can be high and take several days to resolve.

        3. Among the medications causing a fever are diphenylhydantoin, carbamazepine, histamine-2 (H_2) blockers, methyldopa, allopurinol, sulfonamides, cephalosporins, and isoniazid.

    E. Postoperative fever. The temporal relationship of the fever to the surgery may provide a clue to the primary source of the infection (4).

        1. If fever duration is less than 48 hours, consider atelectasis of the lung.

        2. If duration is more than 3 days, consider urinary tract infection or infected intravascular device.

3. If fever has been present more than 5 days, consider wound infection, intraabdominal abscess, or empyema.

F. Hyperthermia. A disruption of thermoregulation can result from excessive heat production, inadequate heat dissipation, or hypothalamus malfunction (5).

References

1. Harper C, Newton P. Clinical aspects of pneumonia in the elderly veterans. *J Am Geriatr Soc* 1989;37:867–872.
2. Mellors JW, Horwitz RI, Harvey MR, et al. A simple index to identify occult bacterial infection in adults with unexplained fever. *Arch Intern Med* 1987;147:666–671.
3. Mackowiak PA, ed. *Fever: basic mechanisms and management.* New York: Raven Press, 1991:239.
4. Mackowiak PA, ed. *Fever: basic mechanisms and management.* New York: Raven Press, 1991:245.
5. Simon HB. Hyperthermia. *N Engl J Med* 1993;329(7):483–487.

2.7 Headache

Robert B. Taylor

Headache is one of the 20 most frequent reasons patients visit primary care providers in the United States. Migraine headache, one of the common causes of recurrent headache, occurred one or more times yearly in 17.6% of females and in 5.7% of males in a study of 20,468 persons (1).

I. **Approach.** In the evaluation of a recurrent headache, the important tasks are to categorize the headache type with as much precision as possible and to eliminate potentially serious causes.
   A. **Headache types.** Basically, two types of recurrent headache are seen: primary headaches and headaches caused by other illnesses (Table 2.5).
   B. **Special concerns include a brain tumor, intracranial bleed, meningitis, or other serious causes.** In primary care patients with "headache" as a presenting symptom, the risk of serious intracranial pathology is less than 1% (2). Generally, such patients have a history of a new onset or worsening headache pattern or an abnormal neurologic finding, which might include a seizure (Chapter 4.7).

II. **History**
   A. **Characteristics of the headache.** What is the type of pain, its location, its duration, and its intensity? What symptoms precede or accompany the pain? Does anything trigger the headache or make the pain better or worse? Tell about a typical headache from beginning to end.

Table 2.5 Types of recurrent headache with selected examples

Primary headaches: Tension-type, migraine, cluster, other.

Secondary headaches *(associated with)*: brain tumor, vascular abnormality, hypertension, infection, chronic daily headache (HA)[a], substance withdrawal, temporal arteritis, neuralgia, sinus HA, metabolic disorders, other.

[a] Chronic daily HA is classified as a secondary HA because it typically presents as a "rebound headache" in a migraineur who overuses analgesics.

1. Migraine food triggers include alcohol, aged cheese, chocolate, and aspartame.
2. Approximately 20% to 30% of migraineurs will report an aura, typically visual in nature.
3. Patients with cluster headache report unilateral temporal headache, occurring generally once daily, usually in the evening and associated with ipsilateral nasal stuffiness and conjunctival injection.
4. Chronic daily headache (CDH) patients will describe headaches at least 10 to 15 days/month and usually report heavy use of relief drugs.
5. Red flags that might suggest intracranial pathology (section **I.B**) include a loss of consciousness, persistent visual loss, seizures, staggering, or hearing loss.

B. **Chronology of the headache**. Most primary headaches recur periodically for years, with only subtle changes over time. If the headache is getting worse, the cause might be psychosocial stressors, medication overuse, or evolving intracranial pathology (Table 2.5). Ask women whether the headache seems related to the menses. Past and current medication use and how they affect the headache can be important clues to headache severity and how the patient may respond to treatment.

C. **Family history.** Migraine headaches often exhibit a familial pattern; the causes of secondary headaches generally do not. Tension headache can represent a family pattern of reacting to stress.

D. **Psychosocial aspects of the headache.** What does the patient believe is the cause of the headache? What life events might be playing a role? How does the patient's family react to the headache? Ask: "If you did not have the headache, how would your life be different?" The key to management of recurrent primary headaches often lies in the responses to these questions, which can reveal unanticipated stressors, secondary gain, or family discord.

E. **Other information.** Important data include use of tobacco, alcohol, or coffee; response to exercise; a history of head trauma; or exposure to toxic fumes or chemicals. Have there been symptoms of fever, or fatigue? Ask about depression, which is often seen in migraineurs.

III. **Physical examination**

A. **Focused physical examination (PE).** This should include vital signs (notably blood pressure) and an examination of the scalp; eyes, including funduscopic examination; ears; nose; paranasal sinuses; throat; and neck. A screening neurologic examination, including cranial nerves, coordination (finger-to-nose test), and deep tendon reflexes, is sufficient in most instances. In the migraineur, the examination findings should be all normal in the absence of a current headache; a positive finding warrants further testing (section **IV**).

B. **Additional PE.** Other PE maneuvers are appropriate if the medical history suggests specific secondary headache causes: palpation of the superficial temporal arteries (temporal arteritis), audiometry (acoustic neuroma), transillumination of the paranasal sinuses ("sinus headache"), or checking for nuchal rigidity plus Kernig's and Brudzinski's signs (meningeal irritation).

IV. **Testing**

A. **Clinical laboratory tests.** For most recurrent headache patients, no blood, urine, or other clinical laboratory tests are needed. Laboratory tests that might be suggested by the clinical history and PE include erythrocyte sedimentation rate (temporal arteritis), hematocrit or thyroid studies (fatigue), cerebrospinal fluid examination (meningeal irritation), and white blood count with differential (systemic infection).

B. **Diagnostic imaging.** In most instances, diagnostic imaging is not needed. In one study, 350 patients with a chief complaint of headache, regardless of the presence or absence of neurologic signs, were referred for computed tomography (CT). Only 2% had clinically significant CT findings, and all patients with significant CT findings had abnormal PE findings or unusual clinical symptoms (3).

1. Diagnostic imaging may be indicated in patients with atypical headache patterns, a history of seizures, or focal neurologic signs or symptoms (4). New onset and "worst ever" headaches are significant complaints (i.e., atypical headache patterns).
2. Despite the greater cost, magnetic resonance imaging (MRI) provides the best imaging for the detection of brain tumors and most other chronic pathologic causes of headache that can be detected by imaging. CT is preferred if acute bleeding is suspected.

V. **Diagnostic assessment.** The key to the diagnosis of headache is the clinical history. A history of an aching, bitemporal headache that is associated with stress and that waxes and wanes is a typical tension headache. Migraine is characteristically a one-sided headache, throbbing in nature, often associated with nausea and vomiting, frequently accompanied by photophobia and sonophobia, and lasting 4 to 12 hours, perhaps longer. It may be "with aura" (classic) or "without aura" (common migraine), with the latter seen in 70% to 80% of migraineurs. Cluster headache is a strictly one-sided, recurring headache that chiefly affects men, and that occurs in "clusters" of 1 to 2 months of episodes. An increasing number of patients have chronic daily headache, often with virtual constant discomfort; many CDHs are the result of "transformed migraine" following daily analgesic use, especially codeine derivatives (5). Because recurrent headache is caused, at least in part, by life stresses and because it also *causes* personal and family stress, the diagnostic assessment is incomplete until this complex relationship has been adequately explored over a series of visits.

References
1. Stewart WF, Lipton RB, Celentano DD, Reed ML. Prevalence of migraine headache in the United States. *JAMA* 1992;267:64–69.
2. Becker L, Iverson DC, Reed FM, et al. Patients with new headache in primary care: a report from ASPN. *J Fam Pract* 1988;27:41–47.
3. Mitchell CS, Osborn RE, Grosskreutz SR. Computed tomography in the headache patient: is routine evaluation really necessary? *Headache* 1993;33:83–86.
4. The utility of neuroimaging in the evaluation of headache in patients with normal neurologic examinations: summary statement. Report of the Quality Standards Subcommittee of the American Academy of Neurology. *Neurology* 1994;44: 1353–1354.
5. Silberstein SD, Lipton RB, Sliwinski M. Classification of daily and near daily headaches: field trials of revised IHS criteria. *Neurology* 1997;49:638–639.

2.8 Hypersomnia

Carol Blenning

Hypersomnia, one of many different types of sleep disorders, accounts for a great number of primary care visits. Patients present with either prolonged nocturnal sleep, excessive daytime somnolence (EDS), or both, and EDS itself affects up to 12% of the general population (1).

I. **Approach.** In evaluating hypersomniacs, it is essential to identify the more common underlying medical causes before making the relatively rare diagnosis of a primary sleep disorder.
   A. **Causes of hypersomnia.** Hypersomnia has four major causes: (a) central nervous system (CNS) abnormality (including narcolepsy, posttraumatic hypersomnia, myotonic dystrophy—CNS mechanism likely—and idiopathic hypersomnia); (b) sleep deficiencies resulting from sleep apnea, mental illness [depression—especially in adolescents, bipolar affective disorder (BAD),

seasonal affective disorder (SAD)], and other causes of reduced nocturnal sleep; (c) circadian rhythm disturbances—primary or environmental (e.g., jet lag or atypical work schedules); and (d) medication effects (1).

B. **Special concerns.** Hypersomnia can be the presenting symptom brought forth by patient or family member in cases of delirium or precoma states. Ominous possibilities include drug toxicities, endocrine and metabolic derangements, sepsis, and aggressive CNS processes. A history of recent or abrupt onset should prompt further investigation. Hypersomnia onset (a) at a young age correlates with narcolepsy and idiopathic hypersomnia; (b) at middle age, it is common because of sleep apnea; and (c) in the elderly, it can have a wide variety of causes, especially medication-related, cardiovascular, and endocrine (2).

II. **History.** The history is the most important influential element in the evaluation of patients with hypersomnia.

A. **Medications.** A careful review of prescription and over-the-counter medications can suggest the basis for hypersomnia. Somnolence is a side effect of many classes of medications, including antidepressants, antihistamines, and beta-blockers. The medical problem for which the drug is prescribed can itself explain hypersomnia; for instance, hypothyroidism or BAD.

B. **Sleep pattern.** A thorough history of the sleep pattern is essential. What time does the patient go to bed, fall asleep, and wake up? How many times does the patient awaken at night? Any obvious reason (e.g., nocturia or paroxysmal nocturnal dyspnea (PND)? Does the patient feel rested on awakening? The bed partner can supply information about snoring and apneic periods. Work schedules and travel history are important for determining environmental causes. Questions specific for narcolepsy should address cataplexy (sudden weakness or loss of muscle tone without loss of consciousness that is elicited by emotion), which is pathognomonic; sleep paralysis; sleep-related hallucinations; irresistible sleepiness; and short and refreshing naps without difficulty awakening (3,4).

C. **Past medical history.** Hypersomnia causes include prior head injury, endocrine abnormalities (e.g., hypothyroidism and glucose or cortisol shifts), chronic pulmonary disease with hypoxia, cardiovascular disease with low output state, and myotonic dystrophy (5).

D. **Mental health.** Depressive symptoms warrant attention, including seasonal patterns and those interspersed with manic episodes (Chapter 3.3).

E. **Family history.** Narcolepsy and idiopathic hypersomnia often have familial patterns.

F. **Social history.** Many substances cause hypersomnia. Alcohol consumed near bedtime causes disrupted sleep; benzodiazepines, opioids and barbiturates obviously cause lethargy; and withdrawal from amphetamines, nicotine, or caffeine can lead to hypersomnia.

III. **Physical examination**

A. **Focused physical examination (PE).** Any derangement of vital signs—blood pressure, pulse, respiratory rate, or temperature—suggests a serious underlying medical disorder, be it cardiovascular, infectious, metabolic, endocrine, pulmonary, toxic, or medication-related. General appearance is important, specifically, level of alertness, affect, and presence of obesity, short neck, jaundice, or muscle atrophy. A focused mental status examination should assess for the possibility of a depressive disorder.

B. **Additional PE.** If history or vital signs warrant, other examination elements can include pulmonary and cardiovascular assessment, checking for evidence of substance use (track marks, pupil dilation, asterixis, and tremor), and other causes (e.g., examination of prostate size in an older man with nocturia and hypersomnia).

IV. **Testing.** Usually, no testing is required in the workup of hypersomnia. A sleep study is useful when considering sleep apnea, narcolepsy, or idiopathic hypersomnia. If the history or examination suggests, several other tests may be needed. Electrolyte abnormalities can be causative (sodium, calcium, magnesium, and bicarbonate in the setting of acidosis). Glucose and thyroid studies cover the major endocrine possibilities. Other tests include hematocrit (anemia), white blood cell count (infection), blood urea nitrogen (dehydration and gastrointestinal bleed), creatinine and uric acid (renal failure), liver function tests and ammonia (liver failure), drug levels (e.g., phenytoin toxicity), toxicology screen with blood alcohol level, pulse oximetry (hypoxia), electrocardiogram (rhythm disturbances), cerebrospinal fluid examination (meningitis), and brain imaging when a structural intracranial process is suspected.

V. **Diagnostic assessment.** A careful history and focused PE almost always reveal the type of hypersomnia and, therefore, its cause. The more evident diagnoses include medication effects and sequelae or complications of a known preexisting condition (e.g., hypothyroidism, chronic hypoxia caused by chronic obstructive pulmonary disease, congestive heart failure, uncontrolled atrial fibrillation, depression, and substance abuse). Patients do not usually present until their hypersomnia has become a chronic problem. When the hypersomnia is more abrupt in onset, however, clinical testing is often indicated. In this setting and without an evident diagnosis by history and PE, chemistry and complete blood cell count tests results often reveal a systemic (i.e., metabolic, infectious, or toxic) cause. Correlation of the sleep study with clinical presentation differentiates the final three diagnostic possibilities: sleep apnea, narcolepsy, and idiopathic hypersomnia (IHS), the last of which is a diagnosis of exclusion. Apneic periods support sleep apnea, episodes of cataplexy cinch the diagnosis of narcolepsy (along with its other more common features as mentioned above), and IHS is diagnosable when the following elements are present: nonimperative sleepiness; long, unrefreshing naps; prolonged night-time sleep; difficult awakening with sleep drunkenness; and prominent mood disturbances.

References

1. Roth T, Roehrs TA. Etiologies and sequelae of excessive daytime sleepiness. *Clin Ther* 1996;18(4):562–576.
2. Vgontzas AN, Kales A. Sleep and its disorders. *Annu Rev Med* 1999;50:387–400.
3. Roth TA, Merlotti L. Disorders of sleep and circadian rhythms. In: Harrisonsonline.com. McGraw-Hill; 1999: ch-027/Page11.html#Sect18.
4. Bassetti C, Aldrich MS. Idiopathic hypersomnia. A series of 42 patients. *Brain* 1997;120(Pt 8):1423–1435.
5. Rubinstein JS, Rubinsztein DS, Goodburn S, Holland AJ. Apathy and hypersomnia are common features of myotonic dystrophy. *J Neurol Neurosurg Psychiatry* 1998;64(4):510–515.

2.9 Insomnia

Charles E. Henley

Insomnia is more than just being unable to fall asleep. It is a subjective condition of insufficient or nonrestorative sleep despite an adequate opportunity to sleep (1). The Institute of Medicine and most current studies place the prevalence of insomnia at 30% to 40% in the general adult population. Although the need for sleep does not necessarily decrease with age, the incidence of sleep disturbances appears to increase with age, particularly among women. Actually, the elderly are more prone to sleep maintenance problems, whereas younger people tend to have trouble falling asleep (2).

I. **Approach.** Insomnia represents a symptom of an underlying problem and is not in itself a disease entity. Sleep and alertness are regulated by a complex interaction between the body's internal biologic clocks, the reticular activating system, and various influences such as light or anxiety that can interfere with the normal sleep cycles. The approach to diagnosis should recognize the potential for various causes and use history and special studies to determine the cause of the insomnia.

A. **Types of insomnia.** Although more than one classification system for insomnia exists, a consensus seems to support dividing insomnia into transient (lasting a few days), short-term (lasting weeks), and long-term or chronic (lasting many weeks to months or years). The Association for the Psychophysiological Study of Sleep has classified insomnia as:

1. Psychophysiologic, which covers the transient and short-term problems associated with situational factors such as concern about an ill family member.
2. Psychiatric, especially depression, which has a very high concordance with insomnia, and which also covers other affective disorders and psychosis.
3. Drugs and alcohol, especially chronic alcoholism, and the use of central nervous system stimulants such as caffeine, nicotine, or other drugs.
4. Sleep-related movements syndromes. These syndromes comprise a special category related to behavioral or motor problems. Periodic limb movements and restless leg syndrome are the most frequent diagnoses.
5. Sleep-induced respiratory problems (e.g., obstructive sleep apnea). With this condition, the patients usually have no trouble falling asleep initially, but have multiple arousals and awakenings during the night.
6. Medical and environmental causes such as repeated rapid eye movement (REM) interruptions from outside noise.
7. Unknown causes—the patient may just be a short sleeper (3).

B. **Special concerns.** Potentially, the most serious problem associated with insomnia is related to obstructive sleep apnea. If left untreated, it is associated with oxygen desaturation, hypercapnia, and hypopnea, which can lead to significant cardiovascular problems (e.g., systemic and pulmonary hypertension, cor pulmonale, and right ventricular failure).

II. History

A. **Characteristics of insomnia.** Insomnia cannot be diagnosed by the amount of time a person sleeps. Rather, it is distinguished by the daytime consequences of unsatisfactory sleep (4). A pertinent history for insomnia would include:

1. A history of restlessness, irritability, daytime somnolence, and impaired work or social functioning, which can lead to situational stress. This may be a transient problem, but it can lead to difficulties with initiation of sleep and early awakenings.
2. Use of caffeine or other stimulants, especially over-the-counter medications (e.g., decongestants) that may contain ephedrine or phenylpropanolamine. Late evening exercise can also be a stimulant. Alcohol may help induce sleep, but it interferes with REM sleep and leads to nonrestorative sleep and early awakenings.
3. Affect changes, sadness, hopelessness, and vegetative signs such as weight loss should suggest depression, the most common psychiatric disorder associated with insomnia (Chapter 3.3). This is especially true if the insomnia persists for weeks. Anxiety disorders cause difficulty with getting to sleep, whereas patients with depression may fall asleep more readily but have early awakening.
4. Medical problems such as peptic ulcer disease and heart failure have been implicated in insomnia (Chapters 7.5 and 9.6). A history of frequent nocturnal urinations can also disrupt sleep and may indicate benign prostate hyperplasia or other prostate problems. Hyperthyroidism can cause irritability and insomnia, as can thyroid replacement therapy for hypothyroidism. Other problems such as asthma, angina, back pain, and sinusitis can also cause sleep disorders.
5. Loud snoring, daytime somnolence, forgetfulness, difficulty concentrating, and a history from the bed partner of periods of discontinuation of

breathing during sleep of 10 seconds or more should suggest a more thorough evaluation for obstructive sleep apnea. Daytime napping, associated findings of gastrointestinal reflux disease, and hypertension are also suggestive associations for sleep apnea.

6. The bed partner is also a good person to ask about leg movements during sleep. This could be suggestive of a periodic limb movement disorder. A similar syndrome, restless legs, is associated with a history of unpleasant sensations in the legs and a persistent desire to move them. Both conditions cause a delay in sleep onset and nocturnal awakenings.

7. Sleep phase disturbances caused by jet lag or shift work can be characterized by early awakening or by awakening later in the day.

III. **Physical examination.** The physical examination for insomnia is more a search for other underlying disease states than for any specific signs for insomnia, although hypertension, obesity, and thick neck suggest consideration of sleep apnea.

IV. **Testing.** The diagnosis of unexplained insomnia may involve testing in a sleep laboratory using polysomnography. This provides the opportunity to monitor such parameters as the electroencephalogram (EEG), breathing, oxygen saturation, and body movements during sleep. Polysomnography can determine the disturbances in chronobiologic rhythms and loss of normal sleep–awake patterns associated with circadian rhythm disorders. The EEG results from the sleep laboratory will demonstrate a patient's ability to progress through the five cycles of normal sleep and where in the process any disturbances may be located. For instance, a short REM sleep latency period from initiation of sleep to actual REM sleep, along with increased REM sleep, and reduced total sleep time with frequent awakenings are all associated with depression.

V. **Diagnostic assessment.** The key to diagnosing insomnia and other sleep disorders is history and sleep laboratory monitoring. Short-term problems related to difficulty with initiating sleep may be situational or environmental. Long-term problems with sleep, lasting weeks to months, may be more psychophysiologic such as with chronic anxiety or depression. A thorough history of personal or job-related issues, caffeine, alcohol and other drug use, related medical problems, abnormal leg and body movements at night, problems with daytime napping and somnolence as well as night time snoring, and apnea spells will all direct the practitioner to the cause of most problems. A good sleep study often confirms the diagnosis and leads to specific interventions.

References

1. Rakel RE. Insomnia: concerns for the family physician. *J Fam Pract* 1993;36:551–558.
2. Rosekind MR. The epidemiology and occurrence of insomnia. *J Clin Psychiatry* 1992;53:4–6.
3. Myer TJ. Evaluation and management of insomnia. *Hosp Pract* (Off Ed) 1998; Dec. 15:75–86.
4. Huari PJ. Insomnia. *Clin Chest Med* 1998:19:157–167.

2.10 Nausea and Vomiting

Eric M. Walsh

I. **Approach.** Nausea and vomiting are common presenting complaints in office practice. An effective diagnostic approach will consider causes both within the gastrointestinal (GI) system, and systemic causes (1–3), as well as paying special attention to the presence or absence of coexisting abdominal pain.

A. Causes originating in the GI system
   1. In the newborn and infant, causes of nausea and vomiting include reflux, pyloric stenosis, meconium ileus, and congenital malformations (e.g., malrotation of the bowel).
   2. In children, consider esophageal reflux, gastritis, peptic ulcer, Crohn's disease, food intolerance or allergy, intussusception, Reye's syndrome, and anatomic disorders (e.g., ileal band).
   3. In adults, the differential diagnosis includes reflux esophagitis (4), gastritis, peptic ulcer, achalsia, malignancy, Crohn's disease, gall bladder disease, liver disease, and pancreatic disease.
   4. GI infections occur in all age groups and include bacterial causes (*Staphylococcus aureus*, *Bacillus cereus*, *Escherichia coli*, and *Campylobacter*, *Helicobacter*, *Salmonella*, *Shigella*, *Vibrio* organisms), viral causes (especially Norwalk agent and rotovirus), and parasitic agents such as *Giardia* organisms.
B. Systemic causes of nausea and vomiting include medications, especially narcotics, oral contraceptives, digoxin, theophylline, nonsteriodal anti-inflammatory drugs, erythromycin, steroids, and iron. Remember, the *Physician's Desk Reference* lists nausea as a potential side effect for many, if not most drugs. Also consider renal disease, electrolyte abnormalities or Addison's disease, pregnancy, central nervous system problems (migraine, bleed, tumor, head trauma, meningitis), and toxins (especially lead, other heavy metals, cholinesterase inhibitors, and methemoglobin formers). Psychiatric problems such as anorexia or bulimia, obsessive compulsive disorder with trichotillomania and bezoar formation, and psychogenic polydypsia can also cause nausea and vomiting (5). Also on the differential diagnosis for infants and children are inborn errors of metabolism, congenital heart disease, and common pediatric infections.

Infections that can cause nausea and vomiting in all age groups include pneumonia, pyelonephritis, pelvic inflammatory disease, and sepsis. Also consider alcohol or drug withdrawal, radiotherapy, chemotherapy, malignancy, thyrotoxicosis, and cardiac causes (e.g., ischemia or congestive heart failure).

II. History. As is usually the case in clinical practice, most diagnoses will be made by history and confirmed by physical examination and laboratory studies. Key points in the history include the following:
   A. Are the symptoms acute, chronic, or recurrent?
   B. If vomiting is the predominant feature, consider GI infection, reflux, gastritis, or ulcer.
   C. Nausea as the predominant feature often results from systemic problems.
   D. Is there a history of travel, drinking unsafe water, or eating unusual or uncooked food?
   E. Is there a history of fevers or chills (Chapter 2.6.)?
   F. Are general systemic symptoms or signs such as edema, discolored urine or jaundice, fatigue, weight loss or anorexia, headache, or blurred vision present?
   G. Are psychiatric symptoms present?
   H. Is the patient taking any medications?
   I. Is diarrhea present?
   J. Is there abdominal pain? The presence of abdominal pain raises some important and potentially serious possibilities:
      1. Common problems presenting with abdominal pain and vomiting include cholecystitis, appendicitis, gastritis or ulcer, hepatitis, small bowel obstruction, inferior myocardial infarction or ischemia, renal colic, peritonitis, pancreatitis, food poisoning, and complications of pregnancy.
      2. Uncommon problems presenting with abdominal pain and vomiting include diabetic ketoacidosis, drug withdrawal, uremia, and vasculitis or abdominal migraine.
      3. Rare problems presenting with abdominal pain and vomiting include porphyria, lead intoxication, adrenal insufficiency, hyperlipidemia, abdominal epilepsy, glaucoma, hypercalcemia, and acute hemolysis.

III. **Physical examination.** A directed physical examination is dictated by the findings on history, but the following are areas of key importance:
   A. **Vital signs.** Focus on presence of fever, pulse, and blood pressure to assess hydration, and respiratory rate to look for acidosis-related hyperventilation.
   B. **Skin, eyes, mucous membranes.** Look for dehydration and signs of jaundice.
   C. **Signs of systemic infection.** Pay special attention to examining the lung and the costovertebral angle for tenderness.
   D. **A detailed abdominal examination** should include inspection, auscultation, palpation, percussion, areas of tenderness, rebound, guarding, hepatomegaly, Murphy's sign, stool for occult blood, and bimanual pelvic examination.
IV. **Testing.** Most cases of nausea and vomiting seen in a generalist's office will not require laboratory testing. If the diagnosis is still unclear after history and physical examination, the laboratory workup can be classified into primary, secondary, and tertiary on the basis of their utility and ability to detect disease with an urgent need for diagnosis.
   A. **Primary tests** include electrolytes, glucose, renal and liver function tests, amylase, urinalysis, stool for white blood cells, pregnancy test, and plain films of the abdomen or abdominal ultrasound if pain is a prominent feature of the presentation.
   B. **Secondary tests** include abdominal ultrasound if not already done, upper GI series or upper endoscopy, stool culture, thyroid-stimulating hormone, electrocardiogram, and chest x-ray study.
   C. **Tertiary tests** include lower endoscopy, computed tomography or magnetic resonance imaging studies, urine toxicology, urine porphyrins, and, in many instances, specialty consultation.
V. **Diagnostic assessment.** The diagnostic assessment of nausea and vomiting will benefit from a structured approach that includes the following:
   A. **A differential diagnosis** based on age and reproductive status.
   B. **Attention to GI versus systemic causes** of nausea and vomiting.
   C. **Special attention** to the potentially more urgent nature of cases of nausea and vomiting that are often accompanied by abdominal pain (Chapter 9.1).

References
1. Avner JR. Vomiting. In: Schwartz MW, ed. *Pediatric primary care—a problem oriented approach*, 3rd ed. Chicago: Yearbook Medical Publishers, 1997:397–406.
2. Sorgel KH, Greenberger NJ. Nausea and vomiting in the diabetic patient. *Hosp Pract* (Off Ed) 1998;33:14–16.
3. Bouchier IAD. Nausea, vomiting. In: Bouchier IAD, Ellis H, Flemming P, eds. *Index of differential diagnosis*, 13th ed. Oxford: Butterworth Heinman Publishers, 1996: 446,710–713.
4. Brzana RJ, Koch KL. Gastroesophageal reflux disease presenting with intractable nausea. *Ann Intern Med* 1997;126:704–707.
5. Withers GD, Silburn SR, Forbes DA. Precipitants and aetiology of cyclic vomiting syndrome. *Acta Pediatr* 1998;87:272–277.

2.11 Night Sweats

Mark Bajorek

Night sweats are drenching sweats that require a change of bedding (1).

   I. **Approach.** The first priority is to exclude night sweats caused by fever. Sweating associated with fever is a separate evaluation (Chapter 2.6). Before the 20th century, night sweats implied infection with tuberculosis. Now, many other ailments are associated with this symptom. Night sweats are often the mark of a known condition such as diabetes (especially with nocturnal hypoglycemia), cancer, head trauma, and rheumatologic disorders. Night sweats can also be a symptom of a new disorder. The investigation of a patient reporting night sweats requires a review of past illnesses and new symptoms.

II. **History.** Night sweats can be characterized by determining onset, frequency, exacerbations, and remissions of symptoms. Question patients about the current state of known disorders. Excessive sweating is associated with poor nocturnal glycemic control (Chapter 14.1). Flares of rheumatologic disorders (rheumatoid arthritis, lupus, juvenile rheumatoid arthritis, and temporal arteritis) cause sweating too. Pregnancy temporarily changes the intrinsic thermostat in many women who perspire excessively (2). Patients who are immunocompromised are at increased risk for infections, especially with atypical agents. Patients with a history of substance abuse need to be asked about needle use and contaminants.

   A. **Review of systems.** Other symptoms that can accompany night sweats include flushing (carcinoid syndrome, pheochromocytoma), joint pain, sleep apnea, menstrual irregularities, reflux, cough, headache, dysuria, dyspnea, rashes, fatigue, palpitations, and weight and bowel habit changes.

   B. **Exposure factors.** Inquire about recent immunizations or new medicines such as antidepressants (3), cholinergics, meperidine, estrogen inhibitors, gonadotropin inhibitors, niacin, steroids, stimulants, over-the-counter preparations, antipyretics, and naturopathic therapies. Question patients about exposure to sexually transmitted diseases (STDs), human immunodeficiency virus (HIV), hepatitis, tuberculosis, or occupational and travel-related exposures. Also ask about increases in general changes in the ambient night temperature.

   C. **Psychological factors.** Anxiety, nightmares, and psychoactive preparations can precipitate night sweats in healthy individuals.

   D. **Family history.** Patients who report a family history of hereditary disorders and possible malignancies should have appropriate screening.

III. **Physical examination.** The physical examination should address the pertinent positives noted in the patient's medical history. Note the patient's weight and temperature. Examination of the head, eyes, ears, nose, and throat (HEENT) should focus on common types of infection: sinusitis, pharyngitis, and otitis. A thorough examination of lymph nodes is helpful to identify infection or lymphatic abnormalities (Chapter 15.1). The cardiopulmonary examination can also signal infection, valvular disease, and stimulant use. Patients should be examined for abscesses, skin ulcers, septic joints, phlebitis, and osteomyelitis.

IV. **Testing**

   A. **Clinical laboratory testing.** For patients with a known condition, testing for exacerbations is appropriate: erythrocyte sedimentation rate (infection, osteomyelitis, and temporal arteritis), C-reactive protein (rheumatologic disorders), and hemoglobin A1C (diabetes mellitus). Depending on the patient's symptoms or exposures, other appropriate tests can include purified protein derivative skin test for tuberculosis, free T_4 level to rule out thyrotoxicosis, complete blood count with differential (infection), and follicle-stimulating hormone to investigate the possibility of menopause. Special tests may be required of patients with travel-related or STD exposures.

   B. **Imaging.** Chest x-ray studies are useful in the evaluation of night sweats in patients with a smoking history, industrial exposure, or a cough. These patients need to be screened for occult malignancy. Computed tomography scans are generally not appropriate unless other signs or symptoms dictate further evaluation.

V. **Diagnostic assessment.** Night sweating as a single entity is not worrisome. Explore the likelihood of exacerbation of known conditions or the onset of a new disease process. The history is the most helpful part of the patient encounter. A new medication, with perspiration as a side effect, is often the culprit. Patients may need cessation of the medication as well as a washout period. Night sweats might be an early symptom of a developing illness so watchful waiting is useful (4). Patients need to be instructed to watch for weight changes, fevers, and sleep and mood changes. Patients can complete a symptom diary, which is very helpful to the clinician in determining the need for additional evaluation. Consider illnesses that tend to be present in the patient's age group. Screening for common malignancies through mammograms, pap smears, and fecal occult blood testing is appropriate health maintenance as well as often being a part of the evaluation of the presenting complaint of night sweats.

References

1. Smetana GW. Diagnosis of night sweats. *JAMA* 1993;70:2502–2503.
2. Lea MJ, Aber RC. Descriptive epidemiology of night sweats upon admission to a university hospital. *South Med J* 1985;78:1065–1072.
3. Babbott SF, Pearson VE. Sertraline-related night sweats. *Ann Intern Med* 1999; 130:242–243.
4. Chambliss ML. Frequently asked questions from clinical practice. What is the appropriate diagnostic approach for patients who complain of night sweats? *Arch Fam Med* 1999;2:168–169.

2.12 Syncope

James C. Chesnutt

Syncope is a common and concerning medical problem, which accounts for 3% of emergency room visits and up to 6% of hospital admissions. Although the cause of syncope can be life-threatening (e.g., ventricular tachycardia) and the result can be devastating (e.g., fractured hip), a definitive explanation for syncope is found less than one half of the time, with an average cost of $16,000/patient (1). Syncope recurrence is approximately 20% per year compared with an incidence of 2% for an initial episode of syncope (2).

I. **Approach.** Syncope is a brief loss of consciousness with collapse resulting from transient brain dysfunction based on decreased blood flow or neurologic insult. Syncope can be categorized based on the causative mechanism (Table 2.6). The most common causes are vasovagal (18%), arrhythmia (14%), neurologic (10%), orthostatic hypotension (8%), and situational (5%) (3).

II. **History**

    A. **What are the symptoms or circumstances related to the syncope?**

        1. Dizziness preceding syncope is highly associated with a psychological cause (24%) versus syncope without preceding dizziness (5%) (3). Dizziness with syncope can also be associated with arrhythmia.

        2. Important history includes palpitation, duration of prodrome and recovery, and presence of postural or exertional symptoms.

        3. Related environmental factors include heat, dehydration, and alcohol.

    B. **Which disease, risk factor, or family history is present?**

        1. Organic heart disease is associated with arrhythmia and increased risk of death.

        2. Psychiatric illnesses most commonly associated with syncope are major depression (12.2%), alcoholism (9.2%), generalized anxiety disorder (8.6%), and panic disorder (4.3%). These correlate with a higher rate of recurrent syncope, younger age, and a more benign course (4) (Chapters 3.1 and 3.3).

Table 2.6 Types of syncope with selected examples

CARDIOGENIC SYNCOPE (CS)
1. Arrhythmia, including ventricular tachycardia, sick sinus syndrome, atrial fibrillation, atrioventricular block and others (See Chapters 7.3, 7.9, and 7.12)
2. Organic heart disease, including coronary artery disease, congestive heart failure, valvular disease, hypertrophic cardiomyopathy, and others

NEUROGENIC SYNCOPE (NS)
1. Seizure disorder
2. Transient ischemic attack and stroke
3. Subclavian steal syndrome and others

NEUROCARDIOGENIC SYNCOPE (NCS)
1. Vasovagal
2. Carotid sinus hypersensitivity
3. Orthostatic hypotension
4. Dysautonomic
5. Postural orthostatic tachycardia syndrome
6. Situational, including micturition, cough, and others

UNCLASSIFIED SYNCOPE
1. Drugs
2. Alcohol
3. Psychogenic
4. Hypoglycemia
5. Pregnancy
6. Hypoxemia, dehydration, and others

---

       3. Older age (>60 years) is more highly associated with arrhythmias, orthostatic hypotension, medication side-effects, and situational (e.g., micturition) syncope.

       4. Ask about diabetes mellitus, neuropathy, anemia, and other chronic diseases.

       5. Inquire about a family history of sudden death, hypertrophic cardiomyopathy, or other organic heart disease.

    C. What medicines does the patient take? The most commonly implicated are antihypertensives and antidepressants. Others include antianginals, analgesics, and sedatives.

III. Physical examination. What are the essential aspects to cover?

    A. General: mental status, temperature, hydration status, pallor, or cyanosis.

    B. Vital signs: tachycardia, bradycardia, irregularity, or orthostatic hypotension.

    C. Cardiovascular: heart sounds, murmurs, bruits, edema, rales, and pulses.

    D. Neurologic: cranial nerves, reflexes, strength and sensation, tremor, Romberg's sign, gait, and cerebellar signs.

IV. Testing. Which tests are useful in diagnosing syncope?

    A. Electrocardiogram (ECG). The most important single initial test to evaluate syncope is the ECG; it is easy and inexpensive and can quickly identify life-threatening arrhythmias or ischemia. Although the diagnostic yield is only 5% (3), if the ECG is normal, ischemia, arrhythmias, and organic heart disease are very unlikely (5). If the ECG is abnormal but does not clearly demonstrate a likely cause for syncope (complete heart block or runs of ventricular tachycardia, for example), other tests are needed to clarify the underlying problem that may be related to the syncope. The result of the ECG, therefore, helps to direct the course of further workup.

    B. Cardiac monitors

       1. Holter monitor or telemetry performed for 24 hours. For patient with organic heart disease, this gives a diagnostic yield of from 2% for arrhythmias correlated to symptoms to 21% with unrelated arrhythmias. Extending this monitoring to 72 hours is not useful (5).

2. A loop event monitor is a portable, prolonged ambulatory event recorder indicating if there is recurrent syncope and no organic heart disease (yield = 24% to 47%) (4).

C. **Electrophysiologic studies.** This invasive cardiac monitoring and arrhythmia induction procedure gives a 50% diagnostic yield for those with organic heart disease or abnormal ECG (compared with 10% if no organic heart disease) (4). This is considered the gold standard for arrhythmia diagnosis but it is expensive and invasive. Powerful predictors of a positive test are an ejection fraction less than 40%, bundle branch block, or atrial fibrillation (5).

D. **Tilt table testing** is indicated for unexplained, recurrent syncope when arrhythmia or organic heart disease is excluded and neurocardiogenic syncope is suspected. In this setting, the sensitivity is 67% to 83% and specificity is 90% (4).

E. **Echocardiogram and stress tests** are used only to evaluate exertional symptoms (echo first in this case) or suspected organic heart disease.

F. **Computed tomography** scan is used to evaluate focal neurologic signs.

G. **Electroencephalogram** is indicated for seizure activity only (Chapter 4.7).

H. **Carotid massage.** Consider this if the patient is aged more than 60 years with unexplained syncope. Perform in the clinic if no bruits, ventricular tachycardia, recent stroke, or myocardial infarction.

I. **Blood tests,** including hematocrit, serum chemistries, and pregnancy test, are not for screening; order only if a specific medical condition is suspected.

J. **Psychiatric evaluation** is useful in the setting of a high recurrence rate in a young patient without resultant injuries and no evidence of organic heart disease.

V. **Diagnostic assessment.** The keys to the diagnosis of syncope are the history, physical examination, and ECG, yielding a diagnosis 45% of the time. The history and physical should focus on cardiac, neurologic, and medication-related issues. Directed testing can add 8% to diagnosis (3). Further classification by age and presence of organic heart disease can help focus evaluation and treatment. If organic heart disease is present or the ECG is abnormal, inpatient telemetry monitoring and electrophysiologic studies are recommended. If organic heart disease is not evident, ambulatory loop ECG and psychiatric evaluations are indicated, as well as possible tilt table testing (4).

Although most syncope patients can be evaluated in the outpatient setting, hospitalization is recommended for those with organic heart disease, chest pain, a history or suspicion of arrhythmia, or presence of neurologic symptoms or signs suggesting transient ischemic attack or stroke. The extent of severity of the organic heart disease is the key determinant of mortality and should direct evaluation and therapy (2). Despite extensive evaluation and testing, the diagnosis may still be elusive in approximately 40% of patients with recurrent syncope, but fortunately these patients have a low incidence of morbidity and mortality.

References

1. Grubb BP, Kosinski D. Neurocardiogenic syncope and related syndromes of orthostatic intolerance. *Cardiology in Review* 1997;5:182–190.
2. Kapoor WN, Hanusa BH. Is syncope a risk factor for poor outcomes? Comparison of patients with and without syncope. *Am J Med* 1996;100:646–655.
3. Linzer M, Yang EH, Estes NA 3rd, et al. Clinical guideline: diagnosing syncope. Part 1: Value of history, physical examination, and electrocardiography. *Ann Intern Med* 1997;126:989–996.
4. Linzer M, Yang EH, Estes NA 3rd, et al. Clinical guideline: diagnosing syncope. Part 2: Unexplained syncope. *Ann Intern Med* 1997;127:76–86.
5. Meyer MD, Handler J. Evaluation of the patient with syncope: an evidence based approach. *Emerg Med Clin North Am* 1999;17:189–201.

2.13 Weight Loss

David B. Graham

Involuntary weight loss is a challenging problem, often surrounded with fears by both patient and physician of an occult malignancy. Although malignancy is an important cause of weight loss, extensive and costly workups for occult cancers are rarely beneficial (1–5). The evaluation of weight loss is accomplished through simple and concise history, physical examination, and laboratory testing.

I. **Approach.** The key to the diagnosis of involuntary weight loss is a careful and complete history and physical examination. The approach begins broadly and then quickly focuses on specifics derived from the initial evaluation.
   A. **Quantify loss.** A loss of 5% of the baseline body weight (not ideal body weight) over 6 months is significant (1–3,5).
      1. Can the weight loss be verified? Serial measurements are best, but other markers include numerical estimates and changes in clothing or belt size.
      2. Up to 50% of patients do not have true weight loss (1), and in up to 25% of cases with documented weight loss and thorough evaluation, no cause is ever found (3,5).
      3. Is there a physical cause? One-third of cases will be caused by depression, dementia, or social factors (1,2) (Chapters 3.3 and 4.4).
   B. **Categories of weight loss.** The evaluation of weight loss can be divided into four major categories: decreased intake, increased nutrient loss, increased metabolic demand, and impaired absorption (Table 2.7).
   C. **Special considerations**
      1. A tailored approach in the elderly includes greater emphasis on social factors.
      2. The approach in human immunodeficiency virus infection and acquired immunodeficiency syndrome is more comprehensive, and special attention is given to disease-specific infections, nutritional changes, and neoplasia.
II. **History: Initial data**
   A. **Is the loss intentional?** Consider dieting, diuretics, and eating disorders.
   B. **What is the patient's average daily or weekly intake?** Consider frequency of meals, appetite changes, and difficulty with food preparation.
   C. **Tobacco, alcohol, and drug histories** are very important and frequently lead to other concerns.

Table 2.7 Major causes of weight loss

DECREASED INTAKE
Malignancy, congestive heart failure, medications, dementia, depression, grief, electrolyte disturbances, poor dentition or taste, gastric or esophageal disease, alcoholism, financial hardship, social isolation, HIV, and AIDS

INCREASED NUTRIENT LOSS
Profuse vomiting or diarrhea, diabetes mellitus

INCREASED METABOLIC DEMAND
Fever, malignancy, tuberculosis, hyperthyroidism, chronic infection, drug abuse (cocaine, stimulants)

IMPAIRED ABSORPTION
Cholestasis, infection (parasitic, other), medications, pancreatic insufficiency, diabetic or HIV enteropathy, inflammatory bowel disease

HIV, human immunodeficiency virus; AIDS, acquired immune deficiency syndrome.

    D. Chronic conditions? Medical, surgical, psychiatric, and family histories are always pertinent.

    E. Social factors include stress, isolation, and the cost and effort required to eat.

III. Basic physical examination

    A. Relevant physical findings will be present in 66% of cases (1,2,5).

    B. Quantify loss by serial weight measurements.

    C. Check the vital signs: temperature, blood pressure, and respiratory and heart rates. Consider determining oxygen saturation.

    D. Perform a physical examination, with emphasis on areas suggested by clues from the history.

IV. Testing

    A. Basic laboratory tests. Debate continues regarding the most useful and cost-effective laboratory testing for involuntary weight loss. A structured approach is best (1–5). Useful tests include:

      1. Complete blood count, thyrotropin assay, urinalysis, and fecal occult blood testing.

      2. Comprehensive chemistry panel including albumin, transaminases, blood urea nitrogen, creatinine, and electrolytes—calcium, magnesium, phosphorus, sodium, and potassium.

      3. Chest radiograph is often useful but not required (1).

    B. Comprehensive analysis. Further testing should be done *only* as directed by the initial findings. Careful observation and follow-up are superior management strategies to undirected diagnostic testing (1–5).

      1. When indicated, upper gastrointestinal radiographs, endoscopy, and colonoscopy are the most useful second-line tests (3).

      2. National Cancer Institute or United States Preventive Services Task Force age-specific screening guidelines should be considered and brought up to date for the patient. These can be accessed on the internet through the National Library of Medicine (http://www.nlm.nih.gov).

      3. Computed tomography and other expensive investigations are seldom beneficial in the absence of a specific (often guideline-based) indication (3,4).

V. Diagnostic assessment. The integration of history, examination, and laboratory data usually reveals the cause for involuntary weight loss.

    A. Cancer, including gastrointestinal malignancies, accounts for 16% to 36% of cases, and other gastrointestinal diseases account for another 14% to 23% (1,3).

    B. If the initial steps are not conclusive, the best approach is careful observation. Follow-up examinations and testing should be done monthly for 6 months. If a physical cause exists, it will almost always be found within this time (1).

    C. If an organic cause is present, this simple approach will find it more than 75% of the time (1–3).

    D. If an organic cause is not identified in 6 months, one is unlikely to be found (1–3). These undifferentiated patients, however, do well and have an excellent prognosis, assuming they do not have continued and progressive weight loss (1).

    E. Malignancy is a significant cause of weight loss; however, a truly occult malignancy is rare and an exhaustive search for one is not supported by the literature (1–5).

References

1. Marton KI, Sox Jr HC, Krupp JR. Involuntary weight loss: diagnostic and prognostic significance. *Ann Intern Med* 1981;95:568–574.
2. Rabinovitz M, Pitlik SD, Leifer M, et al. Unintentional weight loss. A retrospective analysis of 154 cases. *Arch Intern Med* 1986;146:186–187.
3. Thompson MP, Morris LK. Unexplained weight loss in the ambulatory elderly. *J Am Geriatr Soc* 1991;39:497–500.
4. Wise GR, Craig D. Evaluation of involuntary weight loss. Where do you start? *Postgrad Med* 1994;95:143–146, 149–150.
5. Reife CM. Involuntary weight loss. *Med Clin North Am* 1995;79(2):299–313.

3. MENTAL HEALTH PROBLEMS

THOMAS L. CAMPBELL

3.1 Anxiety

Thomas L. Campbell

Anxiety disorders, which are among the most common problems seen in primary care, occur in approximately 10% of patients. Anxiety disorders are associated with significant impairments in physical and emotional health, comparable to the impact of common chronic medical illness (e.g., diabetes and coronary heart disease). Anxious patients are often high utilizers of healthcare services and they generate high healthcare costs. The effective recognition and management of anxiety disorders can reduce medical and psychiatric morbidity and lower healthcare costs (1).

I. **Approach.** Most anxious patients in primary care present with somatic rather than psychological symptoms and may have associated comorbid conditions, either medical or psychiatric illness. These factors can obscure the diagnosis of anxiety and lead to excessive medical workup and improper treatment. For patients who present with chest pain, dizziness, or chronic abdominal pain, it may be particularly challenging to differentiate organic illness from anxiety disorders. Of 40% to 60% of patients with atypical chest pain and normal coronary angiograms, 20% of patients referred for dizziness, and 30% of patients with irritable bowel syndrome have been found to have panic disorder (2).

First, determine whether a patient's anxiety is dysfunctional, that is, whether it is excessive and interferes with normal functioning. "Normal" anxiety is a useful defense that helps us escape from current or future dangers (i.e., fight or flight reaction). Next, determine whether the anxiety symptoms are secondary to organic causes (e.g., an ingested substance such as caffeine or amphetamines) or a medical illness (e.g., hyperthyroidism, hypoxia), or whether they are associated with another psychiatric disorder (e.g., depression, substance abuse). The onset of anxiety symptoms after the age of 35 years, lack of personal or family history of an anxiety disorder, and absence of precipitating events are indicative of a possible organic anxiety syndrome. Of patients with an anxiety disorder, 50% also have major depression.

II. **History.** The most common physical symptoms associated with anxiety disorders include palpitations, shortness of breath, dizziness, sweating, and abdominal and chest pain. Common psychological symptoms can include shakiness, nervousness, fear of dying or going crazy, derealization, or depersonalization. Some patients attribute their anxiety to their physical symptoms ("Of course, I was anxious. I thought I was having a heart attack").

The assessment of anxiety disorders should include the nature, frequency, and duration of symptoms, precipitants, and impact of symptoms. A careful review of all medications (*esp.* stimulants, sympathomimetics, xanthines) and use of legal (e.g., caffeine) and illegal (e.g., cocaine) substances is essential. Comorbid medical and psychiatric illnesses should be assessed. The following symptoms should be specifically solicited: discrete episodes of severe anxiety (panic), intense fear of social settings, specific fears or phobias, obsessions or compulsions, and nightmares or flashbacks.

III. **Physical examination.** The extent of the physical examination or medical workup depends on the age of the patient, severity of symptoms, and presence or suggestion of comorbid medical illnesses (3). Although many patients with chronic medical illnesses may suffer from anxiety, relatively few medical illnesses directly cause anxiety. These include hyperthyroidism, hyperparathyroidism, tachyarrhythmias, and hypoxia from any cause (*esp.* chronic obstructive pulmonary disease).

IV. **Testing.** Laboratory and other medical tests depend on clinical suspicion and the presenting physical symptoms. Hematocrit, thyroid stimulating hormone, and serum calcium are often all the laboratory testing that is necessary. Older patients who present with physical symptoms, especially chest pain, may need more extensive medical evaluation before assuming that the symptoms are caused by the anxiety disorder. For example, an anxious patient with atypical chest pain, aged more than 40 years or with cardiac risk factors, may need an exercise stress test before assuming the chest pain is not cardiac.

V. **Diagnostic assessment.** Once it has been determined that the patient has a primary anxiety disorder, the following specific disorders should be considered (4) (Table 3.1).

A. **Adjustment reaction with anxious features** describes a condition in which the patient is experiencing clinically significant anxiety in reaction to a specific stressor, such as a major life event or interpersonal conflict. This diagnosis, which describes a more severe form of "normal" anxiety, responds to reassurance and short-term anxiolytics.

B. **Panic disorder** is characterized by recurrent, spontaneous, and discrete episodes of intense anxiety associated with symptoms of autonomic arousal (panic attacks). Patients usually present with physical symptoms such as chest pain, dizziness, and shortness of breath. They may also develop anticipatory anxiety or agoraphobia, in which they avoid situations that may precipitate a panic attack (such as crowds). Panic disorder is usually very responsive to medication (antidepressants or benzodiazepines). Panic attacks can also be experienced in association with other anxiety disorders.

C. **Generalized anxiety disorder** (GAD) is a chronic condition of at least 6 months duration, in which exists persistent, excessive worry or anxiety about several areas of life, often including physical health. These patients may be excessively worried about physical symptoms (i.e., hypochondriasis) and become high medical utilizers. Many patients on chronic benzodiazepines have generalized anxiety disorder. Often coexisting with other anxiety disorders, depression, or substance abuse, GAD is difficult to treat, but responds to medication and psychotherapy.

D. **Obsessive-compulsive disorder** is characterized by recurrent, intrusive thoughts (obsessions) and compulsive behaviors or rituals. These symptoms must be specifically elicited, as these patients rarely present with these complaints. Handwashing is a common compulsion, and patients may present with severe hand dermatitis from repeated washings.

E. **Posttraumatic stress disorder** (PTSD) causes persistent reexperiencing of traumatic or violent events through flashbacks or nightmares with associated autonomic arousal. Patients avoid any stimuli that may be associated with the trauma. It is often associated with irritability, hypervigilance, and sleep disturbance. It occurs most commonly in veterans, refugees, and victims of domestic violence and child abuse. Substance abuse, depression, and

Table 3.1 Diagnostic algorithm for anxiety

If the anxiety symptoms:	Consider
ARE DUE TO	
A medication or substance	Substance induced anxiety
A general medical condition	Organic anxiety syndrome
Other primary psychiatric disorder	Depression, substance abuse, psychotic disorder
ARE ASSOCIATED WITH	
A specific stressor	Adjustment disorder
Recurrent discrete, panic attacks	Panic disorder
Persistent chronic anxiety	Generalized anxiety disorder
Reexperiencing traumatic event	Posttraumatic stress disorder
Recurrent, intrusive thoughts and rituals	Obsessive-compulsive disorder
Fear or avoidance of social situation	Social phobia

other anxiety disorders are often associated with PTSD. No reliable effective treatment exists for PTSD, although antidepressants seem to be helpful.

F. **Social phobias** occur in patients who suffer severe anxiety in social settings, especially when they are exposed to unfamiliar people. These patients usually avoid any social situations. Social phobias respond well to cognitive-behavioral therapy and serotonin-selective reuptake inhibitors.

G. **Specific or simple phobias** are characterized by marked and persistent fears of specific situations or objects that interfere with the patient's life. Common phobias include fear of heights, closed spaces, flying, and specific small animals (e.g., spiders, snakes). They often develop in childhood as a result of a traumatic event associated with the situation or object. They are treated by cognitive-behavioral therapy.

References

1. Barlow DH. *Anxiety and its disorders*. New York: Guilford Press, 1988.
2. Stern TA, Herman JB, Slavin PL. *MGH guide to psychiatry in primary care*. New York: McGraw-Hill, 1998.
3. Knesper DJ, Riba MB, Schwenk TL. *Primary care psychiatry*. Philadelphia: WB Saunders, 1997.
4. American Psychiatric Association. *Diagnostic and statistical manual of mental disorders*, 4th ed. Washington, DC: American Psychiatric Association, 1994.

3.2 Confusion

Mark W. Nickels

Acute confusional states represent an etiologically diverse spectrum of disorders that may involve alterations in thinking, perception, memory, orientation, or attention. In addition, present may be physiologic changes, alterations in sleep–wake cycle, or changes in psychomotor behavior. These can be the result of delirium or psychiatric processes, and must be distinguished from dementia. The prevalence of delirium, the most common of these, in general hospital settings ranges between 11% and 16%; it is lower in outpatient practices (Chapter 4.3). This percentage increases significantly in elderly patients, those with preexisting central nervous system disorders, immunodeficient patients, postsurgical and burn patients, substance abusers, those with multiple comorbidities and complex medication regimens, and patients with significant psychosocial stresses.

I. **Approach**. Causative factors include cerebral and metabolic problems and psychiatric disorders. It is important first to consider organic causes.

A. **Organic factors**. The mnemonic **"I WATCH DEATH"** is useful for the differential diagnosis:

1. **I**nfection—sepsis, encephalitis, meningitis, syphilis, human immunodeficiency virus, abscesses
2. **W**ithdrawal—alcohol, sedatives
3. **A**cute metabolic—acid-base or metabolic disturbances, renal or liver failure
4. **T**rauma—head trauma, burns
5. **C**NS pathology—hemorrhage, subdural hematoma, tumors, seizures (nonconvulsive status, postictal states), tumors, hydrocephalus, vasculitis
6. **H**ypoxia—cardiopulmonary failure, carbon monoxide (CO) poisoning, hypotension, anemia
7. **D**eficiencies—B_{12}, folate, niacin, thiamine
8. **E**ndocrinopathies—Addison's or Cushing's diseases, hyper- or hypoglycemia, hypo- or hyperthyroidism, hyperparathyroidism
9. **A**cute vascular—hypertensive crisis, arrhythmia, shock
10. **T**oxins or drugs—medications, illicit drugs, solvents, pesticides
11. **H**eavy metals—lead, mercury, manganese

B. Psychiatric factors. The *Diagnostic and statistical manual of mental disorders*, 4th ed. (1) diagnoses to consider include the acute psychoses of schizophrenia, major depression, or mania; conversion disorder; dissociative episodes; and acute and posttraumatic stress disorders.

C. Special concerns. Urgent attention is required with hypertensive encephalopathy, intracranial bleeds, meningitis, head trauma, seizures, hypoxia, and acute psychiatric decompensations.

II. History. Collateral information is valuable with confused patients.

A. Characteristics. Is there an altered level of consciousness? Is so, consider urgent factors. Is the patient easily distractible or having difficulty keeping track of what is said? Is there an altered sleep–wake cycle; do symptoms fluctuate and are there changes in psychomotor behavior? If so, delirium is likely. Is thinking disorganized or incoherent? Is speech rambling, irrelevant, or frequently switching subjects? Is the patient disoriented? Do memory problems exist? Are there perceptual disturbances, including hallucinations or thought broadcasting, insertion, or withdrawal? The presence of visual hallucinations suggests organic causes. Are delusions present? Is there an indifference to the symptoms? If so, consider conversion disorder. Are there nightmares or increased startle response? If so, acute or posttraumatic stress disorders should be considered (Chapter 3.1).

B. Chronology of symptoms. Is the onset acute? In dementia, a chronic degree of confusion exists; however, acute confusion can herald the onset of delirium, warranting further evaluation (Chapter 4.1). Is the course fluctuating and do symptoms occur more often at night? If so, this suggests delirium. Have such symptoms occurred in the past? If so, what caused them then?

C. Medical history. Confusion is more likely in patients with multiple medical problems, longer lists of medications, or recent medication changes. Medications that can induce confusion include anticholinergics, sedatives, steroids, metronidazole, and digoxin, among others.

D. Psychiatric history. Are there any prior diagnoses and treatments, or a psychotropic medication history? If so, do current symptoms match prior psychiatric episodes? If so, consider a psychiatric recurrence. Have there been any recent psychosocial stressors? If so, consider the possibilities of dissociative and stress syndromes. It is important to note that a prior psychiatric history does not necessarily imply the confusion is caused by a psychiatric exacerbation; conversely, the absence of a psychiatric history does not rule out a psychiatric cause. Psychotic disorders tend to occur in younger patients, whereas delirium is more likely in older patients.

E. Other information. Current or past use of alcohol or drugs, recent injuries (particularly head injuries), and exposure to toxins. A review of systems helps detect organic causes.

III. Physical examination

A. Focused physical examination. This should include vital signs, psychomotor characteristics, assessment of skin, hair, and nail beds; and a funduscopic examination. A screening neurologic examination should include a check for nuchal rigidity, and an assessment of Kernig's and Brudzinski's signs. Positive findings warrant further testing. The Folstein Mini-Mental State examination (2) can help assess cognitive functioning (Chapter 4.5). The Confusion Assessment Method may be used to help detect delirium (3).

IV. Testing

A. Clinical laboratory tests. These should include a complete blood count with differential, urinalysis, toxicology screen, serum chemistry panel, and appropriate medication levels. Vitamin B_{12} and folate levels, serologic test for syphilis, and thyroid function studies can be drawn. As clinically indicated, blood gases can also be checked. Based on history and examination, additional studies may include cerebrospinal fluid examination, heavy metals screen, and erythrocyte sedimentation rate (and others, as needed for vasculitis). An electroencephalogram (EEG) can be particularly useful in distinguishing delirium from psychiatric presentations—in delirium, the EEG will show diffuse slowing, except in cases of sedative drugs and withdrawal when low amplitude fast activity is seen; the EEG is normal in psychiatric syndromes.

B. **Diagnostic imaging.** Magnetic resonance imaging is indicated for first psychotic breaks, new onset of confusion after age 50 years, and in the presence of focal neurologic findings.

V. **Diagnostic assessment**. Assume organic causes until proved otherwise. Delirium is more likely in those populations noted above, and is typically characterized by disorientation, a fluctuating symptom course, and alterations in the sleep–wake cycle. Paranoia may be seen. Be alert to the presence of visual hallucinations, which can suggest the possibility of delirium. A dementia history is typically one of long intellectual decline with usual levels of alertness and attention. Orientation is often impaired, as are recent and remote memory. Perceptual disturbances are often absent, unlike delirium (4). Acute psychoses caused by schizophrenia are often characterized by hallucinations, delusions, and formal thought disorder and do not typically include disorientation or altered levels of consciousness. Symptoms tend not to fluctuate and memory is intact. Psychoses that develop as part of major depression or mania follow the onset of affective symptoms. Conversion disorders can involve hallucinations in the absence of other psychotic symptoms. *La belle indifference* may be present, but no symptom fluctuation or sleep–wake alteration is seen. Dissociative states can include loss of memory, including personal data, and perhaps disorientation, but these are not embedded in other changes. Episodes are usually short and perceptual disturbances are rare. Anxiety-like symptoms may precede dissociation. Acute and posttraumatic symptoms follow traumatic events. Acute stress disorder, by definition, remits within 4 weeks, but has symptoms similar to posttraumatic stress disorder. Orientation is intact, concentration can be impaired, and increased vigilance may be present. Patients may seem detached or in a daze. Nightmares and flashbacks often occur but no perceptual disturbances or thought disorganization is seen. Memory is intact, except perhaps for the traumatic event. Signs of autonomic arousal may be seen, especially with recall of the event. EEG changes are absent in psychiatric disorders.

References

1. American Psychiatric Association. *Diagnostic and statistical manual of mental disorders*, 4th ed. Washington, DC: American Psychiatric Association, 1994.
2. Folstein MF, Folstein SE, McHugh PR. The Folstein Mini-Mental State Examination: a practical method for grading the cognitive state of patients for the clinician. *J Psychiatric Res* 1975;12:189–198.
3. Inouye SK, vanDyck CH. Clarifying confusion: the confusion assessment method. *Ann Intern Med* 1990;113:941–946.
4. Lipowski ZJ. Delirium (acute confusional states). *JAMA* 1987;258:1789–1792.

3.3 Depression

Jeffrey M. Lyness

Depression is a major public health problem because of its high prevalence and attendant morbidity and mortality. Although commonly seen in primary care settings, too often it goes unrecognized or untreated or undertreated.

I. **Approach.** Major (unipolar) depression has a point prevalence of 5% to 10% in adults seen in primary care settings, and a lifetime prevalence of at least twice that figure. The female to male ratio is approximately 2:1, although this ratio lessens with older age. Although major depression has received the most empirical study, so-called "lesser" depressions, including dysthymic disorder, minor depression, and "subsyndromal" depression have even greater combined prevalences and cumulative morbidity. Depressive conditions are a leading cause of functional impairment, including lost time from work, days spent in bed, and greater overall healthcare utilization. They also are risk factors for mortality, including but not limited to death by suicide.

Primary care physicians should evaluate for depression in all patients with any of the following presentations or risk factors (1): chronic medical illness; other psychiatric condition such as an anxiety or substance use disorder; recent psychosocial stressors, especially losses; multiple medical visits or unexplained symptoms; dysfunction at work or in social relationships; complaints of fatigue, sleep disturbance, and sexual dysfunction; or multiple worries. Begin the evaluation by asking the patient, "During the past month, have you been bothered by (a) feeling down, depressed, or hopeless or (b) little interest or pleasure in doing things?" (2) A positive response to either of these queries should lead to a more detailed history and examination.

II. **History and mental status examination (MSE)**
   A. **Symptoms and signs.** The diagnosis of major depression depends on a systematic assessment of psychiatric symptoms and signs (i.e., the history and MSE). At least five symptoms from the following list must be present most of the day, nearly every day, for 2 consecutive weeks or more: depressed mood; decreased interests or pleasure; weight or appetite change; sleep disturbance; psychomotor agitation or retardation; anergia; worthlessness or guilt; trouble thinking, concentrating, or making decisions; or recurrent thoughts of death or suicidal ideation, plan, or attempt. One of the symptoms *must* be depressed mood or decreased interests. Although somewhat arbitrary, the following grouping of symptoms may facilitate their recall.
      1. **Mood**—depressed mood: "How is your mood, your spirits?" "Sad," "blue," "down," crying spells; the patient also may have irritability, anxiety, decreased mood reactivity, and decreased hedonic capacity.
      2. **Ideational or psychological**—decreased interests: thoughts of worthlessness, helplessness, hopelessness, suicide; decreased ability to concentrate; and ruminative thinking (thoughts dwelling on depressive themes). Given the risk of suicide, *all* patients with clinically significant depressive symptoms should be asked about their suicidal thoughts ("Many people who are depressed have thoughts about dying, wanting to be dead, or wanting to kill themselves. What thoughts like this have you had?") (Chapter 3.4).
      3. **Neurovegetative or somatic**—change in appetite and weight: anorexia and weight loss are most common but hyperphagia and weight gain are possible; change in sleep (insomnia, especially early morning awakening is most common but hypersomnia is possible); decreased energy, decreased libido, psychomotor slowing or agitation; diurnal variation (in more severe cases, mornings are worse is the most common pattern).
   B. **Other factors.** In addition to the symptoms that define the condition, other factors should be assessed:
      1. Function. How is the depression affecting performance at work? Interpersonal relations? Attention to grooming and other activities of daily living?
      2. Psychosocial stressors. Both acute life events and ongoing stressors may be relevant.
      3. Prior depressive *episode*. Detailed information about previous episodes and their treatments will guide both prognosis and current treatment.
      4. Family history may reflect genetic vulnerability toward the condition, and also can shape the patient's perceptions about the illness and recommended treatments.

5. **General medical history.** Careful review of past and current illnesses and drugs (including alcohol and other recreational drugs) is needed to identify potential physiologic causes or contributors.
6. **Other pertinent negatives.** A past history of mania or psychosis suggests bipolar or schizoaffective disorder rather than major depression. Objective cognitive deficits (as opposed to merely subjective cognitive complaints) require further evaluation to determine the presence and cause of delirium or dementia, in which depressive symptoms are frequent.

III. **Physical examination.** Any patient with severe depression sufficient to warrant treatment should have both a general screening physical examination, paying particular attention to signs of anemia and endocrinopathies (e.g., hypothyroidism) and a careful screening neurologic examination.

IV. **Testing.** For typical mild major depressions, no tests are routinely indicated except as guided by the general medical history and physical examination. However, the following circumstances do warrant a laboratory workup: first onset of depression in later life; severely debilitating or treatment-refractory depression; or the presence of atypical features (e.g., onset despite the absence of past or family history or psychosocial stressors; severe cognitive complaints). Few empirical data guide the cost-effective use of screening laboratory tests in these cases, but most experienced clinicians would agree with performing most of the following: complete blood count; erythrocyte sedimentation rate; serum electrolytes, glucose, blood urea nitrogen, creatinine, hepatic transaminases, and serologic test for syphilis; and urinalysis. Older patients should also have an electrocardiogram and a chest x-ray study.

V. **Diagnostic assessment.** If the history and mental status examination reveal five depressive symptoms (including either depressed mood or decreased interests) present most of the day, nearly every day for a minimum of 2 consecutive weeks, then the patient has a major depressive syndrome. Such a syndrome can occur in the context of many conditions and not merely idiopathic *major depression*, so definitive diagnosis depends on the larger clinical picture. Depressive symptoms can occur in the context of *delirium* or *dementia*, either of which are evidenced by the presence of cognitive deficits (Chapters 4.3 and 4.4). Prior episodes of mania are indicative of *bipolar disorder*, whereas prior episodes of psychosis in the absence of mood syndrome indicate *schizoaffective disorder*. If the depression is caused by an identifiable physiologic factor (e.g., drugs or a general medical or neurologic disorder), it is a *secondary depression* (formerly known as "organic mood disorder").

Clinically meaningful depressive symptoms that do not meet full criteria for a major depressive syndrome are even more common than full-fledged major depression in the primary care settings. Whereas some such patients are captured by diagnostic concepts such as *dysthymic disorder* or *minor depression*, many elude diagnostic categorization. Making the diagnostic distinction between major depression and other forms is important, because a large body of empirical evidence supports the efficacy of specific treatments for major depression and dysthymic disorder; however, the efficacy of treatments for other depressive conditions is largely unknown.

The following should lead to psychiatric referral sooner rather than later: prominent or imminent suicidality; psychotic symptoms; history of mania; psychiatric comorbidity such as alcohol dependence or a personality, anxiety, or eating disorder; and treatment intolerance or failure to respond to therapy.

References

1. Depression Guideline Panel. Depression in Primary Care: Volume 1. *Detection and diagnosis*. Clinical Practice Guideline, Number 5. Rockville, MD: US Department of Health and Human Services, Public Health Service, Agency for Health Care Policy and Research; April 1993. AHCPR publication 93-0550.
2. Spitzer RL, Williams JBW, Kroenke K, et al. Utility of a new procedure for diagnosing mental disorders in primary care. The PRIME-MD 1000 study. *JAMA* 1994; 272:1749–1756.

3.4 Suicidal Risk

Barbara A. Gawinski

Suicide is the eighth leading cause of death in the United States; every 15 minutes, someone successfully completes suicide. Almost all people who kill themselves carry a diagnosable mental or substance abuse disorder; 80% have depression, 10% have schizophrenia, and 5% have delirium. Because most patients see their primary care provider within a month of their suicide, recognition and treatment of depression is a promising way to prevent suicide (1–6).

I. **Approach.** Suicide is the third leading cause of death between ages 15 and 24 years; it is the fourth leading cause among those aged between 25 and 44 years (7). Four times as many men die from suicide than women. Of people who kill themselves, 60% use firearms (1).

In the evaluation of every depressed patient, consider suicide. Almost every person has an occasional fleeting thought of suicide, but the suicidal patient ruminates about it. Appropriately prescribed serotonin-selective reuptake inhibitors can lessen suicidal tendencies and are markedly safer than the tricyclic antidepressants if taken in an overdose.

II. **History.** The major risk factors for suicidal patients are being male, older, unemployed, unmarried, living alone, having a chronic illness, gay or lesbian, adolescent, and being in a socially alienated group (5). The two major risk factors for child suicide are conflict with parents and an undiagnosed psychiatric disorder. For youth, family and interpersonal conflict were the most prevalent reported precipitating event (4). Drinking alcohol, especially in combination with depression, increases the rate of death; 15% of alcoholics commit suicide. Patients with previous suicidal behavioral are at increased risk for subsequent suicide attempts. Is there a history of previous suicide attempts, explicit statement of suicidal ideas or feelings (such as, "I want to go to sleep and never wake up" or "I'm going away and you won't have to worry about me anymore"), or development of suicidal plan? Some patients may also have a history of self-inflicted injuries, reckless behavior, and unexplained accidents. Clear indication of a suicide plan is the making of a will or distributing personal possessions. All these behaviors lead to increased suicide risk; it is important to assess for them.

III. **Physical examination.** Once a patient is identified as depressed (Chapter 3.3), the clinical interview and the mental status examination (MSE) are the primary methods for assessing severity of suicide risk. To assist the provider in assessing the risk of suicide, Table 3.2 identifies **emotional and behavioral changes associated with suicide.** When these finding are present, the clinician should assess the patient's suicide risk.

IV. **Diagnostic assessment.** All depressed patients need screening for **conditions associated with increased suicide risk** (Table 3.2). If the patient is depressed or has one or more conditions associated with increased suicide risk, ask specific **questions for suicide assessment**. These questions will not increase the patient risk of suicide, but rather will help guide development of a treatment plan. For patients with mild risk—experiencing passive or active suicidal ideation—contract for safety to establish a therapeutic relationship and identify the personal and professional resources for the patient and involved providers to contact if risk increases. The patient at medium risk—suicide plan without means to accomplish the plan—should return to the office frequently with a personal support person to continue to assess suicide risk, assess effectiveness of medication, and receive new prescriptions. Patients who have an active plan and means to carry out that plan are at high risk for suicide and should be transported to a hospital emergency room.

Table 3.2 Recognition of the potentially suicidal patient

Emotional and behavioral changes associated with suicide	Conditions associated with increased suicide risk	Questions for suicide assessment
Depression Declining interests (friends, social activities, sex) Change in sleep habits Change in eating habits Stress around holidays Disregard for medical recommendations	Alcohol abuse Death or terminal illness of a loved one Divorce, separation, or broken relationship Loss of job, home, money, status Exposure to suicidal behaviors of others (family, community) Firearms in the home	**Passive** Have you thought about harming or killing yourself? **Active** Have you ever thought you would be better off dead? **Planning** Have you decided the manner in which you will take your life? **Means to accomplish plan** Do you have the equipment necessary to take your life (pills, gun, car, rope)?

References
1. American Foundation for Suicide Prevention (1998). Suicide facts. www.afsp.org/ suicide
2. Beck AT, Kovacs M, Weissman A. Assessment of suicidal ideation: the scale for suicide ideation. *J Consult Clin Psychol* 1979;47:343–352.
3. Centers for Disease Control and Prevention. Suicide among children, adolescents, and youth: United States, 1980–1992. *MMWR* 1995a;44:289–291.
4. Centers for Disease Control and Prevention. Fatal and non-fatal suicide attempts among adolescents: Oregon, 1988–1993. *MMWR* 1995b;44:312–323.
5. Maxmen JS, Ward ND. *Essential psychopathology and its treatment*, 2nd ed. New York: WW Norton & Co, 1995:23–25.
6. American Foundation for Suicide Prevention. Suicide prevention resources (online). www.afsp.org
7. Ventura SJ, Anderson RN, Martin JA, Smith BL. Births and deaths: preliminary data for 1997. *Natl Vital Stat Rep* 1998;47(4):1–41.

4. PROBLEMS RELATED TO THE NERVOUS SYSTEM

ANNE CATHER CUTLIP

4.1 Ataxia

Robert B. Sammel

Ataxia is the inability to coordinate voluntary movements.

I. **Approach.** Ataxia usually refers to an inability of the cerebellum to coordinate movement, but dysfunction in other regions can also produce ataxia. The many causes of ataxia and the syndromes that mimic it can be narrowed by consideration of the age, acuity, and circumstances of onset, and by associated findings (1–4).

II. **History**

A. **Characteristics of gait and coordination**. Disorders of gait and coordination are common, and many abnormal types of gait can suggest ataxia.

1. Parkinson's disease (and other extrapyramidal syndromes) is characterized by a shuffling gait, deficiencies in movement initiation, *en bloc* movements, and bradykinesia. Normal pressure hydrocephalus and frontal lobe processes (gait apraxias) incorporate some of these features.

2. Hemiparetic and paraparetic gait are seen with unilateral and diffuse spasticity.

3. Motor neuropathies and myopathies interfere with the ability to walk through the limitation of muscular strength.

4. Hysterical gait is typified by a dramatic gait; the patient frequently lurching from point to point, swaying at the waist, and having more normal coordination in supine (astasia-abasia) and nonambulatory tasks.

5. Other neurologic processes (vertigo, myoclonic jerks, petit mal seizures, chorea) can either imitate or coexist with ataxia. Some elderly individuals adapt a wide-based gait because of the fear of repeating a fall, whereas a benign senile gait is also common.

B. **Chronology of ataxia.** The course of symptoms is valuable in the differential diagnosis of ataxia.

1. Acute ataxia can have infectious, neoplastic, toxic, and traumatic causes.

2. Chronic ataxia can be progressive, nonprogressive and persistent, or intermittent.

   a. Chronic progressive ataxia is suggestive of toxins (lead), degenerative diseases, neoplasm, and some metabolic diseases.

   b. Chronic nonprogressive ataxia can be seen with brain malformation (Dandy-Walker syndrome, Arnold-Chiari syndrome), cerebral palsy, and residual damage of past insults (severe hypothermia, hypoglycemia, trauma, infection, toxin).

   c. Intermittent ataxia occurs with some hereditary and metabolic syndromes, migraine, and seizures.

C. **Other history.** Obtain family history, and history of toxin ingestion [lead, thallium, mercury, acrylamide, toluene, and polychlorinated phencyclidine (PCP)], trauma, cancer, and recent infection. The exanthemas are associated with postinfectious ataxia, and varicella is especially associated with a truncal postinfectious cerebellitis. Drugs frequently causing ataxia include anticonvulsants (phenytoin, carbamazepine, and primidone), benzodiazepines, and antineoplastics. Lithium can cause ataxia even with therapeutic serum levels. Alcohol can cause acute Wernicke's encephalopathy or a more chronic or subacute cerebellar degeneration (1–3).

III. **Physical examination**

A. **Neurologic examination.** Evaluate for dysmetria (finger-nose difficulty), saccadic eye movements (differentiated from nystagmus by multidirectionality), titubation (head bobbing), truncal swaying, and dysdiadochokinesia (difficulty with rapid alternating movements). Observe speech patterns (wandering pitch, volume). The typical ataxic gait is wide based. Cerebellar ataxia can be differentiated from sensory ataxia or poor proprioception by Romberg's sign, where the removal of visual input dramatically reduces compensatory ability in sensory ataxia. Unilateral symptoms suggest a focal cerebellar insult (stroke, arteriovenous malformation, tumor), and deviation occurs ipsilateral to the lesion.

B. **Associated symptoms** can reveal specific processes. An older child with intermittent ataxia from basilar migraine, for example, will have a normal neurologic examination, whereas a child with hereditary periodic ataxia can present with nystagmus and more mild symptoms (1). Ataxia can precede the characteristic lesions of ataxia-telangiectasia, which tend to appear around 5 years of age. Opsomyoclonus warrants a search for neuroblastoma. The photosensitive rash of Hartnup's disease and the specific findings of maple syrup urine disease can assist in diagnosis. Look for signs and symptoms of hypothyroidism (Chapter 14.4). Pes cavus and scoliosis are associated with Friedreich's ataxia.

IV. **Testing**

A. **Diagnostic imaging.** Most evaluations should begin with imaging of the brain, because clinical pictures suggest specific diagnoses only on occasion. Magnetic resonance imaging is superior to demonstrate tumors, multiple sclerosis, and malformations. Imaging differentiates between posttraumatic posterior fossa hemorrhage and postconcussion syndrome. Lumbar puncture may be necessary to rule out an infectious cause. An electroencephalogram helps uncover intermittent, seizure-related ataxia ("pseudoataxia").

B. **Clinical laboratory tests.** As indicated, check amino acid screening, toxin screening, and thyroid function. Younger individuals may benefit from testing for IgA, ceruloplasmin, and phytanic acid deficiency to rule out ataxia-telangiectasia, Wilson's disease, and Refsum's disease, respectively. Pyruvate is a marker of mitochondrial disease. Vanillymandelic acid and homovanillic acid levels occasionally help to detect occult neuroblastomas. Paraneoplastic cerebellar degeneration is an immunologic phenomenon, most often associated with small cell lung cancer, for which Hu and Yo antibodies may be diagnostic. Approximately 40% of patients with Friedreich's ataxia have frank or occult glucose intolerance, and there are associated electrocardiogram abnormalities.

V. **Diagnostic assessment.** The list of conditions that cause ataxia is long, but most fall under the categories of neoplastic, infectious or immunologic, hereditary (metabolic or primary cerebellar), structural, degenerative (idiopathic or secondary), toxic, traumatic, or vascular disease. The time course can suggest more or less likely diagnoses. Although degenerative and hereditary diseases occur across the lifespan, certain diseases occur more frequently at certain ages.

References

1. Fenichel GM. *Clinical pediatric neurology: a signs and symptoms approach*, 3rd ed. Philadelphia: WB Saunders, 1997.
2. Lieber CS. Medical disorders of alcoholism. *N Engl J Med* 1995;333:1058–1065.
3. Marsden CD, Fowler TJ. *Clinical neurology*, 2nd ed. London: Arnold Med Publishers, Ltd., 1998.
4. Sudarsky L. Gait disturbances of the elderly. *N Engl J Med* 1990;322:1441–1446.

4.2 Coma

Anne Cather Cutlip

Coma represents a state of unarousable unresponsiveness in which the patient has no evidence of self or environmental awareness (1).

I. **Approach.** A patient presenting with coma should be considered a medical emergency.
  A. **Etiologic categories.** Consider these categories when evaluating a comatose patient.
    1. Traumatic: contusion, intracerebral hemorrhage, diffuse axonal injury.
    2. Metabolic: diabetes; thyroid disease; acid-base or electrolyte abnormalities; hypoxia; hepatic, renal, or adrenal abnormalities; hypo- or hyperthermia.
    3. Vascular: cerebrovascular accident, subarachnoid hemorrhage, aneurysm, hypertensive encephalopathy, eclampsia.
    4. Infectious: meningitis, abscess, subdural empyema, encephalitis.
    5. Toxic: poisoning, overdose, withdrawal syndromes.
    6. Structural: tumor.
    7. Psychogenic: conversion reaction, depression, catatonia, malingering.
  B. **Focal versus nonfocal.** The presentation of coma is typically focal or nonfocal.
    1. Focal: intracerebral hemorrhage, ischemic stroke, demyelinating diseases.
    2. Nonfocal: vascular, toxic, metabolic conditions, nutritional deficiencies, seizures, psychiatric conditions.
    3. Either: trauma, infections, tumors (2).
II. **History**
  A. **Characteristics.** Coma patients essentially behave in a reflex manner without spontaneous or purposeful movements, language cognizance or expression, or specific localizing responses (3).
  B. **Confounding conditions** include some medications, mechanical ventilation, immobilized extremities, facial edema, and diurnal variations.
  C. **Differential diagnosis.** Less severe conditions of altered consciousness include vegetative state, the minimally conscious state, akinetic autism, and locked-in syndrome (3).
III. **Physical examination**
  A. **General examination.** A thorough general examination, including vital signs, helps to establish and rule out potential causes of coma. Look for evidence of head trauma or metabolic encephalopathy.
  B. **Neurologic examination.** A detailed neurologic examination, including mental status; motor, sensory, reflex coordination; gait; and cranial nerve testing, will help distinguish the location and degree of dysfunction. Look for the following important features:
    1. **Level of consciousness.** Is the patient responsive at all? To what degree?
    2. **Brainstem function**
      a. Pupils: assess cranial nerves (CN) 2 and 3 for anisocoria, miosis, pinpoint, mydriasis, or fixed, midposition pupils.
      b. Eye movements: assess conjugate gaze, gaze deviation, nystagmus, and spontaneous movements (CN 3, 4, and 6).
      c. Funduscopic examination: assess for papilledema and underlying diseases. Corneal reflexes (CN 5 and 7); gag and cough reflexes (CN 9 and 10).
    3. **Breathing patterns.** Cheyne-Stokes respiration suggests cerebral hemispheric or diencephalic injury or an encephalopathy (hypoxic or metabolic). Central hyperventilation suggests brainstem injury. Ataxic or Biot's respiration, which can progress to apnea, suggests injury to the reticular formation in the medulla and pons.
    4. **Sensorimotor activity.** Are there spontaneous, volitional movements? Is there other motor activity such as choreoathetosis, decerebrate or decorticate activity, myoclonus, asterixis, or seizure activity? Is the muscle tone flaccid, rigid, spastic, or clonic? Is the response to painful stimuli purposeful, flexion withdraw, abnormal posturing, or no response at all?
    5. **Tendon reflexes.** Are the reflexes asymmetric, increased, or decreased?

6. **Glasgow Coma scale**. Measures the depth and duration of altered consciousness based on the best response to three actions: eye opening, verbal response, and motor response to commands or painful stimulus.

IV. **Testing**

   A. **Clinical laboratory tests.** Complete chemistry profile (including electrolytes, glucose, calcium, magnesium, creatinine, blood urea nitrogen), complete blood count, coagulation panel, arterial blood gas, toxicology screen (blood, urine, gastric contents), thyroid function tests, cortisol level, and select cultures (blood, urine, throat, rectal, spinal fluid). Consider performing lumbar puncture after obtaining a computed tomography (CT) scan.

   B. **Diagnostic imaging.** Cerebral CT findings reliably suggest intracranial hemorrhage, cerebral edema, mass lesions, focal infection, or hydrocephalus as diagnoses. Magnetic resonance imaging is preferred for the detection of abscess, tumor, subdural empyema, inflammatory lesions, or demyelinating diseases.

   C. **Other testing**. Electroencephalography rules out seizures, status epilepticus (SE), and nonconvulsive SE. Lumbar puncture, typically after diagnostic imaging, may help determine increased intracranial pressure as well as infectious causes. Evoked potentials, such as brainstem auditory or short-latency somatosensory, provide information about the physiologic state and response to therapy (4).

V. **Diagnostic assessment.** The prognosis in comatose patients is typically poor except for those that are drug-related or result from traumas. In general, the longer the coma lasts, the poorer the prognosis. Coma rarely lasts longer than 4 weeks, after which, transition into a vegetative state or recovery occurs (3).

References

1. Plum F, Posner JB. *The diagnosis of stupor and coma*, 3rd ed. Philadelphia: FA Davis, 1983.
2. Feske SK. Coma and confusional states: emergency diagnosis and management. *Neurol Clin North Am* 1998;16:237–256.
3. Giacino JT. Disorders of consciousness: differential diagnosis and neuropathic features. *Semin Neurol* 1997;17:105–111.
4. Chiappa KH, Hill RA. Evaluation and prognostication in coma. *Electroenceph Clin Neurophysiol* 1998;106:149–155.

4.3 Delirium

Linda P. Shields

Delirium, as defined by the *Diagnostic and Statistical Manual of Mental Disorders*, 4th edition criterion (1), is a condition involving an acute confusional state recognized by the patient's change in consciousness, attention, cognition, perception, or psychomotor activity level. It is acute in onset, often fluctuates widely throughout the day, and is potentially reversible. Its importance lies in its high incidence (ranging from 5% of young surgical patients to >60% of elderly medical patients) (2,3), increased morbidity and mortality, and the frequency of iatrogenic, and therefore, potentially reversible, causes.

I. **Approach.** Recognition of the risk factors for, and the onset of, delirium is essential for successful management. It is a psychiatric illness that is unique in that it is always associated with underlying medical illness.

   A. **Risk factors.** These include advanced age, preexisting dementia, multiple medications, poor nutrition, history of drug or alcohol use, impaired ambulation or use of restraints, decreased sensory input, pain associated with recent trauma, surgery, or medical conditions.

B. Causes. The precipitating factors in the development of delirium are often multifactorial. Medication, especially anticholinergic and psychotrophic drugs, are the leading cause of delirium. Any medication can be suspect. Common precipitants are infections [urinary tract (UTI), respiratory, human immunodeficiency virus (HIV)]; hypoxemia [congestive heart failure (CHF), myocardial infarction, exacerbation of chronic obstructive pulmonary disease]; and metabolic disorders (abnormalities of electrolytes, thyroid, glucose, renal and hepatic function, calcium, hematocrit, and vitamin B deficiencies). Urinary retention and fecal impaction can present as delirium. Central nervous system sources include meningitis, abscess, stroke, subdural hematoma, and increased intracranial pressure. Withdrawal from alcohol, sedatives, hypnotics or narcotics is a common cause of mental status changes in younger people, but must also be considered in the differential diagnosis for the elderly as well. Finally, remember that sleep deprivation and sudden changes in surroundings, including sensory deprivation, can provoke delirium in all ages.

II. History

A. Baseline. Perhaps the most important aspect of taking the patient's history is establishing the individual's baseline mental status and level of functioning. In addition to interviewing the patient, family, friends, and acquaintances must be interviewed as well. Other healthcare providers, such as nurses and doctors, who have dealt with the patient previously in an office, nursing home, or hospital setting, can be invaluable sources of information. Try to establish the presence or absence of the signs and symptoms of dementia or depression (section **V**).

B. Previous medical history. Look for previously existing medical problems that can precipitate delirium, such as CHF, diabetes, hypothyroidism, benign prostatic hypertrophy or HIV (section **I.B**). Evaluation of the medications is crucial, including prescription and over-the-counter medications. Is the patient taking them as directed? Is the patient on any medications that could be present in toxic levels (e.g., digoxin, phenytoin or theophylline)? Has there been any recent trauma or surgery? Are there symptoms of infection such as UTI or pneumonia? Be sure to interview friends and family.

C. Social history. Does the patient have a history of substance abuse? Is the patient currently using any alcohol or illegal substances? When was their last use? Be aware of potential withdrawal. If the patient is abusing alcohol, is there a history of delirium tremors with previous abstinence? Does the patient live alone? Is the patient at risk for poor nutrition?

III. Physical examination.
Because of the fluctuating nature of delirium, serial examinations are valuable.

A. Mental status. Observe the patient and take note of changes of level of consciousness, orientation, agitation, combativeness, hallucinations, or inability to concentrate. Evaluate the mental status by using the Mini Mental Status Examination (4) or a similar tool to standardize the findings (Chapter 4.5).

B. Physical status. Obtain vital signs and evaluate for clinical signs of dehydration, malnutrition, urinary retention, or fecal impaction. The physical examination should be guided by the history, keeping in mind the multifactorial nature of delirium. Evaluate for signs of infection, look for cardiopulmonary decompensation, and complete a thorough neurologic examination with special attention to identifying any focal neurologic deficit.

IV. Testing

A. Laboratory. All patients should have a complete blood count, serum chemistries including electrolytes, hepatic and renal function, albumin and calcium, and a urinalysis. Additional studies will be directed by clinical suspicions based on the history and the physical examination. These may include thyroid studies, serum medication levels, serum and urine drug screens, lumbar puncture with spinal fluid studies, HIV status, syphilis test, vitamin B_{12} and folate levels, or serum markers of cardiac damage such as creatine kinase-MB or troponin.

B. Additional studies. All patients should have an electrocardiogram and a chest roentgenogram as well as arterial blood gases or oxygen saturation level tests. With no history of trauma or focal neurologic deficit, a computed tomography scan is of limited value. An electroencephalogram is also of limited value unless the diagnosis of seizure is being considered.

V. Diagnostic assessment. Delirium can be a medical emergency, and a high index of suspicion must be maintained to accurately diagnose and treat the condition. Diagnosis is complicated by the similarity of presentation of depression, dementia and delirium, and by overlapping signs and symptoms. It is essential to rule out an underlying dementia or depression before the diagnosis of delirium can be made. This has particular impact on the treatment and prognosis of the illness.

A. Dementia is characterized by a gradual onset of decreased functioning in the areas of memory, execution of the activities of daily living, and social functioning. It is less likely for delirium to cause changes in sensorium, cognition, attention; it is also less likely for delirium to fluctuate from hour to hour. Delirium can coexist with an underlying dementia and should always be considered when a previously diagnosed dementia patient exhibits an acute change in mental status.

B. Depression is characterized by a depressed mood with psychomotor retardation or agitation. Look for a gradual onset of anhedonia, sleep disturbances, fatigue, feelings of guilt or worthlessness, or a previous history of depression (Chapter 3.3).

C. Other diagnoses. Consider in the differential diagnosis functional psychosis and bipolar disease, especially the manic phase. Both can produce hallucinations, although those of delirium tend to be visual or tactile, whereas those of psychosis tend to be auditory in nature. Epilepsy, especially temporal lobe seizures, can mimic delirium. Multi-infarct dementia, with its characteristic labile emotional state, must be considered. Remember that delirium is a complex, multifactorial condition and can present superimposed on a variety of other medical psychiatric conditions. A careful history and physical examination will help clarify the diagnosis and guide the physician and patient toward the correct treatments.

References

1. American Psychiatric Association. *Diagnostic and statistical manual of mental disorders*, 4th ed. Washington, DC: American Psychiatric Association, 1994:129–133.
2. Johnson JC. Delirium in the elderly. *Emerg Med Clin North Am* 1990;8:255–265.
3. American Psychiatric Association Practice Guidelines. *Am J Psychiatry* 1999; 156:S1–S20.
4. Folstein MF, Folstein SE, McHugh PR. Mini-mental status examination: a practical method for grading the cognitive state of patients for the clinician. *J Psychiatr Res* 1975;12:189–198.

4.4 Dementia

Anne Cather Cutlip

Dementia is characterized by a progressive cognitive decline leading to social or occupational disability occurring in a state of clear consciousness. It has an age-dependent epidemiology, occurring in 8% of patients aged 65 years and older in the United States, progressing from 1% to 2% in patients aged 65 to 70 years to approximately 30% in patients aged 80 years and older (1).

I. Approach. A common way to think about the dementias is to consider whether the dementia is either irreversible (90%) or reversible (10%). Among all dementias, Alzheimer's dementia (AD) is by far the most common (50% to 60%). It has been well characterized by the insidious onset of memory loss followed by a decline of other cognitive functions. Personality is preserved.

The vascular dementias (VD), which include multiinfarct dementia and small vessel disease (lacunae), account for 20%. Patients with VD typically have a sudden onset and stepwise deterioration in the presence of cerebrovascular disease (by neurologic examination or imaging). The disease presents with gait disturbances, frequent falls, and personality or mood changes, often in patients with diabetes mellitus, hypertension, or hyperlipidemia. Another 15% of dementias have a coexistence of VD with AD.

A. **Irreversible causes** include AD, VD, intracranial tumor, Pick's disease (PD), Parkinson's disease (30% develop dementia), alcoholism, Lewy body dementia (LBD), Huntington's disease (HD), progressive supranuclear palsy (PSP), Creutzfeldt–Jakob disease (CJD), acquired immunodeficiency syndrome (AIDS), and some metabolic diseases (Gaucher's disease, Niemann-Pick disease, metachromatic leukodystrophy). PD is characterized by socially inappropriate behavior, disinhibition with relatively preserved memory. LBD has features of parkinsonism, hallucinations and fluctuations in alertness and cognition. HD is an autosomal dominant disorder with depression, choreiform movements and dementia. PSP is a parkinsonlike syndrome with gaze paresis. CJD is a fatal viral infection with progressive mental deterioration, myoclonic jerks, blindness, and gait disturbance.

B. **Reversible causes.** About half the cases are caused by depression or drugs and have a fair chance of total recovery. Metabolic disorders, the third most common category of reversible dementia, have less chance of a full recovery. Normal pressure hydrocephalus is the fourth most common cause (2). It should be suspected in the elderly who have dementia, gait disorder, and urinary incontinence. Other diagnoses to consider include psychiatric diagnoses (schizophrenia, malingering), drugs or toxins (alcohol, mercury, lead, lithium), and metabolic conditions (renal disease, hypo- or hyperglycemia, hypo- or hyperthyroidism, hepatic encephalopathy, hyperparathyroidism, Cushing's disease, Wilson's disease, and acute intermittent porphyria). Other common causes include infection (urinary tract infection, pneumonia), anoxia (congestive heart failure, chronic obstructive pulmonary disease, anemia), vitamin deficiency (B_{12}, folic acid, thiamine, niacin), trauma (subdural hematoma, concussion), vascular (ischemic or hemorrhagic stroke), and central nervous system (CNS) infection (syphilis, abscess, chronic meningitis) (3).

II. **History.** A concerned family member will often bring patients into the office when obvious memory impairment occurs. The deficit will be sufficiently obvious to interfere with daily living, work, or social activities. When questioning the reliable historian, ask about the specific cognitive changes (language, judgment, abstract thinking, praxis, visual recognition, and constructional ability). Ask about the duration of symptoms, the mode of onset (insidious or abrupt), and the progression (slow or rapid, gradual or stepwise). Check on general risk factors (e.g., increasing age, atherosclerosis, head trauma, CNS infection), and family history. Specific risk factors for AD include increasing age, lower intelligence, small head size, history of head trauma (4), and Down's syndrome.

III. **Physical examination.** The patient should undergo a thorough general and neurologic examination and Mini-Mental Status Examination (MMSE). Look for focal neurologic deficits and assess cognitive function (memory, language, perception, praxis, attention, judgment, calculation and visuospatial function). Other neuropsychiatric testing is available.

IV. **Testing**

A. **Clinical laboratory tests.** The major value in laboratory tests is to look for potentially treatable causes of dementia. Basic tests should include complete blood count, electrolytes, basic chemistry (glucose, calcium, lipid panel), liver and thyroid function tests, vitamin B_{12}, folate, urinalysis, erythrocyte sedimentation rate, and serologic test for syphilis. In addition, if the history indicates, consider human immunodeficieny virus (HIV) testing as well as heavy metals and toxic screens.

  B. **Diagnostic imaging.** Computerized tomography is usually sufficient to rule out surgical (subdural hematoma, normal pressure hydrocephalus, tumor) and most cerebrovascular causes of dementia. Although more expensive, magnetic resonance imaging is superior to visualize small lacunae and temporal lobe atrophy (2). Positive emission tomography scanning is very expensive and seems to have greater resolution and sensitivity, but for now seems to be more of a research tool.

  C. **Other testing.** Electroencephalography generally shows nonspecific changes except in cases of seizures, CJD, and hepatic encephalopathy. The MMSE, which is a widely used, simple tool that requires less than 10 minutes to perform, enables assessment of cognitive function (Chapter 4.5). Expected results somewhat depend on the patient's educational level.

V. **Diagnostic assessment.** The differential diagnosis in dementia most commonly includes age-associated memory impairment (AAMI), delirium, depression, schizophrenia, chronic alcoholism, and mental retardation. AAMI is a normal aging process with gradual memory loss in absence of dementia or medical conditions. Delirium has a subacute onset with hallucinations, delusions, and psychomotor agitation (Chapter 4.3). Common causes include infection (urinary tract infection, pneumonia), electrolyte imbalance, hypoglycemia, hepatic or renal dysfunction, endocrine abnormalities (thyroid), and medications or toxins (anticholinergics, benzodiazepines, narcotics).

References

1. Richards SS, Hendrie HC. Diagnosis, management, and treatment of Alzheimer dementia. *Arch Intern Med* 1999;159:789–798.
2. Crevel HV, van Gool WA, Walstra GJM. Early diagnosis of dementia: which tests are indicated? What are their costs? *J Neurol* 1999;246:73–78.
3. Weiner MF, ed. *The dementias, diagnosis, management and research*, 2nd ed. Washington, DC: American Psychiatric Press, Inc., 1996.
4. Kaye JA. Diagnostic challenges in dementia. *Neurology* 1998;51(Suppl):S45–S52.

4.5 Memory Impairment

Konrad C. Nau

Memory is the cognitive domain that gives us the ability to store and retrieve information. Up to 80% of community dwelling elderly report subjective memory defects.

  I. **Approach**
  A. **Screening tools** must be used. Significant memory and other cognitive deficits and depression can exist in patients with fully intact doctor's office social skills (1).
  B. **Dementias** are ruled in if memory and other progressive cognitive defects are found (Chapter 4.4)
  C. **Red flags** that signal delirium include acute onset (<1 to 2 weeks), fluctuating levels of alertness, and new urinary incontinence. Medication side effects, serious systemic illness, or intracranial catastrophes are common (2).
  II. **History**
  A. **Presentation.** Dementia patients are brought in by relatives about memory problems; whereas, depressed and age-associated memory impairment (AAMI) patients come in on their own to complain (3).
  B. **Chronology.** Determine if the onset is gradual as in Alzheimer's disease (AD) or abrupt as in multi-infarct dementia (MID), subdural hematoma

(SH), Creutzfeld–Jakob disease (CJD); and steady (AD) or stepwise (MID) deterioration. Check for history of past strokes (MID); head trauma (AD, SH); medication; sexually transmitted diseases; human immunodeficiency virus (HIV) risk; alcohol use; heavy metal exposure; past depression; and many "I don't know" answers (depression).

   C. **Family reports** of change in the patient's judgment and executive functioning indicate other nonmemory cognitive problems (dementia) or visual hallucinations, as in Lewy body dementia (LBD).

   D. **Family history.** Inquire about a possible familial tendency for Huntington's disease (HD), AD, Parkinson's disease with dementia (PDWD), Pick's disease (PD), or alcoholism.

III. **Physical examination (PE)**

   A. **Normal** physical findings are reported in most patients with AD, AAMI, and depression.

   B. **Specific abnormalities that help classify dementias** include resting tremor (LBD, PDWD), myoclonus (CJD, LBD), glabellar reflex (AD), palmomental reflex (AD, PD), cogwheel rigidity (LBD, PDWD), stooped shuffling gait (LBD, PDWD), asterixis (alcoholism), chorea (HD), focal motor or sensory deficits (MID), asymmetric reflexes (MID, CJD), apraxic gait-wide based, feet stuck to floor or magnetic (normal pressure hydrocephalus, NPH), diffuse muscle wasting early in clinical course (CJD, HIV, dementia), and gaze paresis especially downward (progressive supranuclear palsy, PSNP).

IV. **Testing**

   A. **Tests** useful in clinical practice are presented in Table 4.1.

   B. **Clinical laboratory tests** can rule out treatable dementias. Check complete blood count, electrolytes, calcium, phosphorous, magnesium, glucose, blood urea nitrogen, creatinine, liver and thyroid function tests, vitamin B_{12} level, and syphilis test (VDRL). If indicated, test for HIV and heavy metals.

   C. **Cerebral spinal fluid (CSF) examination** is indicated in patients with early onset dementia, metastatic cancer, reactive VDRL, fever, or rapidly progressive dementia. If NPH is suspected, the withdrawal of 30 ml CSF with subsequent clinical improvement may predict therapeutic ventriculoperitoneal shunt success.

   D. **Diagnostic imaging** is indicated in all except perhaps longstanding end-stage dementia. Magnetic resonance imaging is most sensitive but computerized tomography (CT) will suffice to rule out subdural hematoma, central nervous system (CNS) tumor, hydrocephalus, cerebral atrophy, and infarction. Positron emission tomography scans promise to be most specific.

   E. **Electroencephalogram** usually reveals nonspecific slowing, except in CJD (diagnostic high voltage bursts).

V. **Diagnostic assessment**

   A. **AAMI** (benign forgetfulness) is a nonprogressive memory problem with recalling people's names and relatively minor recent events in those aged more than 65 years. Other cognitive domains are intact and this does not appear to predict future acquired dementias.

   B. **Depression** causes a pseudodementia that can be diagnosed using the Mini-Mental Status Examination (MMSE) (score >23) and the Geriatric Depression Scale Short Form (score >4).

   C. **AD** is the leading cause of dementia (127/100,000 population). Gradual onset of a progressive memory impairment along with at least two other cognitive defects that impair social or occupational function, a normal PE and laboratory determinations, and some cerebral atrophy on CT make a probable AD diagnosis. This is substantiated on postmortem examination 85% of the time (Chapter 4.4).

   D. **LBD** is the second leading cause of dementia with a fluctuating course, parkinsonian features, early visual hallucinations, and myoclonus developing within 1 year of the dementia. Patients with LBD are exquisitely sensitive to the extrapyramidal side effects of traditional major tranquilizers and have a two- to threefold increased mortality if on these (4).

Table 4.1 Testing instruments useful in clinical practice (1)

FOLSTEIN MINI-MENTAL STATE EXAMINATION (MMSE)
Validated with dementia/delirium cut off at 23.

	Score	Points
Orientation (disorientation)		
What is the (year) (season) (date) (month)?		5
Where are we (state) (county) (town) (building) (floor)?		5
Registration (memory defect)		
Name three objects, taking one second to say each. Then ask the patient to repeat all three after you have said them. Give 1 point for each correct answer. Repeat until patient learns all three.		3
Attention and calculation (acalcula)		
Serial 7s. One point for each correct answer up to 5. Alternatively: spell "world" backwards.		5
Recall (memory retrieval defect)		
Ask for the names of the three objects repeated in Registration (above). Give one point for each correct answer.		3
Language		
Show the patient a pencil and a watch and ask to name them (agnosia).		2
Repeat the following "No ifs, ands, or buts" (aphasia).		1
Follow a three-stage command: "Take a paper in your right hand, fold it in half, and put it on the floor" (apraxia).		3
Read and obey the following written directions: "Close your eyes."		1
Write a sentence (agraphia).		1
Copy a design of two interlocking pentagons (visual/spatial defect)		1
	TOTAL	**30**

Consider formal neuropsychology testing if MMSE is not conclusive, or if the patient has higher baseline intellect, a more detailed test is needed to detect cognitive defects.

YESAVAGE GERIATRIC DEPRESSION SCREENING SCALE—SHORT FORM
One point for each depressive answer (0–4 = normal; 5–10 = mild depression; 10–15 = moderate or severe depression).

1. Are you basically satisfied with your life? **N**
2. Have you dropped many of your activities and interests? **Y**
3. Do you feel that your life is empty? **Y**
4. Do you often get bored? **Y**
5. Are you in good spirits most of the time? **N**
6. Are you afraid that something bad is going to happen to you? **Y**
7. Do you feel happy most of the time? **N**
8. Do you often feel helpless? **N**
9. Do you prefer to stay home rather than going out and trying new things? **Y**
10. Do you feel you have more problems with memory than most? **Y**
11. Do you think it is wonderful to be alive? **N**
12. Do you feel pretty worthless the way you are now? **Y**
13. Do you feel full of energy? **N**
14. Do you feel that your situation is hopeless? **Y**
15. Do you think that most people are better off than you are? **Y**

Yesavage JA, Brink TL, Rose TL, et al. Development and validation of a geriatric depression screening scale: a preliminary report. *J Psychiatr Res* 1982–1983: 17(1); 37–49, with permission.

E. MID is the third leading dementia type with its stepwise or abrupt history and focal sensor-motor defects.

F. PDWD occurs in 30/100,000 population and develops in up to one-third of Parkinson's disease patients.

G. NPH is suspected with the triad of dementia, urinary incontinence, and an apraxic gait.

H. PSNP is a Parkinson-plus condition with paresis of downward, then later upward and horizontal gaze.

I. HD occurs in 5 to 10/100,000 population with chorea, prominent behavioral problems, dementia, and high suicide rates; onset occurs in individuals in the third and fourth decade of life. It has autosomal dominant heritance on chromosome 4.

J. CJD is a rare (1/1,000,000 population), viral prion CNS infection with rapid progression of dementia, wasting, and myoclonic jerks. Death occurs within 6 to 9 months in these patients aged 40 to 50 years.

K. HIV dementia is rare in the absence of symptoms of systemic infection. Use CSF to rule out CNS infections.

L. PD is rare with psychiatric disorders, blindness, and language defects (compared with more memory defects in AD) (5).

References

1. Gallo JJ, Reichel W, Andersen L. *Handbook of geriatric assessment*. Rockville, MD: Aspen Publishers, Inc., 1988:11–64.
2. Goldmacher DJ, Whitehouse PJ. Evaluation of dementia. *N Engl J Med* 1996; 335:330–336.
3. Robbins LJ. Dementia, delirium and depression: approach to the confused elderly patient. In: *Geriatric medicine for the FP audio CME lectures and workshops*. Kansas City, MO: American Academy of Family Physicians, 1997:9–36.
4. Lapalio LR, Sakala SS. Distinguishing Lewy body dementia. *Hosp Prac* 1998; 33:93–108.
5. Neary D, Snowden JS. *Classification of the dementias*. London: Churchill Livingstone, 1998:717–725.

4.6 Paresthesia and Dysesthesia

Rosemarie Cannarella

Paresthesia and dysesthesia are symptoms of peripheral nerve dysfunction caused by ectopic nerve pulses generated in these fibers. They are unphysiologic evocations of elementary physiologic sensations.

I. Approach. Paresthesias are experienced in the absence of any specific stimuli; dysesthesias are a result of specific stimulus. Patients find these unusual sensations difficult to describe, and may use many descriptions as listed below.

  A. Sensory phenomena can be divided into two categories.

   1. Positive phenomena. These include tingling, pins and needles, pricking, bandlike sensations, lighteninglike shooting feelings (lacinations), aching, drawing, pulling, crawling, tightening, burning, searing, electrical, and raw (1). Pain may or may not be perceived. These sensations are not always accompanied by a sensory deficit on examination.

   2. Negative phenomena describe a decrease or loss of feeling in a particular distribution (1). These sensations are generally accompanied by abnormal findings, and include terms such as hypoesthesia, analgesia, hyperesthesia, and hyperpathia. Dry skin, motor weakness, orthostasis, autonomic dysfunction, and cold extremity are other forms of negative symptoms.

  B. **Special concerns.** Acute onset of paresthesia that persists can indicate a structural problem (transient ischemic attack, stroke).
II. **History**
  A. **Do these sensations occur in a special nerve distribution or in a certain anatomic location?** Do they occur in response to a stimulus? Are they intermittent, or persistent and continuous? Was onset acute or insidious? How have the symptoms progressed? Any chronic medical illnesses?
    1. Glove and stocking distribution: suggests diabetes, vitamin B_{12} or folate deficiency, alcohol, or intoxications (heavy metals, industrial chemicals or medications).
    2. Dermatomal distribution: suggests herpes zoster, vasculitis.
    3. Other distributions: nonspecific pattern suggests idiopathic paresthesia, whereas extremity pattern suggests hyperventilation.
  B. **Is there an exposure** to solvents, pesticides, heavy metals, or recent viral illness? Is there abuse of alcohol or symptoms of systemic dysfunction or chronic illness?
  C. **Would the patient otherwise feel in good health if free of the paresthesia?** The answer to this question provides an idea of the patient's general health and a clue to a systemic illness.
  D. **Is this a sensation that is unfamiliar to the patient** (dysesthesia) or a familiar pain "like a toothache" (nerve trunk pain-aching sensation)?
  E. **What makes it better or worse** (dysesthesia—worse after activity, little makes it better; nerve root pain—better with rest, worse with movement, nerve stretch, or palpation)?
  F. **What is the distribution of the pain** (dysesthesia—cutaneous or subcutaneous; symmetrical distally; nerve trunk origin—deep and relatively proximal) (2)?
III. **Physical examination**
  A. **General examination.** Perform a thorough examination and check for hypertension, tachypnea, and tachycardia.
  B. **Nervous system.** Perform a sensory examination in the area of complaint: touch, pinprick, heat or cold, proprioception, and motor examination, including deep tendon reflexes.
    1. Decreased sharp touch and thermal sensation suggest small fiber neuropathies (spinothalmic tract syringomyelia).
    2. Decreased position sense, vibratory, or motor dysfunction but retention of most other cutaneous sensations are found with large fiber neuropathies.
    3. Sometimes paresthesias alone do not suggest their origins, but when combined with other neurologic deficits, the cause becomes more clear.
    4. Are the signs symmetrical? Do they occur in a graded fashion (polyneuropathy), somewhat asymmetric findings or multifocal signs (multiple mononeuropathy), or damaged individual cutaneous nerves?
  C. **Look for other physical signs of chronic disease** such as alcoholism, diabetes, malnutrition, pulmonary disease, and acquired immunodeficiency syndrome.
  D. **Avoid testing a patient who is extremely fatigued** (unreliable sensory examination). An overly cooperative patient may read too much into an examination and may discern very small differences that are not clinically significant. Do not prompt too much—give general directives.
IV. **Testing** (2–4)
  A. **Clinical laboratory tests** that may be useful include complete blood count; liver, renal, and thyroid function tests; sedimentation rate; antinuclear antibodies; vitamin B_{12}; and folate. Perform heavy metals and toxin assays if the history is suggestive.
  B. **The electromyelogram or nerve conduction study** is the gold standard in assessing the origin of the neuropathy associated with the paresthesia, if indeed one exists. It can differentiate between axonal and demyelinating causes.

C. **A nerve biopsy** is most useful in suspected inflammatory disorders (vasculitis, amyloidosis). It is also useful in suspected, selected small-fiber neuropathies, and in undiagnosed chronic neuropathy where significant debilitation has occurred.

V. **Diagnostic assessment.** The positive phenomena of paresthesia and dysesthesia do not necessarily mean a devastating diagnosis. They can be troublesome with no clinical diagnosis or be harbingers of peripheral neuropathy. The negative phenomena usually are a more ominous sign. Positive phenomena can act as troublesome symptoms that have no clinical diagnosis or as harbingers of more complicated syndromes of the peripheral neuropathies. If there is a documented neurologic deficit, especially once the motor system becomes involved, then it is more imperative to make a diagnosis. The most frequent neuropathy seen in clinical practice is the diabetic neuropathy (5). The real emergent diagnosis is that of Guillian-Barré syndrome, in which paresthesia can rapidly progress to full motor loss within days. Important is the association of symptoms to true sensory or motor deficits, systemic illness, toxin or medication exposure, or the rapidity of worsening symptoms.

References

1. Asbury A. Numbness, tingling and sensory loss. In: Braunwald E, Fauci AS, Isselbacher DL, et al., ed. *Harrison's Principles of internal medicine*, 14th ed. New York: McGraw-Hill, 1998:2457–2469.
2. Asbury AK, Thomas PK. *Peripheral nerve disorders*. Cambridge: Butterworth Heinemann, 1995:8.
3. Bradley W, Daroff R, Fenichel G, Marsden CD. *Neurology in clinical practice*, 2nd ed. Vols. I and II. Boston: Butterworth Heineman, 1996.
4. Haerer AF. *The neurologic examination*, 5th ed. Philadelphia: JB Lippincott, 1992.
5. Poncelet AN. An algorithm for the evaluation of peripheral neuropathy. *Am Fam Physician* 1998;57(4):755–760.

4.7 Seizures

Linda M. Savory

Seizures are a common serious neurologic disorder in the outpatient setting. In the United States, approximately 4 million patients suffer at least one seizure and 2 million have suffered two or more. Approximately 10% of these suffer more than one seizure per month despite treatment. No gender or geographic predominance is seen (1).

I. **Approach.** Seizures must be precisely categorized to be treated. Seizures are categorized as primary or secondary, generalized or focal, and simple or complex.
  A. **Seizure types**
   1. Primary generalized seizures include absence (seconds of staring, lid fluttering with no postictal state); atony (sudden falling); febrile (short seizures associated with rising temperature); myoclonus (short spells of jerking at awakening); and major motor (tonic flexion, followed by rhythmic flexion and extension, and postictal phase).
   2. Simple partial seizures include focal motor seizures (contractions of one limb or side with no loss of consciousness, starting in the frontal lobes).
      a. Complex partial seizures involve a change in sensorium and automatisms (repetitive stereotyped movements), and psychologic phenomena like crying.
      b. Secondary seizures are associated with infectious, metabolic, or structural causes.
      c. Status epilepticus, an unrelenting seizure activity or multiple seizures in rapid succession, is a life-threatening emergency (2).

B. **Special concerns.** Generally, the older the patient, the more chance of structural (tumor) or metabolic brain abnormality (3). Jacksonian march, progressive involvement of one or both lobes of the brain, is strongly associated with tumors.

II. **History.** Seizures can be confused with migraines and syncope.
  A. **Characteristics of the seizure**
    1. What was witnessed? Does the patient fall? Is there urinary or fecal incontinence, tongue biting, or loss of consciousness? Is there a postictal period? Is there staring, lip smacking, or automatisms? Seizure activity in neonates may present with subtle activities such as apnea, tremors, grimacing, or spasms.
    2. What can the patient remember? Are there associated sensations (odors, lights, emotions, tactile input)? Is there an aura?
    3. At what age was seizure onset? What is the frequency of the spells?
    4. What is the setting? Is there evidence supporting anoxia or hypoxia? Was there a sudden rise in temperature (4)? Did the seizure follow flashing lights, exercise, sleeplessness, fasting, or menses?
    5. Red flags include adult age at onset, changing pattern, and regression of motor skills.
  B. **Chronology of the seizure.** Most seizures present a characteristic pattern. A pattern of change or worsening of seizures can indicate new causation.
  C. **Family history.** Febrile, myoclonic, primary idiopathic seizures, and genetic syndromes with seizures often present a familial pattern.
  D. **Psychosocial aspects.** Ask how the family, teachers, employers interact with the patient.
  E. **Other information.** Important data include use of alcohol or drugs, medications that lower seizure threshold, toxic occupational or recreational chemicals, and severe physical [previous head trauma, central nervous system (CNS) infection, chronic illness] or psychosocial stressors.

III. **Physical examination (PE)**
  A. **Focused neurologic examination.** Examine level of consciousness, pupils, fundi, cranial nerves, reflexes, gait, muscle strength, general sensory, coordination, and Romberg's sign (4). Look for abnormal motor activity and test for abnormal reflexes.
  B. **Additional PE**
    1. Look for signs of systemic illness: cardiac disease (cyanosis, pallor, irregular rhythm, cool extremities) and chronic alcoholism (ascites, jaundice, caput medusae, and bruising).
    2. Look for residual signs of trauma or limb asymmetry.
    3. Look for dysmorphic manifestations of heritable disease: vascular malformations (Sturge–Weber), adenoma sebaceum (tuberous sclerosis), or *café au lait* spots and subcutaneous nodules (neurofibromatosis).
    4. Gingival hypertrophy suggests phenytoin therapy.

IV. **Testing**
  A. **Clinical laboratory tests.** Choice of tests is dictated by the patient's age, history, physical findings, and type of seizure.
    1. In evaluating a child, consider a random glucose, calcium, magnesium, electrolytes, and, possibly, a lead level and an electroencephalogram (EEG). In a child aged less than 5 years with one or two short generalized seizures associated with fever, no neurologic abnormality, and normal bloodwork, no imaging study is generally necessary (5).
    2. In adults, obtain glucose, sodium, calcium, and consider thyroid function tests, heavy metal screen, and porphyrins.
    3. Obtain a lumbar puncture when acute or chronic infection of subdural is suspected.
    4. An abnormal EEG supports the diagnosis of seizure and hints at the cause and classification. A normal EEG does not exclude seizure.

B. Diagnostic imaging
   1. In newborns, ultrasound or computerized tomography (CT) imaging may reveal intracerebral hemorrhage or structural abnormality.
   2. Adolescents and adults should have a magnetic resonance imaging scan (or CT) to rule out focal and structural lesions.
C. Special studies include prolonged closed-circuit video EEG to distinguish psychogenic seizures or in a patient with continuing seizures and multiple normal EEGs.
V. Diagnostic assessment. The key to diagnosis is the history and neurologic examination. A history with a focal component indicates a high likelihood of structural pathology. A recent febrile illness with seizure, headache, change in mental status, or confusion suggests acute CNS infection. A history of headache or change in mental function with seizure and abnormal neurologic examination suggests mass lesion. A clear, focal onset of the event (staring or head turning) may aid in distinguishing seizure from syncope. Emotional lability and a history of psychiatric treatment in a patient whose neurologic workup is negative may suggest a diagnosis of pseudoseizures. A pregnant patient near term who seizes may have pregnancy-induced hypertension or declining drug levels.

References
1. Dichter MA. The epilepsies and convulsive disorders. In: Braunwald E, Fauci AS, Isselbacher DL, et al., ed. *Harrison's principles of internal medicine*, 13th ed. New York: McGraw-Hill, 1995:2223.
2. Bradford JC, Kyriakedes CG. Evaluation of the patient with seizures: an evidence based approach. *Emerg Med Clin North Am* 1999;17(1):203–220, ix–x.
3. Hauser WA. Seizure disorders: the changes with age. *Epilepsia* 1992;33(4):S6–S14.
4. Roth HL, Drislane FW. Seizures. *Neurol Clin* 1998;16:257–284.
5. Berg, AT, Shinnar S. The risk of seizure occurrence following a first unprovoked seizure: a quantitative review. *Neurology* 1991;41:965–972.

4.8 Stroke

Gregory A. Doyle

Cerebrovascular disease is the most common acute neurologic illness in the United States. Stroke is defined as a neurologic deficit involving the cerebral circulation that lasts more than 24 hours (1). Transient ischemic attacks (TIA) are deficits that resolve within 24 hours.

I. Approach
   A. Stroke type can be described by circulation:
      1. Carotid (hemispheric)
      2. Vertebrobasilar (brainstem or cerebellar)
   B. Stroke can also be described by cause (2):
      1. Ischemic (85%): atherosclerosis with artery-to-artery embolization.
         a. Cardiac
            (1) Mural hypokinesis with thrombosis, myocardial infarction (MI), cardiomyopathy, atrial fibrillation (arrhythmia)
            (2) Embolism from valvular heart disease (mitral most common)
            (3) Septal abnormalities, including patent foramen ovale, especially in patients aged less than 60 years (3)
         b. Hypercoagulable states: causes include antiphospholipid antibodies, deficiency of protein S or C, presence of antithrombin 3, oral contraceptives

      c. Miscellaneous states include posttraumatic, artery dissection, vasculitis, drugs (cocaine, amphetamines), and fibromuscular dysplasia
    2. Hemorrhagic (15%):
      a. Hypertension: damages putamen, internal capsule, cerebellum, brainstem, corona radiata
      b. Amyloid: lobar (cortical) hemorrhages in elderly
      c. Vascular malformations
  C. Special concerns. The differential diagnosis of stroke includes trauma (subdural hematomas), migraine headaches, focal seizures, metabolic disorders (especially hypoglycemia), Bell's palsy, hyperventilation, hysterical conversion, and tumors. Computed tomography (CT) is valuable in ruling out these lesions.

II. History
  A. Characteristics of the stroke. What is the duration of the deficit? Is the problem acute and lasting several hours? Impaired consciousness can occur in all types of stroke. More specific symptom may help localize the area of stroke:
    1. Carotid circulation: symptoms of hemiplegia, hemianesthesia, aphasia, visual field defects, and loss of spatial function; occasionally, seizures, headache, amnesia, and confusion.
    2. Vertebrobasilar circulation: symptoms of diplopia, vertigo, ataxia, facial paresis, Horner's syndrome, dysphagia, dysarthria, quadraparesis (a component of bilateral arms or legs), and crossed sensory symptoms (ipsilateral face and contralateral body). Cerebellar lesions often display headache, nausea or vomiting, and ataxia.
  B. Past history. A history of trauma, migraine, vasculitis, seizure, and hypoglycemia could produce a condition that can mimic stroke. Fever or infection may suggest abscess. A prior history of stroke or TIA often precedes the presentation of a new stroke. A history of valvular heart disease, atrial fibrillation, or MI is relevant.
  C. Risk factors. Patients need to be assessed for hypertension, cardiac disease (specifically atrial fibrillation), smoking, diabetes mellitus, hypercoagulable states, and hormonal therapy.
  D. Hospitalization. This may be necessary for patients with transient or ongoing ischemic deficits. TIAs can herald a high-grade carotid stenosis or occult left atrial thrombus.

III. Physical examination (PE)
  A. General examination. This should include vital signs (notably blood pressure), Mini-Mental Status Examination, and an examination of the eyes, including funduscopic. A screening neurologic examination of cranial nerves, coordination, muscle strength, sensation, deep tendon, reflexes, and gait is recommended.
  B. Additional PE. Evaluate the heart (arrhythmia, mitral stenosis) and vascular system (carotid bruits), and palpate the scalp and neck (trauma and migraine) and superficial temporal arteries (arteritis).

IV. Testing
  A. Clinical laboratory tests. In most instances, laboratory tests are not helpful in the acute assessment. Laboratory tests that may be suggested by the clinical history and PE include blood sugar, coagulation studies (prothrombin, partial thromboplastin times), platelet count, antiphospholipid antibodies, protein S, protein C, antithrombin III, and toxicology screens (cocaine, amphetamines). C-Reactive protein can be of prognostic significance (4). Additional tests may be relevant, depending on the history and PE, including electrocardiogram, cardiac monitoring, electroencephalogram, and spinal tap.
  B. Diagnostic imaging. In most instances, diagnostic imaging should include an emergent cerebral CT scan of the brain to rule out abscess, tumor, or hemorrhage. A magnetic resonance imaging scan is a better test for aneurysm, arteriovascular malformation, or tumors. Other tests can include transthoracic or esophageal echocardiogram, duplex carotid ultrasonography, cerebral angiography, and magnetic resonance angiography.

V. Diagnostic assessment. The key to the diagnosis of stroke is the duration of neurologic event coupled with the signs and symptoms. The CT scan rules out other serious pathology that can mimic stroke. Specifically, laboratory tests can aid in the workup and are directed by the history and physical examination.

References
1. Schneck MJ. Acute stroke: an aggressive approach to intervention and prevention. *Hosp Med* 1998;34(1):11–28.
2. Graffagnino C, Itaachinski V. Stroke (brain attack). In: Dambro MR, ed. *Griffith's 5-minute clinical consult*, 2nd ed. Philadelphia: Lippincott, Williams & Wilkins, 1999:1014–1015.
3. Nendaz MR, Sarasin FP, Junod AF. Preventing stroke recurrence in patients with patent foramen ovale: antithrombotic therapy, foramen closure, or therapeutic abstention? A decision analytic perspective. *Am Heart J* 1998;135(3):532–541.
4. Muir KW, Weir CJ, Alwan W. C-Reactive protein and outcome after ischemic stroke. *Stroke* 1999;30:981–985.

4.9 Tremor

Peter G. Teichman

Tremor, a rhythmic, involuntary oscillatory movement of a body part, is the most common movement disorder.

I. **Approach.** It is important to classify the tremor based on clinical findings, identify possible reversible causes, and assess the impact that tremor has on the patient's activities. Multiple causative, physiologic, and treatment response classifications have been proposed, although not validated in clinical research. Clinical observation and historical data remain the basis for grouping specific clinical features into tremor syndromes (1).
   A. **Physiologic tremor** is a nonprogressing tremor that occurs in any body part and remits spontaneously with removal of a triggering agent.
   B. **Essential tremor**, the most common type of tremor, is a largely hereditary, mainly postural tremor of the hands and sometimes the head (1). Primary writing tremor (tremor predominantly or only during writing but not during other tasks in the active hand) and isolated voice tremor (tremulous vocalization without involvement of other body parts) are types of essential tremor syndromes (1).
   C. **Parkinsonian tremor** is a tremor at rest that occurs in the setting of other features of Parkinson's disease (PD) such as bradykinesia and rigidity.
   D. **Secondary tremor syndromes.** Many conditions can cause tremor, including drug-induced, toxic, and drug withdrawal tremors; tremor in peripheral neuropathy or dystonia (a syndrome dominated by sustained muscle contractions that cause twisting repetitive movements and abnormal postures) (1); psychogenic tremor; and tremor secondary to specific central nervous system lesions such as stroke or tumor (cerebellar tremor, Holme's tremor, and palatal tremor).
II. **History**
   A. **Tremor characteristics.** Does the tremor occur at rest, with goal-directed movement, or with maintenance of a specific posture? Parkinsonian tremor is a classic resting tremor, whereas essential tremor occurs or increases with maintenance of a posture. Drug-induced, drug withdrawal, and psychogenic tremors can occur at rest, with postural maintenance, or with movement.
   B. **What worsens the tremor?** Parkinsonian tremor increases during mental stress or with movement of other body parts. Observation, stress, anxiety, fatigue, and certain drugs exacerbate essential tremor. Exposure to cold,

fear, pain, caffeine, emotional loss, and stressful situations can initiate and promote physiologic tremors. A complete alcohol and medication history will further elicit possible secondary causes of tremor. Some known tremor-precipitating agents include antidepressants, lithium, neuroleptics, dopamine blocking agents, sympathomimetics, pseudoephedrine, theophylline, caffeine, methylphenidate, and withdrawal of alcohol (1,2).

C. **What inhibits the tremor?** Sleep stops all tremors. Whereas essential tremors increase with movement, Parkinsonian tremors diminish with goal-directed actions of the affected body part. Alcohol ingestion decreases tremor in 75% of patients with essential tremor (3). Physiologic and secondary tremors usually remit with removal of the precipitator or correction of the underlying disorder.

D. **How has the tremor changed over time?** Essential tremor slowly progresses. It can advance to cause social embarrassment, loss of function, and disability. Parkinsonian tremor and secondary tremors parallel the course and treatment of the underlying disease.

E. **Family history.** Only a slight familial relationship is seen with Parkinson's disease, whereas at least 60% of essential tremor patients have a relative with tremor (3).

F. **Onset and progression.** When did the tremor begin? How has the tremor affected your life, your job, and your relationships? Parkinsonian and essential tremors usually occur after the fifth decade. Both can progress to cause decreased function, social embarrassment and isolation, disability, and loss of livelihood. Physiologic and psychogenic tremors rapidly occur and regress.

III. **Physical examination.** A general search for signs of central nervous system involvement, drug use or withdrawal, and peripheral neuropathy may uncover secondary tremor causes. A focused examination of affected body parts, including provocative tests, may distinguish among the tremor types. Essential tremor is usually bilateral, symmetric, and increases with observed provocative testing such as maintaining a posture against gravity, pouring water, or drawing. It most commonly involves the hands and arms. It can also involve the head and voice. In advanced stages, leg and feet involvement can occur.

Parkinsonian tremor, the classic "pill rolling" resting tremor, remits with movement. It can herald the onset of Parkinson's disease, or develop concurrently with rigidity, bradykinesia, and postural instability. Psychogenic tremors appear and remit suddenly, can exhibit unusual combinations of rest and intention tremors, occur in the presence of other unrelated neurologic signs, and diminish with distraction.

IV. **Testing.** The diagnosis and classification of tremor is usually made without laboratory testing or imaging studies, although drug- and disease-specific testing may identify secondary causes. In some cases, electromyographic studies can help distinguish among tremor types; indirectly measure functional disability; and, by repeated testing, assess the progression of the tremor. Clinical functional disability scales may also assess tremor progression. Pharmacotherapeutic challenges (dopaminergic agents in suspected PD and beta-blockers or primidone in suspected essential tremor) may provide further diagnostic insight.

V. **Diagnostic assessment.** In most cases, the diagnosis of tremor is based on specific historical and physical examination findings. Proper treatment depends on classification of the tremor type and the identification of secondary causes. When the cause or classification of tremor is unclear, observation of tremor progression over time may uncover its cause, and guide patient and provider expectations of severity and dysfunction.

References

1. Deuschl G, Bain P, Brin M, et al. Consensus statement of the Movement Disorder Society on Tremor. *Mov Disord* 1998;13(Suppl 3):2–23.
2. Charles PD, Esper GJ, Davis TL, Maciunas RJ, Robertson D. Classification of tremor and update on treatment. *Am Fam Physician* 1999;59:1565–1572.
3. Koller WC, Busenbark K, Miner K, et al. The relationship of essential tremor to other movement disorders: report on 678 patients. *Ann Neurol* 1994;35:717–722.

5. EYE PROBLEMS

JOHN E. SUTHERLAND

5.1 Blurred Vision

Gary K. Phelps

Blurred vision is a common, very nonspecific presenting ophthalmic complaint. Normal visual function requires a sharp image created by the lenses (cornea and crystalline lens) of the eye onto the retina, accurate translation from light to electrical energy by the retina, and transmission of that information through the optic nerve to the chiasm (where the information from each eye is mixed), through the lateral geniculate to the occipital cortex where the image is interpreted and compared with associated information in memory. Failure of any part of the system can be interpreted as blurred vision. Problems anterior to the chiasm cause monocular disturbances, posterior to the chiasm binocular. The critical aspect is to identify the small number of patients requiring immediate intervention to alter the disease course (1).

I. **Approach.** The causes of blurred vision are myriad, but are best considered in three anatomic areas.
   Optical problems include refractive errors, cataract, corneal opacity, and uveitis. Receptor (retinal) problems include macular degeneration, diabetic macular edema, and retinal vascular occlusions. Neurologic pathway problems encompass such entities as optic neuritis and occipital stroke.

II. **History**
   A. **Timing of blurred vision.** Most causes of blurred vision requiring acute intervention are of sudden, recent onset, with the exception of tumor compression, which can be gradual. Episodes of transient duration tend to be more benign, whereas those that are worsening or long term in nature tend to be more ominous.
   B. **Nature of blurred vision.** The monocular, binocular, central, hemianopic, peripheral, color saturation, distortion, or negative nature (loss of area of vision) or positive nature (seeing things that are not there) provides clues to the location and nature of the disease. Binocularity, loss of color saturation, and hemianopic visual loss suggest neurologic disease, whereas monocular, central, and distortion suggest retinal disease.
   C. **Associated symptoms.** Other symptoms, acute or remote in time or location (e.g., hemiparesis, dysarthria, or diplopia) point to neurologic disease (multiple sclerosis, transient ischemic attacks, acute or recurrent stroke, and so on) of which visual blurring is simply one part (Chapter 4.8). Giant cell arteritis, stroke, embolic disease, retinal detachment, and macular degeneration are far more common in the aging population. Diabetes mellitus has a high risk of associated retinal vascular disease, especially in the second decade of duration (Chapter 14.1). Trauma-induced visual blurring is usually self-evident by history or physical examination.

III. **Physical examination**
   A. **Gross examination.** Visual acuity (VA) can be measured at distance or near; it should be done in each eye independently and is best done with spectacles or contact lenses in place. Gross inspecting for visualization of clear iris detail quickly evaluates for corneal clouding or hyphema. Confrontation visual fields (VF) are done by comparing the patient's ability to count fingers in all four quadrants to the examiner. A relative afferent pupillary defect, where light shined into one eye causes both pupils to become smaller than light shined into the other, screens for conduction defects of the optic nerve.
   B. **Instrument-assisted examination.** A clear red reflex with a direct ophthalmoscope eliminates opacities of the cornea or lens and the funduscopic examination identifies a normal macular reflex and a healthy optic nerve. Acute glaucoma is easily screened with a tonometer (Schiotz or Goldman applanation with a slit lamp biomicroscope): a pressure of greater than 30 mm Hg is highly suspicious.

IV. Testing
   A. Laboratory. Erythrocyte sedimentation rate (ESR) and C-reactive protein are pertinent laboratory screens for giant cell arteritis.
   B. Diagnostic imaging. Computed tomography (CT) or magnetic resonance imaging (MRI) scans are useful primarily in cases of trauma to identify disruption of the orbit or orbital hemorrhages or masses, stroke syndromes, or compressive lesions of the optic nerve, chiasm pathways to the occipital lobe, or occipital lobe.
V. Diagnostic assessment (Table 5.1). Transient blurring that clears with blinking is usually tear film-related and can be investigated at leisure. Gradual visual loss, which improves greatly with a pinhole, is almost always optical and can await delayed evaluation. Blurred vision at near can be secondary to aging (presbyopia) or orally or topically administered parasympathomimetic drugs. Sudden monocular loss associated with a relative afferent pupillary defect demands immediate assessment for giant cell arteritis or optic neuritis (vascular or demyelinating). Sudden onset of hemianopic bilateral VF defects, particularly if associated with pain or other neurologic defects, demands immediate evaluation for stroke syndrome (vascular or compressive secondary to tumor). Blurred vision associated with trauma such as corneal foreign body, hyphema, or ruptured globe is usually self-evident. Repeated transient obscurations of minutes in nature, particularly in young and frequently overweight female patients, may indicate optic nerve compression and careful funduscopic examination is necessary to rule out papilledema with increased intracranial pressure (e.g., essential intracranial hypertension). Transient, positive visual disturbances are usually benign (e.g., recurrent migraine scotoma—"scintillating scotoma"—or retinal regenerative phenomena—"after images"). A single episode without ancillary migraine history should arouse suspicion of early stroke syndrome or retinal tear and requires ophthalmic or neurologic workup. Intermittent or persistent episodes of blurred vision, especially combined with a history of pain (sometimes referred to the chest or abdomen), photophobia, halos, red eye, and a duration longer than a few minutes, are diagnostic clues of pupillary block glaucoma or uveitis.

References
1. Glaser JS, Goodwin JA. The visual sensory system. In: Tasman W, Jaeger EA, eds. *Duane's clinical ophthalmology*, Vol 2. Philadelphia: Lippincott, Williams & Wilkins, 1998:(2):1–26.

5.2 Diplopia

Richard C. Mauer

Diplopia, or true double vision, not simply blurred vision, can be a very useful clinical symptom. A range of problems can be limited to the eye or be as severe as an intracranial aneurysm. Evaluation in a systematic manner is critical in coming to the correct underlying cause (1).

   I. Approach. It is critical on evaluation of diplopia to determine if the problem is monocular or truly binocular, as the range of seriousness is directly proportional to whether it falls into one or the other category. It is also important to ascertain whether it is true diplopia or double imaging, simply blurred vision or hazy vision, or floaters in the field of vision. Unless the patient can positively state that actual double imaging is occurring, there is no diplopia (2).
   A. Monocular diplopia. Usually eye-related conditions are the underlying cause here (e.g., cataracts, corneal opacities, and occasionally intravitreous opacity). Monocular diplopia is present when the patient notices diplopia with either the right or left eye being covered.

Table 5.1 Comparison of common causes of blurred vision

Diagnosis	Onset	Duration	Nature	Age	Visual acuity	Fundus	Other
Amaurosis	Fast	1–5 min	Monocular	Adult	Often good	Occasional embolus	—
Fugax amblyopia	Slow	Ongoing	Monocular	Child	6	—	—
Cataract	Slow	Ongoing	Monocular	Adult	5 with pinhole	Variable view	6 red reflex
Drug toxicity	Slow	Ongoing	Binocular	Any	6	Occas macular pigment	—
Giant cell arteritis	Minutes	May fluctuate early	Monocular	Adult	May fluctuate early	Blurred or pale disc	RAPD, ESR and C-reactive protein
Glaucoma, acute	Minutes	Transient to constant	Monocular	Adult	6	Poor view	Red eye, pupil fixed, RAPD often, 6 red reflex
Glaucoma, chronic	Slow	Ongoing	Variable	Adult	Variable	Pale disc, large cup	Paracentral VF defects
Hyphema	Instant	Days	Monocular	Any	6	Poor view	Blood in front of iris, often RAPD
Macular degeneration:							
–Dry	Slow	Ongoing	Distorted	Adult	6	Abnormal macular reflex	—
–Neovascularization	Rapid	Ongoing	Distorted	Adult	6	Abnormal macular reflex	Central scotoma

continued

Table 5.1 *Continued*

Diagnosis	Onset	Duration	Nature	Age	Visual acuity	Fundus	Other
Migraine	Recurrent	10–20 min	Positive scotoma	Any	Good	—	—
Optic neuritis	Hours to days	Days to weeks	Monocular	Adult	6	Normal to blurred disc	Central scotoma, RAPD
Papilledema	Hours to days	Intermittent early	Binocular	Any	Good to variable	Normal to blurred disc	Sometimes RAPD
Refractive error	Slow	Ongoing	Mono-/binocular	Any	6	—	—
Retinal detachment	Minutes to hours	Ongoing	Monocular	Adult/trauma	Poor	Poor view	Superior or inferior VF defect, poor red reflex
Stroke	Rapid	Ongoing	Binocular	Adult	Variable	—	Hemianopic VF defects
Tear film	Intermittant	Minutes	Mono-/binocular	Adult	Good	—	—
Vitreous floaters	Minutes	Ongoing	Monocular	Adult	Good	—	—

RAPD, relative afferent pupillary defect; ESR, erythrocyte sedimentation rate; VF, visual field.

B. **Binocular diplopia.** This is usually secondary to intracranial abnormalities (e.g., aneurysm, stroke, hemorrhage, or increase in intracranial pressure). Binocular diplopia is present when double vision is noted only with both eyes being opened. When the patient closes either eye separately and the diplopia goes away, with each of the right and left eye being occluded, then binocular diplopia is present. In other words, it takes two eyes functioning properly to have binocular diplopia.

II. **History**

A. **Characteristics of the diplopia.** Is it true double vision or simply just blurred or hazy vision? Patients often confuse double vision with blurry vision. Close one eye or the other to test the double vision. If, in the process of covering one or the other eye, double vision is still noted, under the occluded condition, this defines monocular diplopia, a non–life-threatening cause. If double vision goes away when covering the left eye, and again when covering the right eye separately, this is binocular diplopia and the index of severity increases substantially for the underlying cause. Does diplopia get worse looking at a distance and improve when looking up close (i.e., probably a sixth nerve palsy)? Are there any recent headaches associated with this? Is there a problem with balance, coordination, nausea or vomiting, or drooping of the eyes? Is double vision separated horizontally or vertically? A vertical separation suggests either a third or fourth nerve palsy. If there is ptosis with the diplopia, it suggests a third nerve palsy. Is the diplopia sudden in onset? This suggests a vascular event if the headache is binocular.

B. **Concurrent conditions.** Microvascular ischemia is often secondary to diabetes, hypertension, or peripheral vascular disease, which can often cause a third, fourth, or an acute sixth cranial nerve palsy (Chapters 7.8 and 14.1). Thyroid disease can cause a gradually worsening binocular diplopia with a waxing and waning symptom (Chapter 14.8). This is usually associated with obvious proptosis in one or both eyes.

C. **Duration of diplopia.** A chronic subacute intermittent diplopia, with some blurred vision or floaters with decreased vision, usually suggests an eye-related problem such as cataracts, corneal opacity, irregular astigmatism, or vitreous opacity. An acute intermittent diplopia usually represents a cranial nerve palsy and often represents an intracranial condition.

III. **Physical examination. Focused physical examination (PE).** This should include a visual acuity test for each eye. Ask the patient about diplopia being present when covering each eye. If double vision is still present while having one or the other eye covered, by definition, this is monocular diplopia. A rare patient will complain of triplopia, or triple vision. This usually is malingering, but occasionally can be caused by corneal surface irregularity. Other parts of the examination are important: check the ocular rotations; lack of abduction or external rotation of the eye would suggest a sixth nerve palsy. Check for monocular ptosis; if it is present, then a third nerve palsy is suggested. Pupillary responses, if fixed and dilated, suggest an acute pupillary-involving third nerve palsy. An optic nerve where papilledema is present suggests an intracranial-involving process. A red fundus reflex test showing an opacity in the red reflex suggests an ocular cause, such as cataracts or corneal opacity.

IV. **Testing**

A. **Clinical laboratory tests.** For most diplopia workups, no blood, urine, or clinical laboratory tests are needed. The only tests that might be suggested would be a glucose and hemoglobin A1c for those cases in which a suspicion of diabetes exists. An elevated erythrocyte sedimentation rate with temporal tenderness present would suggest temporal arteritis.

B. **Diagnostic imaging.** In monocular diplopia, no diagnostic imaging is necessary. However, with binocular diplopia, diagnostic imaging with a computed tomography scan with and without contrast should be done. With a third nerve palsy present with pupillary involvement, then a magnetic resonance imaging scan would be preferred to look for an aneurysm of the posterior communicating artery. All cases of untreated diplopia should be referred to an ophthalmologist for evaluation. If the diplopia is binocular, the patient needs to be seen on the same day. If monocular, the evaluation should be undertaken within 1 to 3 days.

V. Diagnostic assessment. It is critical in the evaluation to determine whether the problem is monocular or binocular diplopia. In monocular diplopia, there is usually a more vague history; blurred vision is often present, or occasional floaters or lines are noted in the vision. More chronicity is expected of weeks to months with an intermittent presentation. The patient is often more vague about the description of the condition. In true binocular diplopia, the patient classically notes the problem suddenly, is definitely noting two images, which are either vertically or horizontally separated; when covering one and then the other eye, it goes away in each occlusion state. The level of seriousness is markedly increased in binocular diplopia. An ophthalmologic examination is mandated in either scenario (3).

References

1. Brazis PW, Lee AG. Binocular vertical diplopia. *Mayo Clin Proc* 1998:73:55–66.
2. Richardson LD, Joyce DM. Diplopia in the emergency department. *Emerg Med Clin North Am* 1997;15(3):649–664.
3. Spector RH. Vertical diplopia. *Surv Ophthalmol* 1993;38(1):31–62.

5.3 Nystagmus

Michael J. Puk

Nystagmus is an involuntary, rhythmically repeated oscillation of one or both eyes in any or all fields of gaze. Eye movements are coordinated by smooth pursuit and saccadic eye systems (1). An example of these two systems is fixating on a picket fence while moving in a car. Smooth pursuit targets the fence and saccades allow refixation to the next fence post.

I. Approach. Nystagmus can be classified into two basic types, jerk and pendular (2).

  A. Jerk nystagmus consists of an initial slow phase, followed and named by the direction of the fast phase. This is seen in most neuropathologic causes of nystagmus.

  B. Pendular nystagmus consists of smooth back-and-forth movement of the eye and is usually caused by poor vision or it is congenital.

II. History

  A. Age of onset. Congenital nystagmus is either caused by poor vision (sensory) or motor nystagmus. Both develop early in life but sensory nystagmus does not present until 2 to 3 months of age. Nystagmus developing later in life (acquired nystagmus) is neuropathologic.

  B. Family history. Is there a history of nystagmus, strabismus, or visual problem present at an early age in other family members? Hereditary motor nystagmus is not too uncommon.

  C. Associated symptoms. Is oscillopsia (the sensation of environment "jiggling") present? If present, then the nystagmus is likely acquired. Vertigo implies vestibular disease. Previous episodes of weakness, numbness, or loss of vision implicate multiple sclerosis. Associated ptosis suggests myasthenia.

  D. Medications. Medications that can induce nystagmus include lithium, barbiturates, phenytoin, salicylates, benzodiazepines, phencyclidine, and other anticonvulsants or sedatives.

  E. Social history. Alcohol intoxication produces a gaze-evoked nystagmus as well as alcohol-induced thiamin deficiency in Wernicke's encephalopathy.

III. Physical examination

  A. Visual acuity. Visual acuity is more depressed in acquired sensory nystagmus than in congenital nystagmus.

  B. Ocular motility. The direction, plane, and amplitude of the eye movement are described. Nystagmus is conjugate if both eyes demonstrate the same movement and dissociated if they have different movements. Look for a null zone (field of gaze in which the nystagmus is minimal) or a neutral zone (field of gaze where nystagmus reverses direction).

  C. Eye examination. Evaluate for any cause of poor vision that will help confirm sensory nystagmus. Look for aniridia (absence of iris) or iris transillumination as seen in albinism; both are associated with poor vision and nystagmus at an early age. Congenital cataracts or corneal opacities will have poor red reflexes. Analyze the optic nerve to assess for hypoplasia or atrophy. Latent nystagmus (seen only when one eye is covered) is present in congenital esotropia.

  D. Other examinations. Head bobbing is usually present with congenital motor nystagmus and spasmus nutans (see below). A complete neurologic assessment should be done to screen for associated signs seen in cerebellar disease, multiple sclerosis, and so on.

IV. Diagnostic assessment (3,4). An accurate description of the nystagmus will help to categorize the type of eye movement disorder and to determine if any further diagnostic testing is needed.

  A. Congenital nystagmus. The nystagmus develops at birth or in the perinatal period with small binocular and conjugate pendular eye movements. Over the first year of life, a jerk nystagmus develops with a null point. The nystagmus decreases with convergence and is abolished during sleep. Head nodding develops at any point up to age 20 years. Any cause of poor vision can cause sensory nystagmus. Two forms of acquired nystagmus when seen in the young merit concern.

    1. Opsoclonus. Repetitive, irregular, and multidirectional ("dancing eyes" or saccadomania), opsoclonus is associated with cerebellar or brainstem disease, postviral meningitis, or neuroblastoma.

    2. Spasmus nutans. Triad of head turn, nystagmus, and head bobbing that begins between 6 months to 3 years is seen in spasmus nutans. The nystagmus can be monocular or binocular and dissociated; of low amplitude and high frequency; and with horizontal or vertical pendular movements. This usually resolves between age 2 and 8 years. An identical clinical picture can be produced by a glioma of the optic chiasm.

  B. Acquired nystagmus. The following are acquired forms of nystagmus with localized pathology.

    1. See-saw. One eye rises and rotates in whereas the other descends and rotates out. Movements are pendular. This is frequently seen with lesions of the chiasm or third ventricle.

    2. Downbeating. The fast phase of the nystagmus beats down and localizes the lesion at the cervicomedullary junction at the level of the foramen magnum. Arnold-Chiari malformation is the most common cause but spinocerebellar degeneration, brainstem stroke, multiple sclerosis, and platybasia will induce this type of nystagmus.

    3. Upbeat. The fast phase beats up and can be of large or small amplitude. The lesion commonly involves the brainstem or vermis of the cerebellum.

    4. Convergence-retraction. Here, is seen convergence of the eyes with jerk nystagmus and retraction of the globe on upgaze. Eyelid retraction, limitation in upgaze, and large unreactive pupils are associated with the nystagmus. Papilledema may be present. This is caused by midbrain abnormalities loosely correlated with age 10 years, pinealoma; 20 years, head trauma; 30 years, brainstem vascular malformation; 40 years, multiple sclerosis; 50 years, basilar artery stroke.

5. **Periodic alternating.** Jerk nystagmus has the fast phase in one direction with a head turn for 60 to 90 seconds, then reverses direction (neutral zone). The cycles repeat continuously with the nystagmus being horizontal throughout. This can be seen with vestibulocerebellar disease (stroke, multiple sclerosis, spinocerebellar degeneration), severe bilateral visual loss (optic atrophy, dense vitreous hemorrhage), or it can be congenital.

6. **Gaze-evoked.** Jerk nystagmus is present only when eyes look to the side. This is most commonly seen with alcohol or other central nervous system depressants. Cerebellar disease and brainstem disease can be associated with this nystagmus.

7. **Vestibular.** Nystagmus is caused by dysfunction of inner ear, nerve, or central nuclear complex. Peripheral vestibular disease produces unidirectional jerk nystagmus with fast phase opposite the lesion and usually horizontal. This is commonly associated with vertigo, tinnitus, and deafness (Chapters 6.8 and 6.9). It is caused by labyrinthitis, Ménière's disease, neuronitis, vascular ischemia, trauma, or toxicity. Central (nuclear) disease is characterized by uni- or bidirectional nystagmus that may be purely horizontal jerk, vertical, or rotatory. Vertigo, tinnitus, and deafness are mild, if present, and symptoms are not relieved with eye fixation as in peripheral disease. This implies bilateral brainstem disease including demyelinating tumor, trauma, or stroke.

8. **Latent nystagmus.** As discussed, latent nystagmus is found in congenital esotropia.

9. **Dissociated.** The nystagmus in one eye is different than the other. This is seen in posterior fossa lesions; if an abduction nystagmus is present with an internuclear ophthalmoplegia, multiple sclerosis is likely.

C. **Other ocular oscillations**

1. **Ocular bobbing** is characterized by fast, conjugate, downward movement of the eye followed by a slow drift to primary position of gaze. This is seen in comatose patients with large pontine lesions (hemorrhage, stroke, or tumor). Obstructive hydrocephalus or metabolic encephalopathy can cause this type of eye movement.

2. **Superior oblique myokymia** is present with small unilateral, vertical, and rotatory movements of one eye. Symptoms of oscillopsia worsen when looking down and in. This is usually benign and self-limited, but has been noted with multiple sclerosis.

V. **Testing**

A. **Laboratory.** Urine drug screening for alcohol or barbiturates can be helpful in gaze-evoked nystagmus. High serum levels of phenytoin or lithium produce a gaze-evoked nystagmus. Ocular albinism can be associated with a bleeding disorder secondary to platelet dysfunction (Hermansky-Pudlak syndrome) or white blood cell dysfunction with increased susceptibility to infection and lymphoma (Chediak-Higashi syndrome). A bleeding time and a polymorphonuclear leukocyte function test should be ordered in consultation with a pathologist. Urinary vanillylmandelic acid should be obtained in an opsoclonus patient to look for by-products of neuroblastoma.

B. **Imaging studies.** Magnetic resonance imaging (MRI) scan must be obtained for any nystagmus having localized pathology. A child with spasmus nutans must have glioma of the chiasm ruled out by computed tomography (CT) or MRI. For vertical nystagmus, especially downbeating, order an MRI with sagittal views to look for cerebellar vermis herniating through the foramen magnum as seen in Arnold-Chiari malformations. An abdominal or a head CT or MRI should be done to look for neuroblastoma in the adrenal glands or brain in a patient with opsoclonus. Abdominal ultrasound or CT is needed to evaluate the kidneys in aniridia, for which a significant incidence of Wilm's tumor is seen.

References
1. Friedberg MA, Rapuano CJ. *Wills Eye Hospital office and emergency room diagnosis and treatment of eye disease.* Philadelphia: JB Lippincott, 1990:268–271.
2. Bajandas FJ, Kline LB. *Neuro-ophthalmology review manual.* Thorofare, NJ: Slack Inc., 1988:67–75.
3. Vaughn D, Asbury T, Tabbara KF. *General ophthalmology.* Norwalk: Appleton & Lange, 1989:270–272.

5.4 Papilledema

Richard C. Mauer

Papilledema is optic disc swelling produced by increased intracranial pressure. The diagnostic assessment of papilledema is critical in that the underlying cause can range from a subarachnoid hemorrhage to a totally benign optic disc head drusen, giving a pseudopapilledema-type picture (1).

I. **Approach.** In evaluating papilledema, take care first to determine primarily if there is true disc edema or only pseudopapilledema (2).
  A. **True papilledema must have increased intracranial pressure.** A list of the most common underlying causes can be extensive. The most often cited causes include metastatic intracranial tumor, aquaductal stenosis, pseudotumor cerebri (often in young, overweight females), subdural hematoma, subarachnoid hemorrhage, arteriovenous malformations, brain abscess (often with high fevers), meningitis (with fever, stiff neck, headache), encephalitis (often with mental status changes), and sagittal sinus thrombosis.
  B. **Pseudopapilledema** is optic nerve head elevation caused by hyaline deposition within the optic nerve head itself. An elevated nerve exists, but not true disc edema. The vessels will have an anomalous branching pattern and tiny hyaline deposits can be seen in the optic nerve head ophthalmoscopically.
  C. **Disc swelling without increased intracranial pressure** (3,4)
    1. Optic neuritis. An afferent pupillary defect exists along with decreased vision and pain on extraocular movement. Color vision will be decreased in this normally unilateral condition.
    2. Malignant hypertension. Blood pressure is markedly elevated here. The eye findings are characteristic: bilateral prominent disc edema, flame hemorrhages that extend peripherally, and cotton wool spots (Chapter 7.8).
    3. Central retinal vein occlusion is a unilateral disc swelling with very prominent flame and blot hemorrhages, without elevated increased blood pressure.
    4. Anterior ischemic optic neuropathy. Arteritic versus nonarteritic type: usually, in the arteritic type is found headache, stiff neck, temporal tenderness, jaw claudication, elevated sedimentation rate, and severe visual loss in one eye followed by visual loss of the other eye in 60% of cases. In nonarteritic, typically no symptoms are present except decreased vision. Associated systemic findings include systemic hypertension, diabetes mellitus, or collagen vascular disorders.
    5. Infiltration of the optic nerve. Tuberculosis granuloma, leukemic infiltrate, sarcoidosis, and metastatic disease are the more common examples of infiltrative processes. The infiltration can be unilateral or bilateral and can lead to rapid loss of vision. Radiation therapy can be helpful to preserve vision.

6. Leber's optic neuropathy usually affects men in the second or third decade. This is unilateral progressive loss of vision with disc swelling.

7. Diabetic papillitis is an ischemic infarction to the nerve in advanced diabetics. Often this is bilateral and causes mild disc elevation (Chapter 14.1).

II. History. Headache, nausea, vomiting, diplopia, and transient loss of vision lasting seconds, especially with the head in dependent positions, raise the index of suspicion for increased cranial pressure. Mood swings can be present in cases with prolonged increased intracranial pressure. Rarely is a decrease in visual acuity seen in increased intracranial pressure; if truly present, then it would suggest other causes (e.g., vein occlusion, anterior ischemic optic neuropathy, and optic neuritis). The red flags in the history include true binocular diplopia with increasing headache, disorientation, and nausea and vomiting.

III. Physical examination. A focused physical examination should include vital signs, such as blood pressure. Examine the head: check for neck stiffness, temporal artery tenderness, pain in and around the eyes, and pain on ocular rotations, such as occurs in optic neuritis. Afferent pupillary defect is another red flag that almost always signifies an ocular cause of disc edema, retinal vein occlusion, anterior ischemic optic neuropathy, or optic neuritis. Always examine both eyes. Normally papilledema is bilateral, but can be present asymmetrically. In true disc edema, nerve fiber layer swelling is seen, which obscures the margins of the blood vessels. Tiny splinter hemorrhages will be seen in and around the optic nerve. If the other eye has no disc swelling, look for spontaneous venous pulsations (SVP). If these SVPs are present, there is normal intracranial pressure, therefore, no true papilledema. Very prominent retinal hemorrhages suggest malignant hypertension or central retinal vein occlusion, rather than papilledema. Disc elevation can be measured using the diopteric overcorrection in the direct ophthalmoscope. Basically, focus on the retina and add in plus (red) power until the optic nerve blurs. Three diopters equals 1 mm of elevation. Ocular rotations are limited in both third and sixth nerve palsy. Sixth nerve palsies show limited lateral gaze and third nerve palsies have limitation in medial gaze, elevation, and depression. When ptosis and a dilated pupil are seen, suspect an aneurysm at the posterior communicating artery in the circle of Willis as the underlying cause. Decreased visual acuity is another red flag and normally is only mildly depressed in true papilledema. If the vision is decreased severely, look for other causes that are not related to increased intracranial pressure.

IV. Testing

A. Laboratory studies. If disc edema is found, suggested laboratory tests include sedimentation rate and C-reactive protein for temporal arteritis; white blood count to rule out underlying infection and leukemic infiltration of the optic nerve; a computed tomography (CT) or magnetic resonance imaging (MRI) scan to rule out a compressive lesion; cerebrospinal fluid (CSF) examination for signs of meningitis, tumor, or hemorrhage only after ruling out a compressive lesion with a scan.

B. Diagnostic imaging. If true papilledema is suspected, diagnostic imaging is mandatory. A CT scan with and without contrast should be ordered, possibly followed by MRI and MRI angiography, if the CT scan is inconclusive. MRI will be particularly helpful in imaging brainstem and cerebellar lesions, which can obstruct CSF flow. Despite the greater cost of the MRI and the greater specificity of intracranial pathology, the CT scan still is the preferred technique to image acute bleeding intracranially.

V. Diagnostic assessment. The critical workup in papilledema includes an accurate history and assessment of the visual system. Vision is often not significantly impaired in true papilledema; if present, it would suggest seeking other causes. An afferent pupillary defect indicates a localized optic nerve or retinal condition as the cause. A detailed examination of the optic nerve to look for optic nerve drusen or pseudopapilledema is also important. The finding of spontaneous venous pulsation indicates normal intracranial pressure and no imaging is mandatory. However, if absent, this does not rule out normal intracranial pressure. No imaging is mandatory; however, if needed, a lumbar puncture should be performed following imaging. Treatment should be directed toward the underlying cause of the elevated intracranial pressure.

References
1. Gordon RN, Burde RM, Slamovits T. Asymptomatic optic disc edema. *J Neuro-ophthalmol* 1997;17(1):29–32.
2. Hedges TR. Bilateral visual loss in a child with disc swelling. *Surv Ophthalmol* 1992; 36(6):424–428.
3. Moster ML. Unilateral disk edema in a young woman. *Surv Ophthalmol* 1995;39(5): 409–416.
4. Wall M. Optic disc edema with cotton-wool spots. *Surv Ophthalmol* 1995;39(6): 502–508.

5.5 Pupillary Inequality

Gary K. Phelps

Human pupils are generally equal and symmetric, although nearly everyone has a modest degree of difference in pupillary size (anisocoria) at some time during the day; most pupils are in a synchronous but random state of movement (hippus) throughout the day. Pupil size is influenced by the structural integrity of the iris, the amount of electrical energy generated by retinal light stimulation and transmitted along the optic nerves and tracts, the parasympathetic outflow to the iris sphincter from the brainstem via the third cranial nerve, and the sympathetic outflow to the pupillary dilator muscle in the iris via the brainstem and the cervical chain. Multiple central nervous system factors influence pupillary size. Most prominent is the near reflex, a triad of convergence (eyes turn in), accommodation (focus up close), and pupil constriction. Youth and excitement have always dilated the pupils, and age and boredom still constrict them. The critical aspect of unequal pupils is to identify those patients with diseases requiring immediate intervention (1).

I. **Approach.** Asymmetric pupils are best divided into two groups:
   A. **Anisocoria greater in light than in dark** is caused by weakness of the sphincter muscle of the larger pupil, thus the lesion is in the efferent parasympathetic pathway innervating the sphincter or in the muscle itself.
   B. **Anisocoria greater in dark than in light** is secondary to failure of the pupillary dilator muscle, thus the damage is most likely in the sympathetic pathway innervating the dilator.
II. **History.** As anisocoria is a sign, not a symptom, the history of onset is frequently vague, although the duration of the pupillary anomaly can usually be separated into congenital, long-standing, or recent (hours to days) onset (2). A history of previous ocular injury (including surgery), ocular medical disease, or topical drop instillation usually makes the cause of anisocoria self-evident. Associated neurologic symptoms, old or recent, such as altered state of consciousness, hemiparesis, dysarthria, or diplopia point to underlying disease (compressive or ischemic neuropathies, multiple sclerosis, acute or recurrent stroke, and so on) of which anisocoria is simply one part.
III. **Physical examination**
   A. **Gross examination.** The naked human eye is an excellent measuring device for clinical pupillary inequality. A millimeter rule or gauge in half-millimeter steps is useful to estimate the size of each pupil in light and in a darkened room and at distance and near. Differences in size are much easier to detect in small than in large pupils, and area differences are easier to estimate than diameter differences. Either works well. A general neurologic

examination is essential to identify hemispheric, associated long tract signs, or other cranial nerve embarrassment.

B. Slit lamp biomicroscopic examination is the easiest way to identify pupils that are immobile or are irregularly shaped secondary to ocular disease or injury limiting pupil movement.

IV. Testing

A. Pharmacologic. Small amounts of a topically applied weak parasympathomimetic drug (pilocarpine 1%) will cause any healthy pupil to constrict. Topically applied cocaine drops block reuptake of norepinephrine by sympathetic nerve endings, thus causing a normally innervated pupil to dilate.

B. Neuroimaging. Radiographs, computed tomography (CT), or magnetic resonance imaging (MRI) scans are useful primarily when associated symptoms are found; they are directed by the entire constellation of signs and symptoms, not just pupillary signs.

V. Diagnostic assessment

A. Pupillary inequality. Common causes of pupillary inequality are mechanical problems (e.g., pupillary sphincter ruptures secondary to trauma, including previous surgical procedures), or scarring of the iris to the lens behind it following an old inflammatory disease. Acute glaucoma, which attacks with a very high pressure, will also cause a pupil to be fixed; any acute inflammation will cause a pupil to constrict. Thus, a pupil fixed in size, particularly if irregular in shape, should prompt a slit lamp examination for structural factors that restrict its movement. A smaller pupil that fails to dilate with its mate in dark illumination should raise suspicion of Horner's syndrome. This interruption of the sympathetic efferent pathways down the brainstem or back up the cervical chain and to the orbit causes relative pupillary dilator failure and, thus, a smaller pupil. It is variably associated with a mild ptosis and sometimes with a decreased sympathetic tone on the same side of the face. Failure of the small pupil to dilate after topically applied cocaine is diagnostic of Horner's syndrome but should be done with care to ensure accuracy. Congenital Horner's syndromes, which also occasionally have a difference in iris colors, are usually benign. Horner's syndrome in a child can sometimes be caused by a neuroblastoma—a treatable tumor. In adults, anything that can compress the sympathetic pathway can create a Horner's syndrome (lung tumor, cervical disc, cluster headache, carotid dissection, and so on).

1. One fixed and dilated pupil in combination with a major neurologic problem suggests the possibility of increased intracranial pressure with tentorial herniation of the brain and third cranial nerve compression (midbrain pupil, "Hutchinson's pupil"). Anisocoria that is greater in the light (because the larger pupil constricts poorly) should prompt a careful look for associated third cranial nerve dysfunction (e.g., diplopia or ptosis) caused by vascular insult (brainstem stroke or peripheral cranial nerve ischemia) or external compression by aneurysm or tumor. When only the intraocular muscles (pupil and accommodation or ciliary muscle) are involved, it is usually caused by a local ocular problem (see below). A common and intriguing cause of one fixed dilated pupil is pharmacologic paresis with any of many natural or man-made topical drugs that can be accidentally or intentionally instilled for a variety of reasons. Pharmacologically dilated pupils are huge and fail to constrict to instillation of pilocarpine.

2. Adie's syndrome is a common entity is which one pupil is larger than the other. The innervation to the intraocular muscles is damaged so the pupil reacts very poorly to light and at first does not focus well for close vision. Pupil constriction to a near effort is often restored after a few weeks by aberrant regeneration and seems then to move strongly but slowly. Slit lamp examination usually shows that some segments of the iris sphincter are visibly paralyzed. The deep tendon reflexes are often diminished. Adie's syndrome is a benign condition, not associated with

other disease. Rarely bilateral at first, the second eye is often affected later.

B. Pupillary response defects. Pupils that react better to light stimulation than to convergence (light-near dissociation) represent a spectrum of neurologic disease (e.g., Argyll Robertson pupils, pinealoma), but do not cause pupillary inequality. Diseases of the afferent pathways, including those which obstruct large amounts of light from striking one retina (massive intraocular hemorrhage or tumor), retinal detachments, optic nerve damage from ischemia, inflammation, or compression will cause light shined in one eye to cause less pupillary constriction than light shined into the other. This is termed a relative afferent pupillary defect, but will not cause pupillary inequality.

References

1. Slamovits TL, Glaser JS. The pupils and accommodation. In: Tasman W, Jaeger EA, eds. *Duane's clinical ophthalmology*, revised ed., Vol. 2. Philadelphia: Lippincott Williams & Wilkins, 1998:(15):1–24.
2. Thompson HS, Kardon RH. Clinical importance of pupillary inequality. In: *Focal points clinical modules for ophthalmologists*. San Francisco: American Academy of Ophthalmology, December 1992:1–12.

5.6 Red Eye

John E. Sutherland

The most frequent causes of "red eye"—conjunctivitis, trauma, allergies, subconjunctival hemorrhage, and lid problems—are usually benign. Some conditions presenting with a red eye, however, require urgent evaluation and treatment. They include keratitis, episcleritis, scleritis, uveitis, orbital cellulitis, and acute angle-closure glaucoma (1–4).

I. **Approach.** The most important step in evaluating red eye is to distinguish which conditions can be treated by a primary care or emergency room physicia and which should be referred to an ophthalmologist. Symptoms or finding requiring immediate referral to an ophthalmologist are pain, proptosis, per limbal injection, tenderness, photophobia, and decreased or blurred vision.

Diagnostic eye instruments needed for a basic evaluation include topical an thetic drops, Snellen's chart for distant visual acuity (pediatric picture Snel for young children), pinhole card for confirming reduced visual acuity, fluor cein paper strips for staining the cornea, a cobalt-blue penlight, an ophthal scope, a Schiotz tonometer, 0.9% saline for irrigation or to moisten fluoresc and a magnifier instrument. A slit lamp, if available, can also be very help

II. **History**

A. **Overview.** It is important to take a careful history, discriminating bet mild discomforts such as itching, burning, and scratching versus severe or photophobia. A history of trauma or a foreign body is also helpful. S diminution or loss of visual acuity should be considered an ocular emer

B. **Conjunctivitis.** Bacterial conjunctivitis presents with mild discomfor purulent discharge that becomes bilateral within 2 days. Viral conjun is usually bilateral and has a more watery discharge and a burning o sensation, often associated with upper respiratory symptoms. Chlamy junctivitis shows a mucopurulent discharge, whereas gonococcal conj tis is markedly purulent. Both can be associated with symptoms of u or vaginitis, most commonly during the sexually active years and as with sexual abuse. Allergic conjunctivitis is characterized by bilater and tearing, most frequently seasonal and often associated with fever symptoms.

C. Painful red eye. Contact lenses can cause a corneal ulceration, which is painful and usually resolves with removal. Corneal abrasion, the most common urgent eye complaint seen in the primary care setting, is usually associated with a history of a known foreign body or direct trauma to the eye. Intense pain and tearing is usually associated with these injuries. Keratitis presents with pain, photophobia, reduced vision, and tearing. Episcleritis has only mild discomfort and is usually unilateral without discharge. Scleritis usually presents with a slowly progressive unilateral ocular pain. Primary acute angle-closure glaucoma presents with very acute, severe pain and profound visual loss, often with a history of the patient seeing halos around light as a result of corneal edema. Uveitis usually presents over 1 to 3 days of increasing, usually unilateral, pain with mildly decreased vision initially.

D. Other causes of red eye. Blepharitis, an inflammation of the eye lid margin, can be associated with conjunctival injection and a mucous discharge. Orbital cellulitis presents classically as a complication of sinusitis in febrile ill patients. Subconjunctival hemorrhage can come with coughing or straining but often has no associated history. Blood absorbs in 2 to 3 weeks.

III. Physical examination

A. Vision. Visual acuity should be checked; it is usually normal in episcleritis, scleritis, blepharitis, and conjunctivitis unless associated keratitis, such as in epidemic keratoconjunctivitis, is present. Decreased vision is demonstrable in keratitis and acute angle-closure glaucoma, but only mildly decreased in uveitis.

B. Inspection. The location of conjunctival redness is important. It is usually peripheral or diffuse in conjunctivitis, whereas in keratitis it is central or diffuse. It is localized in episcleritis or scleritis. In uveitis, it is central with a "ciliary flush." In glaucoma there is a central perilimbal injection. Tenderness of the globe is usually only present in scleritis or uveitis. Pupillary reaction is normal, except in glaucoma where it is often a fixed mid-dilated pupil and in uveitis where a sluggish, miotic pupil is invariably present. Consensual photophobia is present in uveitis also, because of iris response and movement. The corneal appearance is normal except for scarring and ulceration of *Chlamydia trachomatis* and the haziness or edema of glaucoma.

Special tests. Staining of the cornea with fluoroscein is normal, except with corneal ulceration and abrasion, herpes zoster or simplex keratitis, or a bacterial corneal ulcer. Tonometry will demonstrate increased intraocular pressure in glaucoma. If a slit lamp is available, a narrow chamber angle will be seen with glaucoma. The slit lamp is also helpful to confirm the swelling and inspect scleritis, not present in episcleritis.

crobiology studies. Immunofluorescent tests on ocular scrapings for *achomatis* and culture for *Neisseria gonorrhoeae* are sometimes required. erial cultures are generally reserved for infections of the neonate, in stent conjunctivitis, or with keratitis if a break has occurred in the l epithelium (5). Viral cultures are rarely performed. Gram's stain or a's stain of epithelial scrapings may also be helpful. Urethral cultures indicated. Immunofluorescent detection of the herpes-specific anti- 'so possible.

boratory studies. Additional testing is primarily indicated for r uveitis because of a high frequency of associated rheumatologic Workup should include a complete blood count, sedimentation ctive protein, antinuclear antibodies, rheumatoid factor, and a t for syphilis (VDRL). A spine x-ray study can be helpful in diag- losing spondylitis.

essment. The red eye most commonly results from conjunc- enign. Other causes can threaten sight, so a thorough evalua- e to prevent permanent visual impairment. Chlamydial hronic nature causes trachoma, which is the leading cause ans. The history and physical for both are very important.

The history should include trauma, infectious exposure, and the length of symptoms. The examination should be thorough and methodical as stressed in the introductions. An immediate referral to an ophthalmologist should be made with severe deep pain, proptosis, perilimbal injection, tenderness, photophobia, and decreased vision.

References
1. Bertolini J, Pelucio M. The red eye. *Emerg Med Clin North Am* 1995;13(3):561–579.
2. Davey CC. The red eye. *Br J Hosp Med* 1996;55(3):89–94.
3. Morrow GL, Abbott RL. Conjunctivitis. *Am Fam Physician* 1998;57(4):735–746.
4. Hara JH. The red eye: diagnosis and treatment. *Am Fam Physician* 1996;54(8): 2423–2430.
5. Ruppert SD. Differential diagnosis of pediatric conjunctivitis (red eye). *Nurse Practitioner* 1996;21(7):12–26.

5.7 Scotoma

Michael J. Puk

Scotoma is defined as a blind or partially blind area in the visual field. A basic understanding of neuroanatomy helps to localize the visual field defect. Simply put, pathology anterior to the optic chiasm produces monocular scotomas, whereas chiasmal or posterior chiasmal lesions form binocular field defects (1,2). Caveats apply here: bilateral retina or optic nerve disease will produce scotomas in each eye.

I. **Approach.** Determination of monocular versus binocular vision loss helps to localize the lesion. Patients often confuse a homonymous field loss to one eye (i.e., "can't see in my right eye" with a right homonymous field loss). Inquire about vision loss while each eye is covered. Check for a Marcus Gunn or afferent pupillary defect (APD) to distinguish between an optic nerve or a retina problem. Example: central scotoma in a right eye with a afferent pupillary defect in the same eye equals optic nerve disease; if no prominent APD, then retina disease is more likely.

A. **Special concerns.** Sudden vision loss in one eye with an APD in an elderly patient is giant cell arthritis, unless proved otherwise, which requires immediate treatment. Sudden binocular field loss in a patient is a stroke unless proved otherwise and requires prompt evaluation and treatment by the stroke team.

II. **History**

A. **Nature of the scotoma.** Try to establish whether the field loss is monocular or binocular. Binocular scotomas, which imply chiasmal or posterior chiasmal lesions, are vascular (stroke, transient ischemic attack, migraine, ruptured arteriovenous malformation) or compressive in nature (pituitary mass, meningioma, glioma). Establish with the patient the location of the defect. Scotomas that migrate through the visual field include vitreous floaters, vitreous hemorrhage, scintillating scotoma of migraine, and so forth. An altitudinal field loss is likely a prechiasmal lesion [i.e., optic nerve disease (e.g., ischemic optic neuropathy, glaucoma) or retina disease (e.g., detached retina, retina vascular occlusion)]. Central scotomas are commonly seen in optic nerve and macular lesions with macular degeneration by far the most common in the elderly. Macular holes, optic neuritis, toxic or metabolic optic neuropathy, central serous choroidopathy, maculopathy secondary to medications (hydroxychloroquine, thioridazine, chlorpromazine, quinine, tamoxifen), and others are examples of macular-induced central scotomas. Peripheral vision loss, if bilateral and homonymous, indicates a stroke opposite the side of field loss.

Tumors, arteriovenous malformations, and migraines can cause hemianopias. Glaucoma, detached retina, retinitis pigmentosa, chronic papilledema, and previous laser treatment for diabetes are also common entities affecting peripheral vision.

B. Onset and timing of scotoma. A scotoma of sudden onset will be secondary to some kind of vascular event: embolic, hypoperfusion, inflammatory, or hemorrhagic. Transient vision loss lasting seconds can occur with temporal arteritis, papilledema, or vertebrobasilar insufficiency. Visual loss lasting minutes to hours occurs in temporal arteritis or amaurosis fugax. Visual changes lasting weeks to months represent retinal vein occlusion, expanding compressive lesion, papilledema, and if associated with pain on eye movement, optic neuritis. Gradual progressive visual field loss occurs with compressive masses; however, acute expanding lesions from infectious, inflammatory (e.g., sarcoid, Tolosa-Hunt), aneurysmal, or apoplexy of a pituitary mass can cause rapid vision loss. Monocular vision loss after head trauma suggests injury to the intracanalicular portion of the optic nerve, compressive fracture of the sphenoid bone, or edema to the optic nerve. Emergent computed tomography (CT) scan with neurosurgical or ophthalmic consultation and high-dose intravenous steroids are needed.

C. Associated symptoms. The presence of neurologic signs or symptoms can localize the area of the pathology. Amaurosis fugax implies ipsilateral internal carotid disease or cardiac disease. History of vertigo, diplopia, and urinary incontinence in a young patient with a monocular central scotoma implies multiple sclerosis. Older patients with acute monocular vision loss associated with periorbital pain and headaches, fatigue, jaw claudication, or muscle aches strongly suggests temporal arteritis. Transient dimming or loss of vision in one or both eyes with orthostatic changes can be seen with papilledema of intracranial hypertension. Progressive monocular visual loss with proptosis obviously implies an orbital mass (optic nerve glioma, meningioma, cavernous hemangioma), but asymmetric thyroid-related orbitopathy can present a similar picture. Monocular loss progressing over time without orbital signs can be seen with an intracanalicular or intracranial optic nerve mass.

D. Past medical and social history. Diabetes and hypertension are the two most common causes of ischemic optic neuropathy (ION). ION presents as a sudden painless monocular vision loss, altitudinal in nature, with an APD. The risk of retinal vascular occlusions is much greater in patients with diabetes mellitus or hypertension. The risk is greater with tobacco use. A history of rheumatic fever, heart murmur, or cardiomyopathy is significant for an embolic source. Sudden vision loss without an APD in a diabetic patient is most likely a vitreous hemorrhage. An acquired immunodeficiency syndrome patient with a CD4 count less than 50×10^3 with visual scotomas needs to be evaluated for cytomegalovirus retinitis. A history of alcohol abuse or a psychiatric patient with bilateral vision loss and change in mental status needs urgent chemistries for anion gap acidosis with hemodialysis if methanol ingestion is suspected. An intravenous drug user can suffer a vascular occlusion from talc.

III. Physical examination

A. Visual acuity. The vision of each eye should be assessed with spectacles or contact lenses in each eye independently. Central scotomas are seen with optic nerve, macular disease, or (rarely) an occipital tip lesion; and Snellen visual acuity will be decreased.

B. Visual fields. Confrontation field test is performed with each eye independently. Briefly flash several fingers in each of the four quadrants. Bilateral field loss in the same field of vision in each eye indicates injury posterior to the chiasm. Bitemporal field defects are seen with chiasmal lesions (pituitary masses, craniopharyngiomas, and others). Monocular field defects are seen in retina and optic nerve disease.

C. Pupil examination. The presence of a prominent APD, which implies optic nerve injury, will help to differentiate central scotomas caused by macular disease. An APD is commonly seen with optic neuritis, optic neuropathy (ischemic and traumatic), asymmetric glaucomatous damage, optic nerve tumors, and central retinal artery or vein occlusion. An APD is not seen in early papilledema and minimally with macular degeneration, macular holes, or choroidopathy.

D. **Fundus examination.** Direct ophthalmoscopy can give a quick assessment of the red reflex (i.e., a dim red reflex in a diabetic with vitreous hemorrhage). Vitreous floaters can occasionally be seen as shadows in the red reflex. Examine the nerve for edema, pallor, or glaucomatous cupping. Macular scarring or pigmentary change is most commonly seen with macular degeneration.

E. **Other examinations.** A neurologic assessment is needed for a patient with bilateral field loss, screening for contralateral paresis and other focal deficits, palpation of the temporal artery for tenderness or diminished pulse if the history suggests giant cell arteritis, as is auscultation of the carotids for bruits and the heart for a murmur in a patient with amaurosis fugax or stroke. Glaucoma can be screened with tonometry. Check arms and legs for signs of intravenous drug abuse.

IV. **Testing** (3)

A. **Laboratory tests.** Erythrocyte sedimentation rate and C-reactive protein should be ordered urgently if giant cell arteritis is suspected. Vasculitis workup would include a serologic test for syphilis (VDRL), antinuclear antibody titer, Lyme disease titer, and complete blood count in young patients in whom optic neuritis or ION is suspected. Other laboratory testing is usually not warranted.

B. **Imaging studies.** CT scan to differentiate ischemic versus hemorrhagic stroke is required to promptly institute tissue-type plasminogen activator (tPA) treatment. A magnetic resonance imaging scan is best utilized in correlating demyelinating disease in patients with optic neuritis. Carotid Doppler ultrasound and an echocardiogram are indicated in amaurosis fugax and stroke to look for embolic sources.

V. **Diagnostic assessment.** Ophthalmic consultation can be helpful in confirming and further elucidating the cause of visual scotomas. Suspected giant cell arteritis needs to be aggressively pursued with temporal artery biopsy and steroid treatment. Cerebrovascular accidents, even if vision loss is the only neurologic deficit, need to be evaluated expediently by the stroke team to benefit from tPA treatment (Chapter 4.8). Other visual scotomas can be evaluated with ophthalmic consultation semiemergently.

References

1. American Academy of Ophthalmology. *Basic and clinical science*. Volume 5. 1993–1994. San Francisco: American Academy of Ophthalmology, 1993.
2. Friedberg MA, Rapuano CJ. *Wills Eye Hospital office and emergency room diagnosis and treatment of eye disease*. Philadelphia: JB Lippincott, 1990:1–2, 15–16.
3. Bajandas FJ, Kline LB. *Neuro-ophthalmology review manual*. Thorofare, NJ: Slack Inc., 1988:1–43.

6. EAR, NOSE, AND THROAT PROBLEMS

FRANK S. CELESTINO

6.1 Halitosis

Mark Douglas Andrews

Halitosis (fetor oris) is a common problem, usually thought to be merely a social handicap related to poor oral hygiene or disease of the oral cavity. However, it can represent a marker for a more serious systemic illness that requires diagnosis and treatment (1). In modern society, oral malodor has been continually stigmatized, giving rise to a commercial market for mouthwash and mouth fresheners exceeding $800 million annually (2). Despite this publicity, patients only occasionally present with a primary complaint of halitosis and generally are unaware of the problem, but at some time more than half the population will be affected. Unfortunately, physicians and dentists remain relatively indifferent and unconcerned about this health issue.

I. **Approach.** Persistent or abnormal halitosis (usually noted by persons around the patient) exceeds in severity the more common and benign morning halitosis. The important initial task is to categorize the halitosis as either localized to the oral cavity or originating systemically. In addition, causes of halitosis can be subcategorized into common pathologic and nonpathologic types. The cause of halitosis can be attributed to bacterial activity in disorders of the oral cavity in 80% to 90% of patients, with the remaining 10% to 20% of cases attributed to nonoral or systemic sources (2,3).

A. **Nonpathologic causes**

1. **Morning breath** is caused by decreased salivary flow during sleep associated with increased fluid pH, and resulting elevated gram-negative bacterial growth and volatile sulfur compounds production (4).

2. **Xerostomia**, regardless of cause (e.g., sleep, diseases, medication side effects, mouth breathing), can contribute to halitosis. Age-related changes in salivary gland physiology result in a gradual decline in saliva quantity and quality.

3. **Missed meals.** Dieting or missed meals can lead to halitosis secondary to decreased salivary flow and absence of food's mechanical action on the tongue surface to wear down filiform papillae.

4. **Tobacco or alcohol** use is usually considered to be a contributing cause of halitosis.

5. **Food sources.** Metabolites from ingested food are absorbed into the circulatory system and then excreted through the lungs, thereby contributing to halitosis. Onions, garlic, alcohol, pastrami, and other meats are common offenders.

6. **Medications.** Drugs with anticholinergic side effects can cause xerostomia, especially in the elderly. An assortment of other agents can have a role in the production of offensive breath by a diversity of mechanisms. These agents include amphetamines, anticholinergics, antidepressants, antihistamines, decongestants, antihypertensives, anti-Parkinsonian agents, antipsychotics, anxiolytics, chemotherapeutic agents, diuretics, narcotic analgesics, and radiation therapy.

B. **Pathologic causes**

1. **Local oropharynx.** Chronic peridontal disease and gingivitis are the most common sources caused by the promotion of bacterial overgrowth. Stomatitis and glossitis caused by systemic disease, medication, or vitamin deficiencies can lead to trapped food particles and desquamated tissue. An improperly cleaned prosthetic appliance can be a local contributor as can primary pharyngeal cancer. Also important are conditions associated with parotid dysfunction (e.g., viral and bacterial infections, calculi, drug reactions, systemic conditions including Sjögren's syndrome).

2. **Gastrointestinal tract.** Important sources include gastroesophageal reflux disease (GERD), gastrointestinal bleeding associated with a decayed odor, gastric cancer, malabsorption syndromes, and enteric infections.
3. **Respiratory tract.** Chronic sinusitis, nasal foreign bodies or tumors, postnasal drip, bronchitis, pneumonia, bronchiectasis, tuberculosis, and malignancies may be causative.
4. **Psychiatric causes** are less common, but a complaint of halitosis can represent a delusional syndrome associated with somatization, depression, organic brain syndrome, or schizophrenia. Halitophobia refers to imaginary halitosis (3).
5. **Systemic sources** include diabetic ketoacidosis (sweet, fruity, acetone breath), renal failure (ammonia or "fishy" odor), hepatic failure ("fetor hepaticus"—a sweet amine odor), high fever with dehydration, and vitamin or mineral deficiencies leading to dry mouth.

II. **History.** A focus on the characteristics of the bad breath is critical, although the patient is often unable to self-diagnosis or describe accurately because of olfactory desensitization. Is the odor transient or constant? A constant odor suggests chronic systemic disease or serious disorders of the oral cavity. What are the precipitating, aggravating, or relieving factors? What are the patient's smoking habits, medications, dietary preferences, and brushing and flossing routines?

III. **Physical examination**
   A. **Physical examination should be undertaken with an emphasis on the evaluation of the oral cavity,** particularly looking for ulceration, dryness, trauma, postnasal drainage, infections, cryptic tonsils, or neoplasms.
   B. **Techniques for localizing the odor source** (systemic versus oral cavity).
      1. Seal lips and blow air through the nose. If fetid odor is noted, this is suggestive of a systemic source.
      2. Pinch nose with lips closed. Hold respiration and exhale gently through the mouth. Odors detected in this fashion, generally are local in origin.

IV. **Testing.** For most patients with complaints of halitosis, clinical laboratory testing and diagnostic imaging are unnecessary and should only be pursued on the basis of specific findings indicated by the history and physical examination. The Schirmer's test may be useful in identifying xerophthalmia and associated xerostomia seen with Sjögren's syndrome and some other rheumatologic conditions (Chapter 12.1). If indicated, radiologic studies and imaging procedures of the sinuses, thorax, and abdomen may be used to identify infectious processes, neoplasms, and GERD with its complications.

V. **Diagnostic assessment.** The key to diagnosis and management of halitosis is a thorough history and focused physical examination with a particular emphasis on diseases and disorders of the oral cavity. Because 80% to 90% of all malodorous conditions can be traced to oral causes, simple examination maneuvers as described previously can be diagnostically helpful in excluding the likelihood of more distant or complex systemic sources. Salivation, mastication, and swallowing all lead to a decreased propensity to generate bad breath. Conversely, conditions or medications that reduce salivation or promote masticatory inactivity favor production of fetid breath. Because the key to treatment of halitosis of oral origin, beyond the limitation of aggravating factors, is proper oral hygiene, an evaluation of the patient's toothbrushing and flossing regimens is imperative. Brushing should include gingival, tongue, and palatal surfaces because vigorous tongue brushing twice daily has been demonstrated in several studies to reduce the severity of malodorous morning breath (5).

References
1. Replogle WM, Keebe DK. Halitosis. *Am Fam Physician* 1996;53:1215–1223.
2. Spielman AI, Bivona P, Refkin BR. Halitosis: a common oral problem. *N Y State Dent J* 1996;62:36–42.

3. Ben-Aryeh H, Horowitz G, Nir D, Laufer D. Halitosis: an interdisciplinary approach. *Am J Otolaryngol* 1998;19:8–11.
4. Amir E, Shimonov R, Rosenberg M. Halitosis in children. *J Pediatr* 1999;134: 338–343.
5. Johnson BE. Halitosis, or the meaning of bad breath. *J Gen Intern Med* 1992;7: 649–656.

6.2 Hearing Loss

Mark Knudson

Approximately 28 million Americans have hearing loss. Among individuals aged more than 65 years, 7% to 8% report hearing loss, yet close to 20% will have evidence of hearing loss if screened (1).

I. **Approach.** In the evaluation of an individual with known or suspected hearing loss, separation into sensorineural hearing loss (SNHL), conductive hearing loss (CHL), and mixed hearing loss (MHL) helps in diagnosis (2).
   A. **Sensorineural hearing loss** can be caused by a defect in the inner ear or cochlea, the eighth cranial nerve, or by loss of central nervous system (CNS) function. Common causes of SNHL include acoustic neuroma, multiple sclerosis (MS), hypothyroidism, vertebrobasilar insufficiency, or stroke, Ménière's syndrome, drug toxicity, and idiopathic hearing loss.
   B. **Conductive hearing loss.** Generally less worrisome than SNHL, CHL can result from cerumen impaction, perforation of the tympanic membrane (TM), middle ear effusion, atelectasis, and otosclerosis. In addition, a variety of tumors (e.g., squamous cell cancer, exostoses, or cholesteatoma) can cause CHL.
   C. **Mixed hearing loss.** Presbycusis, medications, and noise-induced hearing loss are examples of mixed loss, where impairment of conduction can complicate a sensorineural component.
II. **History.** Proactive detection of minor hearing alterations is necessary because most patients with hearing loss do not present with a hearing complaint. Many elderly patients, in particular, accept hearing loss as an expected part of aging.
   A. **Presentation.** A small number of patients will present with a complaint of decreased hearing, a few more will admit to abnormal hearing, but most will have no specific hearing concern. A patient's depression, confusion, social isolation, or poor job performance can be caused or complicated by hearing impairment. Family members may describe abnormal, slow, or overly loud answers. A sudden tendency to monopolize or disrupt conversation, or to tilt the head in conversation, may suggest hearing loss.
   B. **Duration.** CHL is often of sudden onset but of a mild degree. Complete occlusion or rapid collection of fluid in middle ear causes abrupt change in hearing. SNHL can be abrupt and severe (stroke, idiopathic, trauma) or gradual (Ménière's syndrome, acoustic neuroma, hypothyroidism). Some forms may be intermittent (such as Ménière's syndrome.)
   C. **Quality of hearing.** CHL often affects quality of hearing first. Described as muffled "like a head in a drum," the patient may lose high frequency and voice discrimination, yet still be able to detect subtle sounds. SNHL, when not associated with tinnitus, can have good quality but diminished hearing that is usually more profound than CHL.
   D. **Associated symptoms.** Tinnitus is classically associated with Ménière's syndrome or disease, but may be seen with other causes of SNHL. Vertigo is associated with inner ear disorders, and is often self-limited (Chapter 6.9).

Associated fluctuating neurologic defects of many sites suggest MS, whereas focal deficits suggest CNS tumors or vascular insufficiency.

E. **Family history.** This may be positive in presbycusis, Ménière's, otosclerosis, and acoustic neuroma.

F. **Social and work history.** Recreational history (loud music or target shooting) or work history (pilots, factory workers, firefighters) can implicate excessive noise exposure. Inquire about use of protective equipment and chronicity of exposure.

III. **Physical examination.** Gross tests of hearing are only helpful to confirm significant hearing asymmetry or to detect profound hearing loss. With one ear covered, the patient tries to hear soft sounds such as the tick of a watch, scratching of two fingers rubbed together, or a softly whispered voice.

A. **Visual examination of ears.** Inspect the canal and TM to rule out obvious causes of CHL. Cerumen impaction is a remarkably common and easily corrected cause of hearing loss. Pneumoscopy to check for normal movement of the TM helps rule out perforation, atelectasis, eustachian tube dysfunction, stiffened TM, ossicular disruption, and middle ear effusion.

B. **Weber test.** With a vibrating tuning fork placed on the top of the head, the patient is asked to describe the sound heard. The patient will perceive the sound to be louder in the affected ear in CHL, because the background noise will be absent on that side. The unaffected ear will be perceived as louder in SNHL.

C. **Rinne test.** With the vibrating tuning fork placed on the mastoid, the patient detects bone conduction (BC). The tuning fork is removed when the patient can no longer hear the sound. Then the tuning fork is held next to the ear to test for air conduction (AC). In an individual with normal hearing, AC is significantly better than BC. CHL will reduce AC, with little effect on BC.

IV. **Testing.** A simple audiogram performed at several frequency responses may detect individuals at risk for hearing loss. Although the sensitivity is good (93% to 95%), the poor specificity (60% to 74%) can result in many false-positive findings (3).

A. **Audiography.** Two forms of testing provide reproducible information about the patient. Pure tone testing documents the exact number of decibels heard at a given frequency. Unfortunately, it describes nothing about the ability to discriminate language. On the other hand, speech detection better estimates impairment of actual language function, but requires a much more cooperative and attentive patient.

B. **Auditory-evoked response.** Able to detect the electroencephalographic stimulation caused by repetitive sounds, this examination is useful in the obtunded, uncooperative, or very young patient.

C. **Computed tomography (CT).** In the setting of traumatic loss of hearing, CT is fast, less expensive than magnetic resonance imaging (MRI), and able to detect abnormalities within the petrous ridge where fractures can affect hearing (4). Likewise, bleeding in the CNS is readily seen. CT is also useful to examine for causes of CHL such as tumors, middle ear anomalies, myringosclerosis, and cholesteatoma.

D. **MRI.** In patients with SNHL, MRI with gadolineum is superior to CT because certain CNS diseases (MS or vascular infarcts) are more easily identified. In addition, acoustic neuromas and labyrinth disorders, often too small to be seen with CT, may be visualized with MRI (4).

V. **Diagnostic assessment.** Separation into CHL and SNHL, and assessment of severity help determine the best diagnostic approach (2).

A. **Conductive hearing loss.** Although bothersome, these disorders are rarely severe or life threatening. Systematic history and physical examination normally will easily localize the site of hearing loss.

B. **Sensorineural hearing loss.** Acoustic neuroma (AN), one of the most feared causes of hearing loss, is actually a nerve sheath tumor accounting for 1% of SNHL; 95% of patients with AN present with gradual progression of unilateral hearing loss (4). Tinnitus and vestibular symptoms are less common. In contrast, Ménière's disease causes a fluctuating but progressive loss of hearing associated with tinnitus and episodic vertigo. Other causes of SNHL can be severe, rapidly progressive, and associated with severe side effects or potential mortality. Rapid systematic evaluation, including MRI in patients aged less than 65 years, should be conducted. For patients over the age of 65 years, exclusion of presbycusis and otosclerosis should prompt the same thorough evaluation.

References
1. Maggi S, Minicuci N, Martini A, et al. Prevalence rates of hearing impairment and comorbid conditions in older people: the Veneto Study. *J Am Geriatr Soc* 1998;46: 1069–1074.
2. Weber P, Klein A. Hearing loss. *Med Clin North Am* 1999;83:125–137.
3. Weissman J. Hearing loss. *Radiology* 1996;199:593–611.
4. Moore A, Siu A. Screening for common problems in ambulatory elderly: clinical confirmation of a screening instrument. *Am J Med* 1996;100:438–443.

6.3 Hoarseness

L. Gail Curtis

Hoarseness (dysphonia) is any change in normal voice quality. It is a nonspecific term with many causes and is the most common symptom of laryngeal disease. Hoarseness occurs early in the process of laryngeal disease and can be readily diagnosed in primary care settings. For a variety of reasons, unfortunately, cancer of the larynx has usually been present for 6 months before a diagnosis is made (1).

I. **Approach**
   A. **Etiologic categories.** In evaluating hoarseness, it is important to decide which of four possible etiologic categories best accounts for the patient's vocal changes: diseases causing inflammation or edema of the larynx; processes affecting position or approximation of the vocal cords; disorders causing malfunction of the larynx; or systemic processes (Table 6.1) (2,3).
   B. **Special concerns.** Laryngeal cancer is suggested by prolonged (>2 weeks) hoarseness associated with dysphagia, pain, alcoholism, or chronic cigarette smoking (3,4). Urgent largyngoscopy is indicated.
II. **History**
   A. **Characteristics of hoarseness.** Short of direct visualization of the larynx, often little exists to distinguish one cause of hoarseness from another based on routine physical examination. Therefore, a thorough history is essential. Patients should be asked about the mode of onset, duration, and consistency of the hoarseness. The voice of patients with myasthenia gravis gets more hoarse as the day progresses. Intermittent hoarseness argues against there being a fixed lesion. Prominent morning symptoms that improve through the day suggest nocturnal gastroesophageal reflux disease (GERD) (Chapter 9.6). Is the hoarseness exacerbated by talking? Is there any pain, dysphagia, or trouble mounting an adequate respiratory force? Surprisingly, pain is a late phenomenon in carcinoma, but prominent in viral or reflux laryngitis (3).
   B. **Other historical information.** The possible role of other medical problems also must be considered. Is there a history of indigestion, heartburn, or regurgitation suggesting reflux laryngitis? Chronic cough, sputum production, or sinus problems with chronic postnasal drainage may also play a role. A history of specific inciting events—upper respiratory infections, sore throats,

Table 6.1 Etiologic categories of hoarseness with selected examples

INFLAMMATION OR EDEMA

Infection (especially viral laryngitis), gastroesophageal reflux disease (GERD), allergies, exposure to irritants (tobacco, alcohol, toxic fumes), voice abuse, aspiration

ABNORMALITIES OF POSITION OR APPROXIMATION OF THE VOCAL CORDS

Vocal polyps, vocal nodules, contact ulcers, granulomatous disease (tuberculosis, syphilis, fungal, sarcoid, autoimmune), neoplasms (benign—hemangioma, papilloma; malignant—usually squamous cell carcinoma)

ABNORMALITIES CAUSING MALFUNCTION OF THE LARYNX

Intubation, trauma (direct or hemorrhage), recurrent laryngeal or vagus nerve lesions (tumor, neck surgery, aortic aneurysm), aging changes (muscle atrophy, loss of moisture, bowing of the cords)

SYSTEMIC PROCESSES

Hypothyroidism, rheumatoid arthritis, Parkinson's disease, multiple sclerosis, acromegaly, myasthenia gravis, psychogenic/psychiatric

fevers, myalgias, fatigue or other infectious exposures (tuberculosis)—need to be explored. Has there been exposure to dust, fire, smoke, or noxious fumes? Smoking and alcohol use are well-known laryngeal irritants as well as carcinogens, and they must be asked about in detail. Is there any history of intubation, prior neck surgery, or neck mass.

   C. **Voice use and abuse information.** It is important to establish an individual's pattern of voice use. Specifically, does the patient raise his or her voice over crowds or machinery, or by yelling? Does his or her profession involve voice overuse or abuse (e.g., singers, politicians, preachers)?

III. **Physical examination**

   A. **Voice quality.** Begin the physical examination by listening to the patient's voice while obtaining the history. No specific features of hoarseness are definitively diagnostic, but a *raspy voice* suggests cord thickening caused by edema or inflammation; a *breathy voice* indicates poor vocal cord position or approximation; and a *high, shaky or soft voice* is more likely caused by malfunction of the larynx (2).

   B. **Focused physical examination (PE).** Obtain vital signs with attention to temperature and weight. Completely examine the scalp, neck, thyroid gland, cervical nodes, ears, nose, sinuses, and oral cavity. Tender neck adenopathy suggests infection, whereas painless enlargement may imply malignancy (Chapters 15.1 and 15.2). Unless a diagnosis is obvious from the history and initial PE, visualization of the larynx is required. Using one of the techniques described below (section III.C.), carefully inspect the posterior nasopharynx, tongue, lymphoid tissue, and entire larynx. Perform vocal maneuvers while directly observing vocal cord movement. Assess for mucosal and cartilagineous lesions, edema, erythema, and excess mucus—the latter finding suggesting prominent allergies. Edematous vocal cords and glottis with hyperemia suggests GERD or laryngitis.

   C. **Techniques for laryngeal visualization**

      1. **Indirect laryngoscopy** is performed by placing a laryngeal mirror (warmed to prevent fogging) against the soft palate while grasping the tongue with gauze. A bright light source and head mirror, or a headlight, is focused on the laryngeal mirror to reveal an image of the larynx. This technique, although simple, can prove difficult secondary to a strong tongue or gag reflex.

      2. **Fiberoptic laryngoscopy** provides an excellent view of the larynx and avoids the problems noted above in III.C.1. The scope is placed via one nares after topical anesthesia is applied intranasally (e.g., 2% lidocaine

gel). The larynx is visualized while the patient swallows and phonates. The procedure is quick and painless and allows a thorough evaluation of the larynx.

IV. **Testing**
   A. **Clinical laboratory tests.** Routine blood testing is not helpful, unless dictated by features of the history or PE.
   B. **Imaging.** If indicated by history or PE, magnetic resonance imaging is used to assess the extent of serious laryngeal or neck disease.
V. **Diagnostic assessment.** The key to diagnosis is a thorough history combined in most cases with visualization of the larynx. Hoarseness of less than 2 weeks duration is considered acute and is usually self-limited. Chronic hoarseness (>2 weeks duration) suggests a more serious cause and a laryngeal examination is critical (2–4).

Some laryngeal lesions have a pathognomonic appearance (3). *Vocal polyps* are benign and result from chronic voice abuse or direct trauma. They occur on the anterior portion of one vocal cord. *Vocal nodules* result from poor voice use (e.g., singers, preachers) and always occur at the junction of the anterior and middle third of the vocal cords bilaterally. *Contact ulcers* present as bilateral ulcerations at the tips of the laryngeal cartilages and are the only common lesion other than cancer that causes throat pain. *Leukoplakia* presents as a raised, white plaque at the anterior extremity of one vocal cord. It is usually premalignant, related to alcohol use or smoking, and needs to be biopsied.

Although most causes of hoarseness are benign, laryngeal cancer produces early changes in voice quality and is the most serious cause of hoarseness. This cancer presents as persistent hoarseness with a lesion in the hypophyarnyx, glottis, or supraglottis. Any suspicious lesion seen on laryngoscopy needs to be referred for biopsy.

References

1. Yanagisawa E. The larynx. In: Lee KJ, ed. *Essential otolaryngology—head and neck surgery*, 5th ed. Norwalk: Appleton & Lange, 1995:757–800.
2. Rosen CA, Anderson D, Murry T. Evaluating hoarseness. *Am Fam Physician* 1998;57:2775–2782.
3. Garrett CG, Ossoff RH. Hoarseness. *Med Clin North Am* 1999;83:115–123.
4. Vaughan C. Glottic carcinoma. In: Gates G, ed. *Current therapy in otolaryngology—head and neck surgery*, 5th ed. St. Louis: Mosby, 1994:288–298.

6.4 Nosebleed

Douglas G. Browning and Stephen H. Keiser

Nosebleed, or epistaxis, is a common otolaryngologic problem, with 15/10,000 persons requiring physician care annually for this problem, and 1.6/10,000 requiring admission to the hospital for a persistent nosebleed. Most cases occur in patients aged less than 10 years, and the incidence decreases with age (1).

I. **Approach**
   A. **Etiology.** Epistaxis results from an interaction of factors that damage the nasal epithelial (mucosal) lining and vessel walls. The causative factors or processes include:
      1. **Environmental:** lack of humidity, warm ambient temperature.
      2. **Local:** direct or indirect trauma, anatomic abnormalities (especially deviated septum), inflammation, allergies, iatrogenic (surgery), neoplasms.
      3. **Systemic:** hypertension, platelet and coagulation abnormalities, blood dyscrasias, disseminated intravascular coagulation, renal failure, alcoholism.

4. **Drugs affecting clotting:** aspirin, warfarin, heparin, ticlopidine, dipyridamole, NSAIDS, and so on.
5. **Other drugs:** steroid nasal inhalers, thioridazine, anticholinergics (drying).
6. **Hereditary:** hereditary hemorrhagic telangectasia (Osler-Weber-Rendu).
7. **Idiopathic**

Cold, dry air increases cases of epistaxis as demonstrated in countries with seasonal climates where hospital admissions for nosebleed increase significantly during the winter months (2). Regarding the importance of anatomic abnormalities, a study of recurrent epistaxis showed that 81% of patients had septal deviation versus 31% of the control group (3). Although hypertension is often cited as a cause of epistaxis, studies have not usually supported this association (4) (Chapter 7.8). Medications that interfere with clotting, especially aspirin and nonsteriodial antiinflammatory drugs (NSAIDs), are particularly common contributors to epistaxis with up to 75% of patients in some series using them versus less than 10% of controls (5).

B. **Special concerns.** Rare causes of epistaxis include potentially life-threatening posttraumatic pseudoaneurysm of the internal carotid artery. This entity presents from days to weeks after initial trauma to the base of the skull with a classic triad of unilateral blindness, orbital fractures, and massive epistaxis. Optimal management demands rapid recognition and treatment to give the best functional outcome. Also, epistaxis is the presenting complaint in four of five cases of the rare, but less life-threatening, hereditary hemorrhagic telangiectasias (Osler-Weber-Rendu disease) (5).

II. **History.** An assessment of the amount of blood lost is made from the history, including the onset of the bleeding, precipitating factors (including any acute or subacute injury to the nares or cranium), duration and quantity (i.e., number of soaked towels), past history of epistaxis and treatment, and history of blood dyscrasias. In adults, a history of medication use (including NSAIDs, anticoagulants), allergic rhinitis, hypertension, liver disease, ischemic heart disease, diabetes mellitus, and alcohol abuse may influence management. A family history of problems with epistaxis should be obtained. Be alert to the possibility of an intranasal foreign body in children with epistaxis with unilateral nasal discharge or foul odor.

III. **Physical examination.** The blood supply to the nose arises from the internal maxillary and facial arteries via the external carotid artery and the anterior and posterior ethmoid arteries via the internal carotid. The anteroinferior septum (Little's area) is supplied by a confluence of both systems known as "Kiesselbach's plexus." Little's area is a common site of epistaxis because it is ideally placed to receive environmental irritation (cold, dry air, cigarette smoke) and is easily accessible to digital trauma. Fortunately, this area is easy to access and treat. However, approximately 5% of nosebleeds originate from a posterior nasal source (5); it can be much more difficult to identify a source of epistaxis in this area. Providing effective treatment for obstinate bleeding in this area may also be more uncomfortable for the patient and much more formidable for the health provider.

A. **Focused physical examination (PE).** When examining the epistaxis patient, first assess vital signs for hypotension, orthostasis, and hemodynamic instability. After examining the face for any obvious signs of recent injury, it is important to visualize as much of the nasal vestibule as possible. It is imperative to keep the patient's head upright, for if he or she tilts backward, then only the roof of the nasal cavity will be seen. The nasal speculum should be held in a horizontal position to allow an optimal view of the nasal septum, which is the site of most bleeding.

Visualization of the bleeding can be done by direct illumination of the area, or sometimes more easily by indirect illumination using a head mirror. Suction may be needed to remove clots, fresh blood, or mucous to visualize the bleeding. Direct nasopharyngoscopy with endoscopy (using a topical anesthetic such as Cetacaine or lidocaine gel) may be necessary, especially if the source of the bleeding is extremely posterior. Topical vasoconstrictors such as phenylephrine or oxymetazoline can be useful in decreasing the rate of bleeding in order to visualize the area (and may sometimes help achieve long-term cessation of the bleeding).

   B. General PE. Depending on the patient's history, it may be important to proceed to a more general PE with a special focus on the skin to look for petechiae, telangectasias, hemangiomas, and ecchymoses (Chapter 15.3).

IV. Testing

   A. Clinical laboratory tests. If bleeding is minor and not recurring, no testing is needed. For more vigorous bleeding or recurrent epistaxis, consider a complete blood count (CBC) with platelet count, bleeding time, prothrombin time, partial thromboplastin time, and possibly blood type and crossmatch for hypovolemic shock or severe anemia. Testing stool for occult blood may help to assess chronicity as will assessing the red cell mean corpuscular volume. The CBC can detect blood dyscrasias as well as anemia. An elevated bleeding time may imply aspirin use, von Willebrand's disease, and many platelet-based bleeding disorders. Coagulation times can be elevated in coagulation factor diseases, but more often they implicate liver disease.

   B. Imaging. Sinus radiographs or a limited CT scan of the sinuses may also be considered if concern exists for benign neoplasms or malignancy. Rarely, angiography may also be indicated for diagnosing (and treating) vascular lesions.

V. Diagnostic assessment. For most cases of acute epistaxis, treatment should occur simultaneously with the diagnostic assessment. However, for persistent or recurrent nosebleeds, it is important to look further for the underlying cause of the problem by performing a careful history and evaluating the problem with expedient laboratory evaluations, appropriate imaging, or further consultation when necessary to rule out more malignant causes.

References
1. Pfaff JA, Moore GP. Epistaxis. In: Rosen P, Barkin R, Danzl DF, et al, eds. *Emergency medicine: concepts and clinical practice*, 4th ed. St. Louis: Mosby-Year Book, Inc., 1998:2725–2727.
2. Tomkimon A, Bremmer-Smith A, Craven C, et al. Hospital epistaxis admissions and ambient temperature. *Clin Otolaryngol* 1995;20:239–240.
3. O'Reilly BJ, Simpson DC, Dharmeratnam R. Recurrent epistaxis and nasal septal deviation in young adults. *Clin Otolaryngol* 1996;21:82–84.
4. Weiss NS. Relationship of high blood pressure to headache, epistaxis and selected other symptoms. *N Engl J Med* 1972;287:631–633.
5. Tan LK, Calhoun KH. Epistaxis. *Med Clin North Am* 1999;83:43–56.

6.5 Pharyngitis

Frank S. Celestino

Nearly 5% of all primary care office visits are for "sore throat" (ST) or pharyngitis (1). Only a small minority (10% to 20%) of ST patients are infected with group A β-hemolytic streptococci (GABHS) (2–4). However, to minimize potential adverse effects of inappropriate antimicrobial therapy, it is important to accurately identify GABHS infection because it is the only commonly occurring form of pharyngitis for which antibiotic therapy is definitively indicated (3). Early identification and treatment of GABHS will help prevent rheumatic fever, provide symptom relief, reduce suppurative complications, and decrease infectivity.

I. **Approach**
  A. **Causes of ST.** The differential diagnosis is extensive, but viruses and GABHS predominate in primary care as shown in the following list of likely causes of pharyngitis (2–5).
    1. Viral: 50% to 80%
    2. GABHS: 5% to 30% (mean 15%)
    3. Epstein-Barr virus: 1% to 10%
    4. *Chlamydia pneumoniae*: 2% to 5%
    5. *Mycoplasma pneumoniae*: 2% to 5%
    6. *Neisseria gonorrhoeae*: 1% to 2%
    7. Other bacteria, fungi, parasites: all rare
    8. Noninfectious causes (allergic rhinitis with postnasal drip, gastro-esophageal reflux, foreign body, burns, neoplasms, radiation, inhaled or swallowed toxins, dryness, psychogenic, dust): all rare, except perhaps rhinitis and psychogenic
    9. Referred pain (thyroiditis, dental): rare
  B. **Seasonality.** Visits for ST occur year round but peak in winter. GABHS infection peaks in late winter and early spring (1).
  C. **Age distribution.** Data show that the probability of GABHS pharyngitis in primary care by age is: 0 to 2 years (<1%), 2 to 4 (14%), 5 to 9 (34%), 10 to 19 (16%), adult (9%) (2). Infectious mononucleosis (IM) as a cause of ST peaks between ages 15 and 30 at a probability of 5% to 10%.
  D. **Chronicity.** Most pharyngitis is acute and self-limited. When ST lasts longer than 2 to 3 weeks, consider noninfectious causes or atypical bacterial causes (e.g., chlamydia or mycoplasma) (4).
  E. **Special concerns** include peritonsillar or retropharyngeal abscesses, epiglottitis, palatal cellulitis, toxic shock syndrome, Kawasaki's disease, Stevens–Johnson syndrome, and Behçet's syndrome.

II. **History.** Is there any history of seasonal allergies, trauma, malignancy, radiation therapy, inhalation, ingestion, thyroid dysfunction, or significant psychiatric illness? If so, then the possibility of a noninfectious cause of ST exists. How severe is the ST and how abrupt was the onset? Is there accompanying rhinitis, nasal congestion, cough, malaise, myalgias, rash, diarrhea, conjunctivitis, fever, tender or swollen "neck glands," pain on swallowing, headache, nausea, vomiting, or abdominal pain? Classically, GABHS pharyngitis is severe and of acute (<1 day) onset and accompanied by fever (temperature >101°F), painful swallowing, tender anterior cervical adenopathy and myalgias, but not cough or rhinitis. Headache, nausea, vomiting, and abdominal pain may be seen as well, especially in children. Conversely, the gradual onset of mild ST accompanied by rhinorrhea, cough, hoarseness, conjunctivitis, or diarrhea in an afebrile patient speaks strongly for a viral cause. Despite these broad generalizations, classic symptom complexes alone are neither sensitive nor specific enough to rely on for judging the need for antibacterial treatment (2–5). For example, the symptoms most likely to predict the presence of GABHS infection—fever and lack of cough—have sensitivities of 0.58 to 0.72 and specificities of only 0.43 to 0.67 (2). Additionally, the presence of a positive throat culture in the prior year or recent exposure to GABHS has high specificity, 0.90, but low sensitivity, 0.23 (2,3).

III. **Physical examination**
  A. **Focused physical examination (PE).** This should include assessing vital signs (especially temperature) and examining the head, eyes, ears, nose, throat, neck, and skin. Findings classically associated with GABHS infection include palatal petechiae, intense ("beefy red") tonsillopharyngeal erythema with exudates, tender anterior cervical adenopathy, and a scarlatiniform rash (Chapter 13.5). Conversely, absence of these features together with the presence of rhinitis, hoarseness, conjunctivitis, stomatitis, discrete ulcerative lesions, or a typical viral exanthem point toward a viral cause. In IM, the classic GABHS features are often combined with posterior cervical or generalized lymphadenopathy and hepatosplenomegaly. However, once again

none of these physical findings in and of themselves have sufficiently high
sensitivity and specificity to rely on for accurate diagnosis (2–4).

   B. Additional PE. Abdominal examination is dictated by either gastrointestinal
symptoms or the presence of severe fatigue with posterior cervical adenopathy
(suggesting IM). Cough or fever should lead to pulmonary examination. Cardiac examination is important for toxic appearing patients.

IV. Testing

   A. Clinical laboratory tests. Because even experienced clinicians are unable to
use the clinical presentation of pharyngitis to reliably predict the causative
agent (because of inadequate sensitivity and specificity), accurate diagnosis
should be based on results of a throat culture (TC) or rapid streptococcal antigen detection test (RSADT). In an untreated patient with streptococcal pharyngitis, a properly obtained (vigorously swabbing both tonsils and posterior
pharynx) TC is almost always positive (sensitivity 90% to 95%) (3,4). Unfortunately, the culture does not reliably distinguish between acute GABHS infection and streptococcal carriers with concomitant viral infection. Streptococcal
pharyngeal carriage, unfortunately, is a common finding particularly in school-
aged children (20% to 30%) (2,3,5). A negative TC does permit the withholding
of antimicrobial therapy (i.e., specificity = 0.99) (3–5).

      Although methods vary, RSADTs do have high degrees of specificity (92% to
95%) (3,4). Unfortunately, their sensitivity in routine clinical practice is un-
acceptably low (60% to 85%) (3,4). Therefore, a negative antigen test does not
exclude GABHS and a back-up throat culture must be obtained. Also, RSADTs
suffer the same limitation as TCs because of the presence of carrier states.

      Streptococcal antibody titers are of no immediate value in the diagnosis
of acute GABHS pharyngitis.

      If IM is suspected, a complete blood count and heterophil antibody testing
can confirm the diagnosis reliably if the patient is in the second week of illness.

   B. Imaging studies. None are usually necessary unless a serious suppurative
sequela is suspected (e.g., retropharyngeal abscess).

V. Diagnostic assessment. Researchers have tried to incorporate clinical and
epidemiologic features of acute pharyngitis into scoring systems that attempt
to predict the probability of GABHS (2–5). Unfortunately, even the best of these
predict positive TCs less than 70% of the time. Most scoring systems have incor-
porated the cardinal features such as fever, tender cervical adenopathy, tonsillar exudates, and lack of cough or rhinitis. Patients, especially adults, who have
none of these features have a very low (<5%) probability of GABHS and no further testing is advised. For most other patients, who have varying numbers of
cardinal features, the probability of GABHS is either intermediate (10% to 30%)
or high (40% to 60%) and further testing is necessary, usually first with a
RSADT and, if negative, a follow-up TC. Only in patients, usually children, with
all the cardinal features plus a history of recent GABHS exposure or culture-
proved recurrent streptococcal illness, can further testing be eliminated and
empiric therapy begun.

References

1. *National Ambulatory Medical Care Survey*. Hyattsville, MD: National Center for
   Health Statistics, 1993.
2. Ebell MH. Sore throat. In: Sloane PD, Slatt LM, Curtis P, et al., eds. *Essentials of
   family medicine*, 3rd ed. Baltimore: Williams & Wilkins, 1998:632–634.
3. Bisno AL, Gerber MA, Gwaltney JM, Kaplan EL, Schwartz RH. Diagnosis and
   management of group A Streptococcal pharyngitis: a practice guideline—Infectious
   Disease Society of America. *Clin Infect Dis* 1997;25:574–583.
4. Komaroff AL. Sore throat and acute infectious mononucleosis in adult patients. In:
   Black ER, Bordley DR, Tape TG, et al., eds. *Diagnostic strategies for common medical problems*, 2nd ed. Philadelphia: American College of Physicians, 1999:229–242.
5. Perkins A. An approach to diagnosing the acute sore throat. *Am Fam Physician*
   1997;55:131–138.

6.6 Rhinitis

Gail S. Marion

No universal system of definition or classification exists for rhinitis—a common presenting symptom. Rhinitis connotes inflammation of the nasal mucosa, but also commonly refers to a constellation of rhinopathy symptoms, including mucus drainage, stuffiness, sneezing, and itching. Rhinitis currently affects about 40 million Americans with annual costs to society of more than $15 billion dollars (1). Considered a minor complaint, it is frequently untreated. Proper evaluation and treatment of rhinitis is not only economically important, but also improves health outcomes and quality of life for patients (2–4). An important example is increasing evidence that aggressive allergic rhinitis management improves the management of asthma because the nose serves as a filter for inhaled air (2,5).

I. **Approach.** Evaluation of rhinitis requires determining whether the symptoms are caused by (a) allergy; (b) infection; (c) anatomic defect; (d) serious systemic illness; or (e) some combination of these (Table 6.2).

    A. **Etiology.** Allergic rhinitis (seasonal and perennial), which causes most recurrent or chronic rhinitis, is increasing in children and adults (2). Infections (viral and bacterial) are the second most common cause. Allergy and infection produce bilateral nasal complaints, whereas most rhinitis relating to structural problems of the nose is unilateral.

    B. **Special concerns.** Approximately 1% of rhinitis is caused by foreign bodies, anatomic defects, trauma, drug side effects, idiopathic syndromes, systemic diseases, and neoplasm (Table 6.2). In such patients, recent onset of persistent symptoms is present with other associated symptoms.

II. **History**

    A. **Characteristics of rhinitis.** What are the specific symptoms (i.e., stuffiness, itching, clear or purulent drainage)? Are symptoms unilateral or bilateral? When did the symptom(s) begin? Ask what the patient believes caused the symptoms.

Table 6.2 Rhinitis etiologies

COMMON

Allergic: seasonal, perennial

Infection: acute vs. chronic, bacterial vs. viral

LESS COMMON (SELECTED EXAMPLES)

Nonallergic perennial rhinitis: eosinophilic, noneosinophilic

Miscellaneous: foreign body, nasal polyp, septal deviation, neoplasm (primary or secondary), enlarged adenoids or tonsils, recent head trauma (with cerebrospinal fluid leak), autonomic, vasomotor rhinitis

Drug-induced: oral contraceptives, hormone replacement therapy, antihypertensives (several classes), ophthalmic beta-blockers, local decongestants (rhinitis medicamentosum), aspirin and nonsteroidal antiinflammatory drug, cocaine

Atrophic rhinitis: extensive surgery

Physical/chemical exposures: occupational, pollution, gustatory, dry air, bright light

Associated with a systemic disorder: hormonal, hypothyroidism, pregnancy, acquired immune deficiency syndrome, immunological, systemic lupus, rheumatoid arthritis, Sjögren's syndrome, primary mucus or ciliary defect, cystic fibrosis, antibody deficiency, granulomatous disease

B. **Chronology.** How often and when do symptoms occur? Do they predominate at certain times of the year?

C. **Associated symptoms.** What other symptoms are associated? What makes the symptoms better or worse? Associated complaints (e.g., frank fatigue, irritability, depression, or chest symptoms) tend to point to untreated allergic causes, systemic disease, or drug-induced illness (Table 6.2).

D. **Pertinent medical history.** Include questions about atopic disease, upper respiratory allergies, asthma, nasal surgery, serious infections, and current prescription medication use.

E. **Lifestyle history.** This discussion should address tobacco (personal use or use by those at home), alcohol or other recreational drug use, over-the-counter medication, herbal remedies, and pets in the home.

F. **Family history.** Is there a family history of allergies or other relevant systemic diseases?

G. **Occupational history.** Are there suspected environmental irritants?

III. **Physical examination**

A. **General inspection** of the patient frequently offers clues to the cause of the rhinitis. For example, "allergic shiners" (infraorbital, bluish discoloration of the skin) or a crease at the lower part of the nose from repeated rubbing are common physical findings of allergic rhinitis.

B. **Focused physical examination (PE).** Evaluate vital signs (especially temperature) and the ears, nose, and throat, including examination for lymphadenopathy and thyroid disease. A competent examination of nasal passages requires a nasal speculum (a 4–5 mm ear speculum on a handheld otoscope is acceptable for children) and a good light source. Carefully place the nasal speculum vertically into each vestibule. Insert a handheld otoscope light source through the speculum to survey for nasal patency, mucosal color (pale, red or bluish), degree and location of edema, presence and type of nasal drainage (thin, clear, thick, purulent, unilateral, or bilateral), anatomic deformities (bone spurs, septal deviation), and the presence of polyps or other masses. If swollen nasal turbinates block the view, apply a short-acting decongestant spray, then reexamine in 10 minutes. Evaluation of the posterior portion of the nose is often difficult or impossible with a nasal speculum and light source. A flexible nasopharyngoscope permits examination of the structures between the nasal vestibule and the larynx (1).

Assess the lungs and skin for signs of atopic disease (wheezing or eczema) (Chapters 8.9 and 13.4).

C. **Additional physical examination.** If systemic illness is suggested after the focused examination, a thorough multisystem PE is necessary (Table 6.2).

IV. **Testing**

A. **Clinical laboratory tests.** After a thorough history and focused physical examination, most common causes of rhinitis will not require additional testing to initiate effective treatment. Microscopic examination of nasal secretions can be done to help define uncertain allergic or bacterial causes of rhinitis, although most primary care clinicians often leave these tests to an otolaryngologist because these are usually done to clarify less common causes of rhinitis (3). Prompt referral is indicated if doubt exists, serious pathology is suspected or found, PE is difficult secondary to nasal obstruction, or symptoms do not improve with treatment.

B. **Diagnostic imaging.** If an anatomic abnormality or sinus pathology is suspected, limited computerized tomography (CT) of the sinuses is recommended (1,3,5).

V. **Diagnostic assessment.** The patient's story is critical to determining an accurate diagnosis. Additionally, purulent nasal drainage implies an infectious cause, whereas clear discharge suggests a noninfectious cause. Viral infection will create whitish to pale yellow drainage with associated symptoms of generalized head or body aches, nasal congestion, and sneezing. Bacterial infection will cause yellow or green drainage with focal sinus pain, upper teeth complaints, and possibly fever. Look for edematous, erythematous turbinates. Other less common infectious sources (fungal or parasitic) should be suspected if treatment fails or the patient has a suggestive medical or travel history (5).

To distinguish between allergic and nonallergic rhinitis, focus on symptoms of sneezing, clear drainage, postnasal drip, itching, nasal congestion, generalized sinus pressure, specific irritants or allergens, and family and personal history of atopy and allergy. Next, consider seasonal, perennial, or geographic relationships. The presence of blue or pale boggy turbinates with clear drainage suggests an allergic process.

After a thorough history is taken, the physical examination should confirm the patient's story and help identify any anatomic defects or systemic disease. Several follow-up visits may be necessary to assess, treat, and educate those with allergic rhinitis and to confirm any need for further evaluation or treatment by an otolaryngologist or allergist (4).

References

1. Fornadley JA. The stuffy nose and rhinitis. *Med Clin North Am* 1999;83:211–224.
2. Hadley JA. Evaluation and management of allergic rhinitis. *Med Clin North Am* 1999;83:13–25.
3. Galen BA. Rhinitis. *Lippincott's Primary Care Practice* 1997;1:129–141.
4. Leopold D, Ferguson BJ, Piccirillo JF. Outcomes assessment. *Otolaryngol Head Neck Surg* 1997;117:S58–S68.
5. Benninger MA, Anon JB, Mabry RL. The medical management of rhinosinusitis. *Otolaryngol Head Neck Surg* 1997;117:S41–S49.

6.7 Stomatitis

John G. Spangler

Stomatitis represents a broad category of oral mucosal infections and inflammatory lesions that are more common in the adult population than tension headaches, phlebitis, or arthralgias. In one large survey, the 30 most common lesions accounted for 93% of all oral lesions (1).

I. **Approach**
   A. **Stomatitis categories** include the following: (a) premalignant or malignant lesions; (b) human immunodeficiency virus (HIV)-related lesions (e.g., Kaposi's sarcoma, oral hairy leukoplakia); (c) infections that may be bacterial (e.g, necrotizing ulcerative gingivitis), viral [e.g., herpes simplex virus (HSV), hand-foot-mouth disease], or fungal (e.g., thrush, angular cheilitis); (d) ulcerative and erosive conditions (e.g., Behçet's disease, autoimmune disorders); (e) traumatic and irritant lesions; and (f) drug-related eruptions (Stevens–Johnson syndrome, chemotherapy-associated mucositis).
   B. **Special concerns.** Treatable infections such as thrush should be recognized promptly and in certain clinical situations may raise the suspicion of underlying immunosuppression. Premalignant and malignant disorders need prompt diagnosis and treatment to optimize survival. Oral signs of some systemic diseases, such a Behçet's disease or drug-related Stevens–Johnson syndrome, may be life threatening and require urgent attention. **In general, any oral ulceration, patch, or plaque that does not heal within 2 weeks needs referral for definitive diagnosis and treatment (2).**
II. **History**
   A. **Characteristics of the oral lesion.** Describe the onset: Was it abrupt, suggesting infection; or insidious, suggesting inflammatory or neoplastic origin? Are there associated signs and symptoms? Many oral infections are associated with pain, malaise, and fever. Behçet's disease has associated

ocular and genital lesions, whereas other autoimmune diseases such as systemic lupus erythematosus (SLE) or ulcerative colitis may have systemic symptoms (3). Describe the lesions: Are they painful or painless? Infections? Inflammatory lesions and aphthous ulcers are usually painful (3), whereas premalignant and malignant lesions may be painless (2,4). Are there vesicles or bullae? Pemphigoid and pemphigus can cause bullae or ulcers. HSV starts as vesicular lesions, then ulcerates. Varicella zoster lesions can occur in the mouth (3,5). Did vesicles precede the lesions, suggesting HSV, or was there ulceration without vesicles, suggesting aphthous ulcers (3)? Are the lesions white and will they not wipe off of the mucosa? Leukoplakia, a premalignant lesion, is white and will not wipe off. Any coexisting red component, called erythroplakia, greatly increases the malignant potential of the lesion (2,4). Lichen planus also produces a striated white lesion, usually on the buccal mucosa (3). Where are the lesions? HSV tends to occur on periosteally bound mucosa (gingiva, hard palate), whereas recurrent aphthous ulcers occur on nonperiosteally bound mucosa (buccal, lip, or tongue mucosa) (3). The floor of the mouth under the tongue, the lateral aspects of the tongue, the retromolar regions, and the soft palate are worrisome areas for malignancy to develop (4), but malignancy can occur anywhere.

B. Past medical history. Does the patient have systemic inflammatory conditions such as SLE or lichen planus? Has the patient had the lesions previously? Aphthous ulcers and HSV tend to recur. Does the patient wear dentures making him or her more susceptible to denture stomatitis or angular cheilitis, both caused by *Candida* species (5)? Are HIV-risk factors present, making oral hairy leukoplakia, Kaposi's sarcoma, and severe oral candidiasis more likely (5)? Do family members or other close associates have similar symptoms, suggesting enteroviral infections (e.g., herpangina and hand-foot-mouth disease) (Chapter 13.3)? Is the patient on any medications known to cause oral drug-related eruptions? Sulfonamides and many other drugs can cause Stevens–Johnson syndrome, whereas recent cancer chemotherapy can produce severe mucosal inflammation.

C. Social history. Does the patient use alcohol or tobacco, thus increasing the risk for premalignancy or malignancy (2,4)? Has there been exposure to known oral irritants such as foods or spices or potential irritants such as chemicals or new mouth care products? Is the patient sexually active and has there been oral–genital contact? Syphilis and gonorrhea can both occur in the oropharynx.

III. Physical examination

A. Head, eyes, ears, nose, and throat (HEENT). Based on the history, a focused physical examination of the HEENT is necessary. Look for signs of trauma. Examine the conjunctiva and nasal mucosa for inflammatory changes or ulcerations. Evaluate the patient for coexisting upper respiratory signs and symptoms such as rhinorrhea, sinus tenderness to palpation, and otitis media. Inspect facial skin for vesicles from HSV or varicella-zoster or other lesions such as echymoses, malar rash, or viral exantham. Look for facial asymmetry. Varicella-zoster can cause facial nerve paralysis, called the "Ramsay Hunt syndrome." Evaluate preauricular, postauricular, and cervical lymph node chains. Finally, evaluate the oral cavity, documenting the size, location, and appearance of the lesion.

B. Additional physical examination. Based on findings from the HEENT examination, additional physical examination might include (a) pulmonary examination for viral pneumonitis or pulmonary findings in autoimmune diseases; (b) abdominal and rectal examination for Crohn's disease or ulcerative colitis; (c) genitourinary examination for mucosal ulcers in Behçet's disease and Stevens–Johnson syndrome, and for signs of syphilis or gonorrhea; (d) a general skin examination looking for viral exanthemas, drug eruptions, lichen planus, pemphigus, pemphigoid, and SLE; and (e) a musculoskeletal examination for signs of SLE, Reiter's syndrome, or other autoimmune diseases (3).

IV. **Testing**
- A. **Clinical laboratory testing** should be guided by history and physical findings. A potassium hydroxide wet mount is useful in the diagnosis of candidiasis. Viral and bacterial cultures can be obtained from swabs of oral lesions, but viral cultures are usually more helpful than bacterial cultures. Darkfield microscopy can be performed from swabs of syphilis chancres or plaques. Cytologic scrapings of premalignant or malignant lesions, prepared in a manner similar to a Pap smear, are not a substitute for biopsy of suspected oral neoplasia (2,4).
- B. **Diagnostic imaging** is indicated only in selected cases such as coexisting sinus disease ["mini" sinus computed tomogram (CT)], coexisting neck mass or lymphadenopathy suggestive of malignant disease (head and neck CT), suspected metastatic disease (chest x-ray study; CT of the head, abdomen, and chest), or trauma (cervical spine series; cranial CT; dental Panorex films). If HSV is suspected, cranial magnetic resonance imaging (MRI) may be useful to evaluate the temporal lobes. A chest x-ray study is also indicated in suspected lower respiratory tract disease such as viral or autoimmune pneumonitis or secondary bacterial pneumonia. If a severe lip laceration has occurred, plain films can help to rule out mandibular condylar fractures or tooth fractures.

V. **Diagnostic assessment.** The diagnosis of stomatitis depends on synthesis of the aforementioned key historical, physical examination, laboratory, and imaging elements. **All oral ulcers that do not heal, as well as white or reddish-white lesions that do not resolve in 2 weeks, need biopsy to rule out malignancy (2,4).**

References

1. Yeatts D, Burns JC. Common oral mucosal lesions in adults. *Am Fam Physician* 1991;44:2043–2050.
2. Silverman S. *Oral cancer*, 4th ed. Hamilton, Ontario: BC Decker, 1998.
3. Salisbury PL, Jorizzo JL. Oral ulcers and erosions. *Adv Dermatol* 1993;8:31–79.
4. Mashberg A, Samit A. Early diagnosis of asymptomatic oral and oropharyngeal squamous cell cancer. *CA Cancer J Clin* 1995;45:328–351.
5. Laskaris G. Oral manifestations of infectious diseases. *Dent Clin N Am* 1996;40: 395–423.

6.8 Tinnitus

Sara Lynn Neal

Tinnitus, which has been described as "ear noise," consists of sounds heard by the patient with no sound source external to the head. Although infinite variations can occur, most commonly patients will describe ringing, buzzing, clicking, hissing, or humming. Of the population, 10% to 14% will complain of prolonged, recurrent tinnitus, with 20% of these people having symptoms that have a significant impact on their quality of life (1,2). In the United Kingdom, 7% of the population will at some time seek evaluation in primary care for tinnitus (2).

I. **Approach.** Tinnitus is not a disease, but an indication of some other ongoing process, pathologic or not. The first clues to diagnosing which process is responsible for the tinnitus are the type of sound heard and any relationship to the pulse or respiration. These clues subdivide tinnitus into two general categories, vibratory and nonvibratory.
- A. **Types of tinnitus**
    - 1. **Vibratory (objective, pseudotinnitus).** These sounds are often synchronous with the pulse. They are real sounds and mechanical in ori-

gin; they can sometimes be heard by the examiner as well as the patient who may describe the sound as pulsatile. Sources, either vascular or muscular, include:

    a. Venous hum: caused by eddy currents in the jugular vein and exacerbated by concurrent conductive hearing loss.

    b. Arteriovenous malformations: most commonly between the occipital artery and the transverse sinus.

    c. Arterial bruits: most commonly from the petrous carotid system.

    d. Myoclonus of nearby structures, most commonly the palate, stapedius muscle, or tensor tympani. These are usually asynchronous with the pulse.

    e. A patulous or abnormally patent eustachian tube can cause chronic or intermittent tinnitus. Sometimes related to respirations, it is frequently described as a "hissing" sound.

  2. Nonvibratory (subjective). This type is more common. Subdivision into central versus peripheral tinnitus is helpful.

    a. Central tinnitus is caused by any eighth nerve or cortex lesion, including multiple sclerosis (MS).

    b. Peripheral tinnitus has many perpetrators including metabolic disorders (hyperlipidemia, thyroid disease, zinc deficiency), infection, medications (section **II.E.**), cerumen impaction, sensorineural hearing loss (especially presbycusis or noise-induced), Ménière's disease, temporomandibular joint dysfunction, otosclerosis, and spontaneous cochlear emissions.

  B. Special concerns. Tinnitus can be a component of several conditions that threaten hearing such as Ménière's disease, acoustic neuroma, or Cogan's syndrome. Special attention should be paid to patients presenting with unilateral tinnitus, associated vertigo, unilateral sensorineural hearing loss, and eye inflammation.

II. History. Important features of the history should include:

  A. Date of tinnitus onset, particularly any relation to an illness or change in drug regimen.

  B. A description of the tinnitus may help subdivide into vibratory and nonvibratory sources. Are there any exacerbating or ameliorating factors? An association with respirations or pulse points to a vibratory source. Positional change (such as lowering the head between the knees causing venous engorgement), variation with respirations, or distortion of one's own voice can point toward a patulous eustachian tube as the mechanism for tinnitus.

  C. Fluctuation of symptoms. This is commonly associated with Ménière's disease.

  D. History of noise exposure or hearing loss. Noise-induced hearing loss usually causes high-pitched tinnitus, whereas Ménière's disease usually produces a lower-pitched sound. Conductive hearing loss from cerumen impaction, otitis media, or otosclerosis can heighten the awareness of internal vibratory sounds such as a venous hum or myoclonus. Presbycusis, or degeneration within the organ of Corti, is frequently seen in the elderly. It is associated with high-frequency hearing loss and high-pitched tinnitus (Chapter 6.2).

  E. Medication history. Drugs can be a major contributor to tinnitus (e.g., salicylates, caffeine, aminoglycosides, alcohol, quinidine, nonsteroidals, carbamazepine, levodopa, propranolol (Inderal), and aminophylline) (3). Some hormonal preparations have also been implicated as has the postpartum state.

  F. Significant weight loss can be associated with a patulous eustachian tube (Chapter 2.13).

  G. Concurrent medical conditions to be considered include hypertension, diabetes mellitus, thyroid disorders, hyperlipidemia, and infection. Arteriovenous sounds will be heightened by increased cardiac output. Vascular disease can cause ischemia of the auditory organs, including the cortex. Neural impulses can be affected by diabetes or MS.

       H. **Psychiatric disturbances** can affect sound perception. Ask about anxiety or depression, which can heighten awareness of internal auditory sounds. In turn, tinnitus can exacerbate these underlying conditions. Auditory hallucinations can be assessed by mental status testing.

       I. **Psychological effects.** Ask about impact on sleep, concentration, hearing, memory, irritability, and sense of well-being.

III. **Physical examination.** Focus on the head, ears, eyes, nose, throat, and neck as well as the cardiovascular and neurologic systems. Assess vital signs and perform a complete ear examination, including evaluation for obstruction of the external auditory canal. Look for tympanic membrane landmarks, tympanic pulsations, or signs of tumor. Auscultate the external auditory canal for transmitted sounds and use tuning forks to assess air and bone conduction. Observe the neck for thyroid masses and auscultate for thyroid or carotid bruits. Evaluate extraocular movements, speech discrimination, and the integrity of the central nervous system (gait, equilibrium, sensation). If appropriate, include evaluation of mood, affect, and perception (e.g., hallucinations).

IV. **Testing**

       A. **Clinical laboratory tests.** Most tinnitus patients will need only audiometry (4,5). If indicated by history and physical examination, consider thyroid functions, electrolytes, lipids, sedimentation rate, toxicology, syphilis serology, or rheumatology screen. A complete audiometric evaluation (pure tone and speech thresholds, speech discrimination, acoustic reflexes, and impedence testing) should always be done, especially to search for sensorineural hearing loss (4,5). A tympanogram may reveal pulsations coincident with the heart rhythm or respirations.

       B. **Imaging.** Plain radiographs are rarely useful. Evaluation for neoplasm, especially an acoustic neuroma, is best done with magnetic resonance imaging (MRI), which will also delineate eighth nerve lesions and cortex damage. Computed tomography (CT) with contrast is superior to MRI in suspected lesions of the temporal bone and mastoids (5). Auditory brainstem-evoked responses can help to localize cortical lesions or MS (1,5). Duplex ultrasound will reveal carotid stenosis. An angiogram may be necessary to examine vasculature near the inner ear. Patients with pulsatile tinnitus may need MRI, CT, and angiography before a definitive cause is found (5).

V. **Diagnostic assessment.** Because tinnitus is a symptom, not a disease, the focus of evaluation should be on identifying those few patients with serious or treatable causes and convincing the remaining patients of the nonthreatening nature of the symptom. The key to diagnosing tinnitus is determining if it is vibratory or nonvibratory. If vibratory, search for a structural source (e.g., vascular complex, muscular component, eustachian tube) of the sound through audiometry and imaging. Nonvibratory tinnitus, although more common, often has a less easily definable cause. Consider drug effects and hearing loss first, then search for altered metabolic states (e.g., diabetes, hyperthyroidism, or infection), not forgetting psychiatric causes. Evaluate for neurologic conditions (acoustic neuroma, damage to the organ of Corti or a brain lesion) as indicated.

References

1. Pfeifer KJ, Rosen GP, Rubin AM. Tinnitus: etiology and management. *Clin Geriatr Med* 1999;15:193–203.
2. Vesterager V. Fortnightly review: tinnitus—investigation and management. *BMJ* 1997;314:728–731.
3. Seligmann H, Podoshin L, Ben-David J, et al. Drug-induced tinnitus and other hearing disorders. *Drug Saf* 1996;14:198–212.
4. Seidman MD, Jacobson GP. Update on tinnitus. *Otolaryngol Clin North Am* 1996; 29:455–465.
5. Fortune DS, Haynes DS. Tinnitus—current evaluation and management. *Med Clin North Am* 1999;83:153–162.

6.9 Vertigo

Frank S. Celestino

Dizziness accounts for 1% to 2% of all office visits, 7% of visits by patients aged more than 80 years and 20% to 25% of all non–pain-related emergency room visits (1–3). Dizziness and vertigo are usually benign, self-limited processes not associated with excess mortality, although some individuals suffer impaired quality of life because of recurrent or persistent symptoms (4) (Chapter 2.2).

I. **Approach**
   A. **Classification of dizziness.** Careful interviewing allows placement of patient complaints into one of four categories, each implying certain pathophysiologic mechanisms and, thus, specific differential diagnoses (2,4).
      1. True vertigo. This is an hallucination of movement—a feeling that the body or environment is moving. Patients often report rotation or spinning. It often begins abruptly and, if severe, is accompanied by nausea, vomiting, and staggering gait. True vertigo most often implies a disturbance of the peripheral vestibular system (labyrinth and its connections to the brainstem) or, less commonly, of the central vestibular apparatus (brainstem or cerebellum) (2,3,5).
      Peripheral causes of vertigo (in approximate order of frequency in primary care) include viral labyrinthitis or vestibular neuronitis (acute unilateral vestibulopathy), benign paroxysmal positional vertigo (BPPV), serous otitis, perilymphatic fistula, Ménière's disease, and drugs (alcohol, aminoglycosides) (4,5). Central causes of vertigo include vertebrobasilar transient ischemic attack, cerebellar infarction or neoplasm, demyelinating disease, brainstem infarction or neoplasm, cerebellopontine angle tumors, migraine, hyperventilation, seizures, spinocerebellar degeneration, and certain systemic disorders (infections, vasculitis, syphilis) (2,4). Rarely, the cervical spine is the source of vertigo, by either osteoarthritic spur occlusion of vertebral arteries or proprioceptive overstimulation by facet joint arthropathy (2).
      2. Presyncope is a sensation of impending faint ("severe lightheadedness") implies a temporary decrement of cerebral circulation. Common causes include postural hypotension, vasovagal reactions, impaired cardiac output, and hypoglycemia (Chapter 2.12).
      3. Disequilibrium is a feeling of unsteadiness of gait or imbalance in the absence of any abnormal head sensation indicating a disturbance of the motor control system. Causes include alcoholism, drugs, cervical facet joint arthropathy, multiple sclerosis, and multiple neurosensory deficits (e.g., a combination of visual impairment, vestibular hypofunction, deconditioning, peripheral neuropathy, and medications).
      4. Other or atypical. Often described as a vague or mild wooziness, lightheadedness or heavy headedness, this category has a high association with psychological disturbances such as anxiety, depression, and panic (2,4).
   B. **Patient's age.** In young adults (<30 years) psychological causes predominate, whereas vestibular disorders do in middle age. In the elderly, cerebrovascular and cardiac disorders, combined with multiple sensory deficits, outweigh simple vestibular causes (1,5).
   C. **Special concerns.** These include potentially life-threatening central nervous system (CNS) neoplasms, brainstem ischemia, and cardiac dysfunction manifest by focal neurologic and cardiovascular abnormalities.
II. **History.** The patient's age, underlying comorbidities, and symptom classification category will help limit the diagnostic possibilities. Further specificity is gained by eliciting the following:

A. **Temporal pattern.** Are the symptoms episodic or continuous? If episodic, how long do they last? Peripheral origin vertigo is often intermittent and of sudden onset compared with the usual, more gradual onset of central vertigo. A continuous history suggests CNS pathology, drug or toxin effects, metabolic dysfunction, or psychiatric disease. BBPV episodes last less than a minute; vertebrobasilar transient ischemic attacks last minutes to an hour; Ménière's disease persists 1 to 24 hours; and vestibular neuronitis or acute labyrinthitis continues several days.

B. **Precipitating or exacerbating factors.** Has there been recent head trauma (implying perilympathic fistula) or viral illness (labyrinthitis)? What is the relationship to sudden head movement or turning over in bed (BPPV), coughing or sneezing (perilymphatic fistula), postural changes (orthostasis), exercise (arrhythmias), foods (salty meals exacerbating Ménière's), walking and turning (multiple sensory deficits), micturition or pain (vasovagal reaction), and emotional upset (hyperventilation)?

C. **Associated symptoms.** Marked nausea, vomiting, diaphoresis, aural fullness, and recruitment (perception of sounds being too loud) are typical of peripheral vestibular disorders. Episodic vertigo associated with tinnitus and gradual (unilateral) hearing loss involving low frequencies preferentially suggests Ménière's disease. Asymmetric weakness, cranial nerve or cerebellar dysfunction, diplopia, or dysarthria suggests brainstem or CNS disease. Headache, scotomata, or tunnel vision points to migraine. Numbness or paresthesias may indicate neuropathy contributing to multiple sensory deficits (Chapter 4.6). A single, abrupt episode of severe vertigo with negative Dix-Hallpike (DH) testing (section **III.A**) that gradually subsides over days implies labyrinthitis (if hearing is affected) or vestibular neuronitis (if hearing is unaffected). Mild vertigo with prominent tinnitus, unilateral hearing loss, and loss of corneal reflex is worrisome for an acoustic neuroma.

D. **Medications or toxins.** Many medications can cause "dizziness," although few (aminoglycosides, lead, mercury) cause vertigo. Assess toxin exposure by exploring job and recreational activities.

III. **Physical examination (PE).** This will emphasize orthostatic vital signs, the eyes, ears, and neurologic and cardiovascular systems.

A. **Detection of nystagmus** is critical because it is the only objective sign of vertigo (5). Nystagmus can occur spontaneously or in response to changes in eye or body position. Peripheral vestibular disorders usually cause horizontal or rotatory nystagmus, whereas CNS pathology is reflected by vertical nystagmus—an ominous sign. In true vertigo caused by BPPV, DH maneuvers will often confirm the diagnosis (sensitivity 60% to 90%, specificity 90% to 95%) (2,3). The patient is moved rapidly from a sitting to a supine position with the head turned at a 30-degree angle, first to one side and then to the other. A positive DH test includes precipitation of vertigo, latency of onset by a few seconds, rotational nystagmus, resolution within a minute, and lessened symptoms and nystagmus with prolonged latency on repeated testing (i.e., fatiguability). Lack of latency and fatiguability characterize vertigo caused by serious central lesions.

B. **Neurologic examination** serves to detect brainstem or CNS pathology.

C. **Otoscopy** can detect otitis media or cholesteatoma. Nystagmus with vertigo following positive or negative pressure applied to the tympanic membrane (pneumatic otoscopy) suggests a perilymphatic fistula.

D. **Other provocative tests** (forced hyperventilation, vestibulo-ocular reflex testing, vigorous horizontal head shaking) are not routinely helpful.

IV. **Testing**

A. **Clinical laboratory tests.** Most (80% to 90%) patients will need no laboratory testing (2,4,5). Audiometry is suggested if tinnitus or hearing loss is present. Blood tests are dictated by appropriate clinical indications only. Brainstem auditory-evoked responses can help elucidate multiple sclerosis. Holter monitoring is indicated if arrhythmias are suspected. Specialized testing—posturography, rotational chair testing, electronystagamography—is best ordered by a consultant.

B. Diagnostic imaging. Consider Doppler ultrasound for suspected transient ischemic attack and magnetic resonance imaging if CNS lesions are suspected.

V. Diagnostic assessment. A comprehensive history can categorize the patient's problem as one of vertigo, presyncope, disequilibrium, or other (atypical). PE maneuvers (especially DH testing), detection of nystagmus, and assessment of neurologic function will further pinpoint the likely diagnosis. It is helpful to remember that true vertigo results most often from peripheral vestibular disorders, presyncope from cardiovascular dysfunction, disequilibrium from neurologic disorders, and other (atypical or vague) symptoms from psychological or psychiatric disease.

References

1. Sloane PD. Dizziness in primary care: results from the National Ambulatory Medical Care Survey. *J Fam Pract* 1989;29:33–38.
2. Derebery MJ. The diagnosis and treatment of dizziness. *Med Clin North Am* 1999;83:163–176.
3. Walker JS, Barnes SB. Dizziness—the difficult diagnosis. *Emerg Med Clin North Am* 1998;16:845–878.
4. Sloane PD. Evaluation and management of dizziness in the older patient. *Clin Geriatr Med* 1996;12:785–801.
5. Drachman DA. Clinical crossroads—a 69-year-old man with chronic dizziness. *JAMA* 1998;280:2111–2118.

7. CARDIOVASCULAR PROBLEMS

JIM NUOVO

7.1 Chest Pain, Atypical

Jim Nuovo

Atypical chest pain is defined as pain that does not have a characteristic anginal quality (heaviness or squeezing sensation), precipitating factors (e.g., exertion), or location (substernal and radiating).

I. **Approach.** The highest priority is generally given in distinguishing cardiac from noncardiac causes. Studies have demonstrated that 10% to 30% of patients with chest pain who undergo coronary arteriography have no arterial abnormalities.

   A. **Common noncardiac causes.** The most common diagnostic findings in those whose pain is not likely to have a cardiac cause include:

      1. Gastrointestinal (gastritis, esophagitis, and esophageal motility disorders).

      2. Musculoskeletal (costochondritis).

      3. Psychiatric (panic attacks, major depression, or both). Be wary for warning signs for less-common, life-threatening conditions such as pulmonary embolism, aortic dissection, and pneumothorax.

II. **History**

   A. **Characteristics of the chest pain.** Important questions to ask: What is the quality of pain? Where is it located? What is its duration and intensity? What symptoms accompany the pain? Does anything trigger the chest pain or make the pain better or worse? Is there any relationship between exertion and the pain?

   B. **Determining the likelihood of ischemic heart disease.** Four major features in the initial history and physical examination can be used to determine the likelihood of IHD. They are in order of importance:

      1. Angina description (definite angina, probable angina, probably not angina, and not angina).

      2. Prior myocardial infarction [by history, or electrocardiographic (EKG) findings].

      3. Age (risk of IHD increases with age).

      4. Number of risk factors (e.g., diabetes, smoking, hypercholesterolemia, and hypertension).

   C. **Features suggesting nonanginal pain.** Features suggesting nonanginal pain include pleuritic pain (sharp or knifelike pain brought on by respiratory movements or cough), pain localized with one finger, pain reproduced by movement or palpation of the chest wall or arms, constant pain lasting for days, and very brief episodes of pain lasting a few seconds (1).

   D. **Other key considerations.** Key considerations in the history include the following:

      1. All presentations of chest pain should be taken seriously until proven to be benign.

      2. The description of pain can be greatly influenced by socioeconomic status, education, culture, and personality.

      3. A review of cardiac risk factors is appropriate for all patients who present with chest pain.

      4. Red flags suggesting a noncardiac, life-threatening condition include tachypnea, dyspnea, and hypoxemia.

      5. Sharp, stabbing, or pleuritic qualities do not completely exclude an ischemic cause (Chapter 8.5). In the Multicenter Chest Pain Study, IHD was diagnosed in 22% of patients coming to the emergency room with a sharp quality pain (2).

III. **Physical examination**. No reliable physical signs can be used to determine whether a patient with atypical chest pain has ischemic heart disease. The main purpose of the examination is to assess the patient for evidence of complications from atherosclerotic disease (e.g., peripheral vascular disease, cerebrovascular disease, and congestive heart failure). Pay attention to findings on the vascular examination (e.g., peripheral artery bruits, retinal arteriolar changes, the presence of a cardiac gallop) and for signs of the consequences of diminished myocardial contractility (e.g., lower extremity edema or pulmonary crackles) (Chapter 7.5).

IV. **Testing**

A. **Probability of IHD based on history.** Prior to testing, the probability of IHD can be inferred by the estimates made by Diamond and Forrester (3). Examples of these estimates include (a) high probability situations (probability > 75%)—men aged more than 40 years and women aged more than 50 years with typical anginal symptoms; (b) moderate probability situations (probability > 50%)—men aged more than 40 years and women aged more than 60 years with atypical features; (c) low probability situations (probability < 20%)—men aged less than 40 years and women aged less than 50 with atypical features.

B. **Response to nitroglycerin (NTG).** Response of chest pain to sublingual NTG can be used (with caution) as an adjunct for determining whether a patient's chest pain is from IHD. For example, a prompt response (< 3 minutes) increases the probability of IHD; however, it should be noted that esophageal spasm and biliary colic may also respond favorably to this intervention. Conversely, failure to respond to NTG should not be used to exclude the possibility of IHD.

C. **Response to a gastrointestinal (GI) cocktail.** It is common practice in many emergency room and urgent care settings to give a patient a GI cocktail that typically contains a liquid antacid, xylocaine, and an antispasmodic. No reliable studies exist on the diagnostic accuracy of this intervention.

D. **Resting ECG.** A normal resting ECG cannot be used as the sole criterion to rule out the presence of ischemic heart disease.

E. **Exercise testing.** The standard provocative test for patients with atypical chest pain who have at least a moderate risk for IHD is the exercise treadmill test. During exercise, the patient is monitored for symptoms of chest pain, heart rate, blood pressure response to exercise, arrhythmias, and ST-segment changes. A significant test includes an ST-segment depression of at least 1.0 mm below the baseline. It is important that the patient achieve a vigorous heart rate response to exercise. Approximately 20% of patients with an abnormal exercise tolerance test (ETT) have significant ST-segment changes occurring only at maximal or near-maximal heart rate changes. Therefore, when reviewing an ETT report, if the maximal heart rate achieved was less than 85% of the predicted heart rate, the results of the test should be interpreted more cautiously.

F. **Other diagnostic tests.** Some patients should not undergo the standard ETT for a number of reasons. These include the inability to exercise because of gait or instability problems and underlying ECG abnormalities that make the standard ETT unreadable (e.g., left ventricular hypertrophy with strain and left bundle branch block). If the patient is able to exercise, the preferred test will be either an exercise echocardiogram or an exercise thallium test. If the patient is unable to exercise, test options include a dobutamine echocardiogram and a dipyridamole (Persantine) thallium test. A divergence of opinion is seen as to which of these tests is best; however, each has higher sensitivity and specificity than the standard ETT.

V. **Diagnostic assessment.** The key to the diagnosis of atypical chest pain remains in the clinical history. An assessment of the probability of ischemic heart disease should be made on all patients. Those with a very low probability of IHD should not undergo diagnostic testing because, given the problems of sensitivity and specificity, the results will have little or no impact on the management of the patient. Critical pathways for triage have been proposed to help identify inter-mediate and high risk patients (4,5).

References

1. Panju AA, Hemmelgard BR, Guyatt GH, Simel DL. Is this patient having a myo-cardial infarction? *JAMA* 1998;280:1256–1263.
2. American College of Emergency Physicians. Clinical policy for the initial approach to adults presenting with a chief complaint of chest pain, with no history of trauma. *Ann Emerg Med* 1995;25:274–299.
3. Diamond GA, Forrester JS. Analysis of probability as an aid in the clinical diagno-sis of coronary-artery disease. *N Engl J Med* 1979;300:1350–1358.
4. Nichol G, Walls R, Goldman L, et al. A critical pathway for management of patients with acute chest pain who are at low risk for myocardial ischemia: recommendations and potential impact. *Ann Intern Med* 1997;127:996–1005.
5. Braunwald E, Mark DB, Jones RH. *Diagnosing and managing unstable angina: quick reference guide for clinicians*, Number 10. AHCPR Publication No.94-0603. Rockville, MD: US Department of Health and Human Services, Public Health Ser-vice, Agency for Health Care Policy and Research and National Heart, Lung, and Blood Institute; 1994.

7.2 Chest Pain, Substernal

Marie K. Yamamotoya

Substernal chest pain requires a rapid and accurate assessment to identify potentially life-threatening events. Substernal chest pain of cardiac origin encompasses the entire clinical spectrum from typical angina to unstable angina and ultimately to myocardial infarction (MI) (Chapter 7.1).

  I. **Approach.** In the evaluation of substernal chest pain, the initial step involves estimating the likelihood of coronary artery disease (CAD) with a thorough his-tory, physical examination, electrocardiogram (ECG), and other potentially diagnostic tests. Serious noncardiac conditions that must be considered on ini-tial presentation include aortic dissection, pericardial tamponade, pulmonary embolism, and tension pneumothorax.
 II. **History**
   A. **Characteristics of pain in stable angina**
      1. **Quality.** The pain of angina pectoris is often not described as a pain at all. Instead, it is frequently referred to as a squeezing, heaviness, or pres-sure sensation lasting 5 to 10 minutes. Diaphoresis, dyspnea, nausea, and vomiting often accompany the discomfort. Pain that is sharp, stabbing (especially if exacerbated by deep inspiration), pain reproducible with chest wall palpation, and pain lasting seconds or days to weeks is less likely to be from CAD.
      2. **Location.** Generally, angina is poorly localized in the retrosternal area, anterior chest, or epigastrium and typically radiates to the left arm, neck, or jaw.
      3. **Precipitating and alleviating factors.** Angina is often precipitated by conditions that increase myocardial oxygen demand, most com-monly physical exertion, emotional stress, or cold weather. It is relieved promptly with rest or sublingual nitroglycerin.
   B. **Characteristics of pain in unstable angina.** According to the clinical practice guidelines recently developed by the Agency for Health Care Policy (1), unstable angina is defined as:
      1. Angina at rest lasting greater than 20 minutes.

2. New onset angina (< 2 months) precipitated by walking one to two blocks or by climbing one flight of stairs at a normal pace.

3. Angina that is more frequent, longer in duration, or occurring at a lower threshold.

C. **Risk factors.** The Framingham Heart Study along with numerous other large epidemiologic studies has established the following risk factors for CAD (2):

1. Sex and age: men aged 45 years or older; women aged 55 years or older; women with premature menopause without hormone replacement.

2. Family history: MI or sudden death occurring in a first-degree male relative aged 55 years or younger or in a first-degree female relative aged 65 years or younger.

3. Smoking: in men who smoke one pack per day, a three- to fivefold risk for CAD compared with nonsmokers. Those who quit smoking can reach the same risk level of nonsmokers within 2 years of stopping.

4. Hypertension: blood pressure greater or equal to 140/90 (Chapter 7.8).

5. Cholesterol: total cholesterol greater than 200; low-density lipoprotein (LDL) greater than 130; high-density lipoprotein (HDL) less than 35. An HDL level above 60 is protective.

6. Diabetes mellitus: a twofold increase in CAD, compared with nondiabetics (Chapter 14.1).

III. **Physical examination**

A. **Focused physical examination.** This should include vital signs (notably blood pressure). During a symptomatic episode, the finding of a mitral regurgitation murmur, S_3 or S_4 gallop, bruits or precordial lift all suggest a high likelihood of CAD. Findings of xanthelasma, tendinous xanthomata, tobacco-stained teeth and fingernails, and decreased or asymmetrical peripheral pulses indicate the likely presence of cardiac risk factors.

IV. **Testing**

A. **ECG.** Despite the availability of a number of tests, the history remains very important in determining the likelihood of CAD in a patient with substernal chest pain. It is important to avoid using a normal ECG as "rule out" criteria, as many patients with unstable angina or even an acute MI may initially have a normal ECG. The diagnosis of CAD can be based on characteristic changes in the ST-T wave morphology during a symptomatic episode. Specifically, ST segment elevation greater than or equal to 1 mm in two or more consecutive leads is highly suggestive of an acute MI and is associated with the highest morbidity and mortality rate (3). ST segment depression of greater than or equal to 1 mm or T-wave inversion in two or more contiguous leads also strongly suggests ischemia or acute MI. The presence of Q waves greater than or equal to 0.04 seconds indicates previous MI. However, Q waves occurring in lead III alone may be a normal finding. As patients with initially normal ECG are still at risk for life-threatening complications and death (3% and 1%, respectively), it is important to follow serial ECGs for any evolution (3).

B. **Creatinine kinase.** The most widely used laboratory test for the detection of MI is the creatinine kinase enzyme. The isoenzyme, CK-MB, is abundant in the myocardium and, therefore, is sensitive and specific for myocardial injury. With acute MI, the MB fraction typically begins to rise within 6 hours of symptom onset, peaks at 18 hours, and falls after 24 hours. Total CK and CK-MB should be measured every 6 to 8 hours for a 24-hour period.

C. **Troponin I and T.** Both troponin I and T proteins are located on the contractile apparatus of the myocardium. These proteins are highly sensitive for myocardial injury. The prospective study conducted by Hamm et al. showed that in the 47 patients diagnosed with acute MI, 94% were positive for troponin T and 100% for troponin I (4). In addition, the negative predictive value of troponin T was 98.9% and that of troponin I was 99.7% (4).

D. **Noninvasive and invasive testing.** Both exercise and pharmacologic stress tests are used to assess for CAD in patients with stable angina. Unstable angina, uncontrolled hypertension, severe aortic stenosis, unstable arrythmias, and recent MI (4–6 weeks) are contraindications to stress testing.

1. Exercise ECG is a relatively inexpensive test with an overall sensitivity and specificity of 50% to 70%. It is most useful for those patients with a moderate pretest probability. Protocols are used to incrementally increase treadmill speed and elevation until the maximal heart rate for age is achieved. The ECG is monitored for ST depression and any ventricular arrythmias. The patient is also monitored for any fall in blood pressure or complaints of chest discomfort or dyspnea.

2. Exercise ECG with thallium or technetium sestamibi. The use of these radioisotopes improves the sensitivity and specificity of exercise ECG to approximately 90%. Thallium is distributed in proportion to blood flow. Areas of decreased uptake during exercise followed by normal uptake at rest suggest ischemia, whereas areas of persistent defect indicate infarction. Technetium is a newer agent with the advantage of a slow washout and added contrast, which results in fewer false-positive findings than thallium.

3. Exercise echocardiogram. This method detects wall motion abnormalities during exercise and has comparable sensitivity and specificity to exercise ECG. It is preferred in patients with abnormal resting ECGs and in patients with a low pretest probability. The disadvantages include difficulty imaging obese patients and the need to image as close to peak exercise as possible.

4. Dipyridamole or adenosine stress testing. The use of intravenous coronary vasodilators (dipyridamole or adenosine) in combination with a radioisotope (thallium or technetium sestamibi) is useful in patients who are unable to exercise. Areas of redistribution suggest ischemia, whereas areas of persistent defects indicate infarction. The use of phosphodiesterase inhibitors and the presence of reactive airway disease are contraindications.

5. Dobutamine echocardiogram. This method is also used for those who are unable to exercise. Dobutamine increases myocardial oxygen demand by increasing contractility and essentially "exercises" the heart. The echo monitors for any wall motion abnormalities.

6. Coronary angiography. Considered the "gold standard" test, this procedure provides the most detailed structural information of all the tests discussed. It is indicated in those patients who are at high risk for CAD by noninvasive tests and for those with persistent symptoms despite medical therapy. As diagnosis is closely tied to therapy, only those patients who are candidates for invasive procedures (e.g., percutaneous transluminal coronary angioplasty or coronary artery bypass graft) should be considered.

V. **Diagnostic assessment.** In patients presenting with substernal chest pain, the key to diagnosis involves quickly and accurately assessing for the likelihood of myocardial ischemia or infarction. An initial history, physical examination, and ECG will help in the risk assessment of the patient for significant CAD. Those who are at high to intermediate risk need to then be evaluated for presence of unstable angina. Once established, further steps involve the simultaneous evaluation with serial ECGs and enzymes along with therapy to reduce ischemia. Cardiac angiography is the final step in evaluation and treatment. For those at low risk for CAD and not meeting criteria for unstable angina, further evaluation involves noninvasive diagnostic testing with the possibility for cardiac angiography and revascularization.

References

1. Braunwald E, Mark DB, Jones RH. *Unstable angina: diagnosis and management.* Clinical Practice Guideline Number 10. AHCPR Publication No. 94-0602. Rockville, MD: Agency for Health Care Policy and Research and the National Heart, Lung, and

Blood Institute, Public Health Service, US Department of Health and Human Services, March 1994.
2. Anderson KM, Wilson PWF, Odell PM. An updated coronary risk profile. A statement for health professionals. *Circulation* 1991;83:356–362.
3. Karlson BW, Hallgren HP, Liliequist JA. Emergency room prediction of mortality and severe complication in patients with suspected acute myocardial infarction. *Eur Heart J* 1994;15:1558–1565.
4. Hamm CW, Goldmann BU, Heeschen C. Emergency room triage of patients with acute chest pain by means of rapid testing for cardiac troponin T or troponin I. *N Engl J Med* 1997;337:1648–1653.

7.3 Bradycardia

Paul C. Riggle and Richard W. Harper

Bradycardia, which is defined as a heart rate below 60 beats/minute, results from abnormalities in impulse formation or failure of atrioventricular (AV) conduction. As with all arrhythmias, the physician managing bradycardia must simultaneously address resuscitation and other management issues while identifying the specific cause.

I. **Approach.** In the evaluation of bradycardia, focus on the clinical status of the patient and not on the absolute heart rate. The important tasks in managing bradycardia are to treat life-threatening symptoms, identify the specific bradyarrhythmia, and determine the underlying cause.
   A. **Symptomatic bradycardia.** Manifestations include hypotension, pulmonary edema, altered mentation, myocardial ischemia, or acute myocardial infarction (MI) (1).
   B. **Bradycardia can be classified as primary or secondary.** Primary bradycardia, which is seen 15% of the time, is caused by an intrinsic defect in the generation or conduction of an impulse. Secondary causes, which are seen 85% of the time, result from to factors extrinsic to the conduction system (2).
      1. Primary bradycardia is encountered more often in elderly patients and may be a manifestation of sick sinus syndrome.
      2. Secondary bradycardia can be caused by the following:
         a. Acute coronary ischemia
         b. Nonischemic cardiovascular disease (e.g., dilated cardiomyopathies and cardiac tamponade)
         c. Metabolic derangements (e.g., hypothyroidism, hypoadrenalism, hyperkalemia, hypercalcemia, hypermagnesemia)
         d. Pharmacologic effects (β-adrenergic blockers, calcium channel blockers, digoxin, α-adrenergic agonist, and cholinergic agents)
II. **History**
   A. **Symptoms.** Bradyarrhythmias may or may not cause symptoms. When symptoms do occur, they are caused by either an awareness of the irregular rhythm (palpitations) or a reduced cardiac output (lightheadedness, syncope, fatigue, shortness of breath, or chest pain) (3) (Chapter 7.9).
   B. **Exercise tolerance.** Ask patients about their level of physical fitness. In the well-conditioned patient, impulse generation in the sinus node is often slowed.
   C. **Underlying conditions.** It is important to determine any underlying medical conditions that can cause bradycardia [e.g., ischemic heart disease (IHD), cardiomyopathies, previous arrhythmias, rheumatic heart disease, or thyroid disease].

  D. **Medications.** Typical medications associated with bradycardia include digoxin, phenothiazines, quinidine, procainamide, beta-blockers, calcium channel blockers, clonidine, reserpine, methyldopa, flecainide, encainide, propafenone, and lithium.
  E. **Cardiac risk factors.** Elicit risk factors for coronary heart disease (family history, tobacco use, hypercholesterolemia, diabetes, or hypertension).
III. **Physical examination**
  A. **Vital signs.** Heart rate and blood pressure determine the immediacy of treatment.
  B. **Inspection, palpation, and auscultation.** Bradycardia is best revealed on physical examination by inspection of the jugular pulses, palpation of the arterial pulse, and auscultation of the heart. Inspection of the jugular pulses is vital in the evaluation of bradycardia, and they often reveal atrial activity. For example, cannon waves are seen intermittently in complete heart block as the atrium contracts against a closed tricuspid valve. Palpation of the arterial pulse establishes the conducted ventricular rate. Auscultation establishes ventricular rate and rhythm. The intensity of S_1 is an important heart sound in the evaluation of bradycardia. A soft S_1 suggests a first-degree AV block. A variation in S_1 intensity suggests second- or third-degree AV block. In third-degree AV block, the intensity of heart sounds is augmented when an atrial systole immediately precedes ventricular contraction.
  C. **Associated conditions.** The physical examination should include an assessment for evidence of cardiac decompensation (e.g., jugular venous distension, pulmonary crackles, lower extremity edema, gallops, murmurs), and thyroid disease.
IV. **Testing**
  A. **Electrocardiogram (ECG).** It is essential to obtain an ECG when evaluating a patient with bradycardia. Usually, a resting ECG is sufficient, but occasionally an ambulatory (Holter) monitor or exercise ECG is indicated. Atrial activity is best assessed in leads II, III, aVf, and V_1. The presence of P waves, their configuration, and their relationship to QRS complexes must be established. Normally, the PR interval is between 0.12 and 0.20 seconds and each QRS complex is preceded by a P wave (5).
  B. **Laboratory.** The following tests should be considered when appropriate:
    1. Electrolytes: potassium, calcium, and magnesium
    2. Drug levels: digoxin, quinidine, and procainamide
    3. Thyroid function tests
V. **Diagnostic assessment.** The key to the diagnosis of bradycardia is a focused history, physical examination, and an ECG. No specific symptoms will separate the various causes of bradycardia.
  A. **Sinus bradycardia**
    1. **Etiology.** Normal (well-conditioned athletes), sleep, carotid sinus massage, glaucoma, increased intracranial pressure, and an acute inferior wall myocardial infarction.
    2. **ECG.** Normal P-QRS-T sequence at a rate less than 60 beats/minute (5).
  B. **Sinus node exit block (sinoatrial node block, SA block).**
    1. **Etiology.** Medications (digitalis, quinidine, procainamide, salicylates), hyperkalemia, cardiomyopathy, IHD, and vagal stimulation or increased vagal tone.
    2. **ECG.** A missing P wave is the hallmark of SA block. The prolonged PP interval must be a multiple of the baseline PP interval; otherwise it is called a sinus pause.
      a. Incomplete SA block: occasional absence of P-QRS-T sequence.
      b. Complete SA block: P waves absent, QRS-T sequence present but at a slow rate, QRS interval varies depending on the origin of the escape pacemaker (5).

C. **Sick-sinus syndrome** is a generalized abnormality of cardiac impulse formation and intraatrial and AV conduction abnormalities that can be manifested by various combinations of brady- and tachyarrhythmias (4).
   1. **Etiology.** Idiopathic fibrosis or degeneration of sinoatrial and AV conduction system, IHD, amyloidosis, surgical injury, and hypertension. More prevalent in the geriatric population (4).
   2. **ECG.** The hallmark is sinus nodal depression, including sinus bradycardia, sinus arrest, and sinoatrial exit block. Also seen are AV node dysfunction, and atrial fibrillation or atrial tachyarrhythmias with slow ventricular response (5).
D. **First-degree AV block** is defined as a prolonged PR interval. The block may be caused by a prolongation of conduction in any of the structures between the SA node and His bundle.
   1. **Etiology.** Found in well-conditioned people (long distance runners, heavy laborers), elderly patients; other causes include increased vagal tone (pain, vomiting, vasovagal syncope), medications (digitalis, quinidine, procainamide, propranolol, verapamil), acute rheumatic fever, myocarditis, and congenital heart disease (4).
   2. **ECG.** PR interval greater than 0.20 seconds. Each P wave followed by a QRS complex (5).
E. **Second-degree AV Block, Mobitz I (Wenckebach)**, is characterized by intermittent failure of conduction from atria to ventricles with progressive lengthening of the PR interval, eventually leading to a nonconducted P wave.
   1. **Etiology.** Normal variant occurs in well-conditioned people; causes include medications (digitalis, beta-blockers, calcium blockers, clonidine, methyldopa, flecainide, encainide, propafenone, lithium), MI (especially inferior MI), acute rheumatic fever, and myocarditis (4).
   2. **ECG.** PR interval progressively increases and the RR interval shortens until a nonconducted P wave occurs. Typically, small groups of beats occur, such as pairs and trios (5).
F. **Second-degree AV Block, Mobitz II**, is characterized by intermittent failure of conduction from atria to ventricles where appropriately timed P waves fail to conduct and no pattern is seen of progressive PR lengthening.
   1. **Etiology.** Almost always secondary to organic heart disease (4).
   2. **ECG.** PR interval is fixed with intermittent, nonconducted P waves. Conducted P waves with the same PR interval. Often it is associated with a bundle branch block (5).
G. **Third degree block** is defined as no atrial impulses reaching the ventricle through the AV conduction system.
   1. **Etiology.** Causes include congenital heart block (maternal anti-Ro antibodies), cardiomyopathy, IHD, aortic valve disease, endocarditis, Lyme disease, infiltrative processes (amyloid, sarcoid), medications (digitalis, quinidine, procainamide), hyperkalemia, connective tissue disease, trauma, and acute rheumatic fever (4).
   2. **ECG.** No AV conduction occurs. The atrial rate is faster than the ventricular rate. PP and RR intervals are constant: numerous P waves are seen, which occur at all phases of the ventricular cycle (5).

References

1. Emergency Cardiac Care Committee and Subcommittee, American Heart Association. Guidelines for cardiopulmonary resuscitation and emergency cardiac care. *JAMA* 1992;268:2171–2302.
2. Brady Jr WJ, Harrigan RA. Evaluation and management of bradyarrhythmias in the emergency department. *Emerg Med Clin North Am* 1998;16:361–388.
3. Alexander RW, Schlant RC, Fuster V. *Bradydysrhythmias in the heart.* New York: McGraw-Hill 1998:927–941.

4. DiMarco JP. Cardiac arrhythmias and conduction disorders. In: Freed M, Grimes C, ed. *Essentials of cardiovascular medicine*. New York: Physician's Press 1994:137–138, 168, 181–185.
5. Marriott HJL. *Practical electrocardiography*, 8th ed. Baltimore: Williams & Wilkins, 1988:371, 353–376.

7.4 Cardiomegaly

John Coe and Ron Sand

Cardiomegaly is a common, nonspecific finding that can be detected by physical examination, electrocardiogram (ECG), chest radiograph, or echocardiogram. With rare exceptions, it is a sign of organic heart disease. The absence of cardiomegaly does not rule out significant cardiac pathology. Cardiomegaly, especially in the elderly and those with coronary artery disease, is associated with a poor prognosis (1).

I. **Approach.** Cardiomegaly can be caused by chamber dilation, wall hypertrophy, or both. The underlying causes can be grouped into three categories: volume overload, pressure overload, or cardiomyopathy. The false impression of cardiomegaly can be seen with pericardial effusion or thickening, mediastinal mass, thoracic deformities, or faulty radiographic technique.

II. **History**
   A. **Presenting symptoms.** As congestive heart failure (CHF) and cardiomegaly represent the final common path for many patients with these common conditions, the typical symptoms are exertional dyspnea, syncope, fatigue, and angina. Many patients are asymptomatic at the time of diagnosis and sudden death can be the presenting event (2) (Chapter 7.5).
   B. **Etiology.** The most common conditions that result in cardiomegaly include hypertension, coronary artery disease, rheumatic and degenerative valvular heart disease, anemia, alcoholism, endocrinopathies, and infectious and inflammatory conditions.
   C. **Family history.** Premature atherosclerosis and ischemic cardiomyopathy can be caused by familial dyslipidemia. A family history of early CHF may indicate familial dilated cardiomyopathy and premature sudden death may indicate familial hypertrophic obstructive cardiomyopathy.

III. **Physical examination.** The typical signs of CHF are usually noted on examination. A decreased arterial pulse with narrowed pulse pressure is common. Cyanosis is rare. Significant cardiac enlargement should be evident on physical examination. Examples of these finding include the following:
   A. **Lung sounds.** Rales or pleural effusion with dullness to percussion and decreased breath sounds may be indicative of left ventricular failure.
   B. **Heart sounds.** Gallops, soft heart sounds, and regurgitant heart murmurs are nonspecific findings of advanced CHF. Alterations in S_1 or S_2, specific murmurs, (e.g., a Valsalva-enhanced systolic murmur in hypertrophic obstructive cardiomyopathy), and muffled sounds with pericardial effusion, all indicate specific underlying pathology.
   C. **Cardiac pulsations or point of maximal impulse (PMI).** Visible pulsations seen lateral to the midclavicular line signify cardiac enlargement unless is found a thoracic deformity or congenital absence of the pericardium.
   D. **Apical beat or PMI.** The apical beat, or PMI, which is typically palpable in only 40% of cases, is highly dependent on body habitus. Use the flat of the hand to palpate the PMI. Time the pulsations using the carotid pulse or auscultated heart sounds. The left lateral decubitus position increases the palpability of both normal and pathologic apical beats.
   A PMI within or superior to the fifth intercostal space is normal. Left ventricular enlargement displaces the PMI laterally and downward. A PMI lateral to the midclavicular line or more than 10 cm lateral to the midsternal

Table 7.1 Common causes of cardiomegaly

Pathologic condition	Typical symptom pattern	Physical findings	Radiographic findings	Sonographic findings	Common underlying causes
CHF—volume overload	Exertional dyspnea, syncope, angina	Diffuse PMI	Prominent hilar vessels	Chamber dilation	VSD, valvular insufficiency, thyrotoxicosis, anemia
CHF—pressure overload	Same	Lateral, downward displaced PMI, sustained	Prominent hilar vessels, isolated chamber enlargement	Thickened chamber walls early, dilation later	Aortic/pulmonary stenosis, hypertrophic cardiomyopathy (chronic), HTN, coarctation of the aorta
CHF—cardiomyopathy/myocarditis	Same	Diffuse PMI, hypokinetic	Prominent hilar vessels, global dilation	Chamber dilation, global	Viral, ischemic idiopathic, alcoholic, peripartum
Pericardial effusion	Symptoms of pericarditis and/or underlying disease	Muffled heart sounds, blunted PMI, narrowed pulse pressure	Flask-shaped heart, obscured hilar vessels, widened epicardial stripe	Pericardial fluid accumulation	Pericarditis, penetrating trauma
Mediastinal mass	Vascular/airway obstruction	—	Widened mediastinum	Normal cardiac findings	Thymus, tumor, vascular

CHF, congestive heart failure; PMI, point of maximal impulse; HTN, hypertension; VSD, ventricular septal defect.

line is a sensitive but nonspecific indicator of left ventricular enlargement. An apical impulse of more than 3 cm diameter is an accurate sign of left ventricular enlargement.

With moderate or severe left ventricular hypertrophy, the outward systolic thrust persists throughout ejection, often lasting up to the second heart sound. In patients with volume overload or sympathetic stimulation, the left ventricular impulse is brisker and larger than normal but is hypokinetic in patients with reduced stroke volume (e.g., acute myocardial infarction or dilated cardiomyopathy). Large left ventricular aneurysms are palpable above and medial to the apex beat. Thoracic deformities—particularly scoliosis and pectus excavatum—can laterally displace a normal heart.

E. **Percussion.** In the absence of an apical beat, as in patients with pericardial effusion or with dilated cardiomyopathy and a markedly displaced, hypokinetic apical beat, the left border of the heart can be outlined by means of percussion. Percussed dullness in the left fifth intercostal space more than 10.5 cm from the midsternal line is sensitive and specific for cardiomegaly (3).

IV. Testing

A. **Radiographs.** The cardiothoracic ratio is quick to measure and relatively reliable as an indicator of cardiomegaly on an adequate, upright, posterior–anterior chest film. Watch for rotation and adequate inspiration: the diaphragm should be lowered to at least the posterior portion of the ninth rib. Calculate the ratio by first measuring the transverse cardiac diameter horizontally through the widest part of the cardiac silhouette. Divide this by the chest diameter measured at the widest part between the inner surface of the ribs. A ratio of 0.5 to 0.55 or less can be considered within the limits of normal for an adult. Ratios of up to 0.6 are normal in children and infants. Fluid accumulation in the pericardium causes distention, enlarging the cardiac silhouette and overlapping and obscuring the hilar vessels. In CHF, the vessels become congested and appear more prominent than normal. Also, the epicardial fat line (radiolucent stripe) on the lateral chest film between the anterior surface of the heart and the retrosternal mediastinal fat should be no more than 1 to 2 mm. Widening beyond this is a reliable indicator of pericardial effusion.

B. **Sonography.** An echocardiogram is generally considered the standard in assessing cardiac dimensions. With evidence of cardiomegaly on physical examination, an echocardiogram is appropriate if clinically useful in the patient's care.

C. **ECG.** The ECG is almost invariably abnormal in true cardiomegaly. Common findings are premature ventricular contractions, atrial fibrillation, atrioventricular and intraventricular conduction abnormalities, and nonspecific ST segment and T-wave changes. Left ventricular hypertrophy and atrial enlargement can be diagnosed by morphology and voltage, but the ECG is rarely diagnostic of a specific underlying cause. Pericarditis causes ST elevation with flat or concave ST segments. Pseudoinfarction patterns are seen in hypertrophic obstructive cardiomyopathy (4).

V. Diagnostic assessment. The significance of cardiomegaly is determined by the underlying pathology. The most common presenting conditions to consider are listed in Table 7.1.

References

1. Frishman WH. Cardiomegaly on chest x-ray: prognostic implications from a ten-year cohort study of elderly subjects: a report from the Bronx Longitudinal Aging Study. *Am Heart J* 1992;124:1026–1030.
2. Craddock LD. Cardiac enlargement and the cardiomyopathies. In: Friedman HH, ed. *Problem oriented medical diagnosis*, 5th ed. Boston: Little, Brown and Company, 1991:67–71.
3. Heckerling PS. Accuracy of precordial percussion in detecting cardiomegaly. *Am J Med* 1991;91:328–334.
4. Kamiyama N. Electrocardiographic features differentiating dilated cardiomyopathy from hypertrophic cardiomyopathy. *J Cardiol* 1997;30:301–306.

7.5 Congestive Heart Failure

Anthony F. Jerant

Congestive heart failure (CHF) is the most frequent reason for hospitalization among older adults in the United States. Nearly one-third of a national cohort of 170,239 Medicare enrollees hospitalized for the first time with CHF died within a year of discharge (1).

I. **Approach.** CHF is a syndrome, not a disease. Attempt to elucidate which type of CHF is present and search for causes and exacerbating factors to optimize therapy.
   A. **Types of CHF.** Two types of CHF are seen, each with many potential causes (Table 7.2).
   B. **Special concerns: CHF associated with hypoxia, hypotension, angina, myocardial infarction (MI), florid pulmonary edema, or severe complicating illness (e.g., pneumonia).** Emergent stabilization and hospitalization are indicated in such cases (2).

II. **History**
   A. **Common presenting symptoms.** Does the patient have orthopnea, paroxysmal nocturnal dyspnea, or dyspnea on exertion? How much exertion triggers dyspnea? These are *relatively specific symptoms* for CHF. *Less specific symptoms* include swelling of the legs, increasing weight, and generalized fatigue. Older patients with CHF may not have dyspnea on exertion because of a sedentary baseline status; they often present with *atypical symptoms* such as dry cough, daytime oliguria with nocturia, and confusion (3).
   B. **Past medical history.** Are conditions present that can cause CHF (Table 7.2)? If so, are they well-controlled with lifestyle changes, medications, or both? Uncontrolled hypertension, myocardial ischemia, and medication noncompliance frequently trigger CHF.
   C. **Psychosocial history.** Is there current or previous heavy alcohol use, tobacco use, or stimulant drug use? Is the patient consuming too much dietary sodium (> 2 g/d)? Are symptoms hindering the patient's ability to perform daily activities? Is the patient depressed? How is the family coping? Poor understanding of lifestyle factors, depression, and limited family resources can lead to noncompliance and frequent CHF exacerbations.

Table 7.2 Types and causes of congestive heart failure (CHF)

CHF WITH LEFT VENTRICULAR (LV) SYSTOLIC DYSFUNCTION
Causes include:
Ischemic heart disease, hypertension, alcohol toxicity, obesity, valvular disease (e.g., aortic stenosis), or chronic tachydysrhythmias.

CHF WITH PRESERVED LV SYSTOLIC FUNCTION
Subtypes and causes include:
Transient systolic dysfunction due to acute myocardial ischemia.

Left atrial hypertension due to high-output states (e.g., thyrotoxicosis), volume excess, or mitral stenosis.

LV diastolic dysfunction due to hypertension, ischemia, aging, obesity, or sustained tachydysrhythmias.

Miscellaneous disorders such as restrictive cardiomyopathy due to infiltrative diseases (e.g., amyloidosis), constrictive pericarditis and pericardial tamponade, and pure right-sided heart failure.

III. Physical examination

A. Focused physical examination. In general, the physical examination is more sensitive in detecting acute CHF than it is in detecting chronic CHF. Evaluate the following:

1. Vital signs. Note the blood pressure; hypertension with acute CHF suggests diastolic dysfunction (4). Obtain pulse, respiratory rate, and pulse oximetry to detect hypoxia.
2. Neck. Look for jugular venous distension, one of the more reliable physical examination indicators of CHF (4).
3. Lungs. Rales are commonly heard, but wheezing ("cardiac asthma") can also appear.
4. Heart. Palpate the apical impulse. If laterally displaced, diffuse, and especially of sustained duration, CHF caused by reduced left ventricular (LV) systolic function is likely (4). Listen for murmurs, gallops, and rubs. An S_3 gallop is generally suggestive of CHF (4), whereas an S_4 gallop may be a nonpathologic, age-related finding in elderly patients (3).
5. Abdomen. Assess for hepatosplenomegaly and try to elicit abdomino-jugular reflux.
6. Extremities. Look for leg edema (pitting in acute CHF, brawny in chronic CHF).

B. Additional physical examination. Further examination is appropriate if the history suggests specific causes for CHF: funduscopic examination to search for hypertensive retinopathy; thyroid palpation and auscultation; palpation of peripheral pulses; and carotid palpation and auscultation for evidence of stenosis, a marker of coronary atherosclerosis.

IV. Testing

A. Preliminary evaluation. Obtain the following when acute CHF is suspected to assess for confirmatory signs, triggers, and associated conditions: electrocardiogram (MI or ischemia, dysrhythmia; chest radiograph (cardiomegaly, pulmonary vascular redistribution, alveolar edema); serum electrolytes, albumin, blood urea nitrogen, creatinine (hypokalemia, hypoalbuminemia, acute renal failure); complete blood count (anemia); and urinalysis (nephrosis).

1. In the setting of suggestive symptoms, anterior Q waves and left bundle branch block on electrocardiography are each nearly 90% specific for LV systolic dysfunction (4).

B. Confirmatory evaluation. Echocardiography (ECHO) should be expeditiously obtained in all patients when new-onset CHF is suspected clinically. An LV ejection fraction (EF) $\leq 40\%$ indicates systolic dysfunction, whereas a normal EF accompanied by findings suggestive of increased LV end-diastolic pressure suggests diastolic dysfunction. ECHO is technically inadequate in up to 18% of patients (2). Radionuclide ventriculography can be used in such cases, but it is less able to detect valvular disease and LV hypertrophy.

C. Additional testing. Because of frequent comorbid lung disease, pulmonary function testing should be considered in older patients before dyspnea is attributed to CHF. The need for other tests (e.g., thyroid-stimulating hormone) is determined by findings on the history and physical examination.

V. Diagnostic assessment. The two keys to the diagnosis of CHF are:

A. A high index of suspicion in patients with potential causes and suggestive symptoms. However, findings on history and physical examination are neither sensitive nor specific. Half of all CHF diagnoses made in the primary care setting using clinical indicators alone are inaccurate (5).

B. ECHO. This critical diagnostic study may also indicate which type of CHF is present which, in turn, facilitates the selection of an appropriate therapeutic regimen. Nevertheless, ECHO has some limitations. Current techniques cannot provide definitive proof of diastolic dysfunction, so a thorough search for other causes of CHF with preserved systolic function should be conducted before accepting this diagnosis. Furthermore, LV systolic dysfunction can be a transient phenomenon in patients with acute myocardial ischemia. Therefore, a repeat ECHO should be obtained after stabilization of such patients.

References
1. Croft JB, Giles WH, Pollard RA, Keenan NL, Casper ML, Anda RF. Heart failure survival among older adults in the United States. *Arch Intern Med* 1999;159:505–510.
2. Agency for Health Care Policy and Research. Clinical practice guideline. *Heart failure: evaluation and care of patients with left-ventricular systolic dysfunction*. Silver Spring, MD: Agency for Health Care and Research, 1994.
3. Tresch DD. The clinical diagnosis of heart failure in older patients. *J Am Geriatr Soc* 1997;45:1128–1133.
4. Badgett RG, Lucey CR, Mulrow CD. Can the clinical examination diagnose left-sided heart failure in adults? *JAMA* 1997;227:1712–1719.
5. Vasan RS, Benjamin EJ, Levy D. Congestive heart failure with normal left ventricular systolic function. *Arch Intern Med* 1996;156:146–157.

7.6 Heart Murmur, Diastolic

David E. Anisman and Gerald F. Farnell

A diastolic murmur is a finding that provides a clue to an underlying disease process. Unlike their systolic counterparts (Chapter 7.7), diastolic murmurs almost always indicate underlying heart disease.

I. **Approach.** Given the broad range of factors that may cause diastolic murmurs, a two-part scheme is used to narrow the differential diagnosis. First, the timing of the murmur (early, mid-, or end-diastolic) helps in localizing the anatomic abnormality to a specific valve or other heart structure. Second, historical features such as congestive heart failure, rheumatic disease, congenital abnormalities, or connective tissue and collagen vascular disease further characterize the underlying cause.

II. **History**
   A. **Symptoms.** Many patients with diastolic murmurs will not present with specific complaints; rather, the murmurs will be found in the course of a routine medical examination. With symptomatic lesions, the patient may experience dyspnea, chest pain, or palpitations. Pulmonary regurgitation (PR) is usually asymptomatic except in its most severe forms. More specific symptoms include chest or neck pounding in aortic regurgitation (AR); hemoptysis, embolism, or hoarseness (left recurrent laryngeal nerve compression from the left atrium) in mitral stenosis (MS); failure to thrive or frequent respiratory infections with congenital MS; edema in tricuspid stenosis (TS); and fever, anemia, weight loss, embolism, digital clubbing, arthralgias, syncope, rash, and Raynaud's phenomenon with an atrial myxoma (1).
   B. **Past medical history.** Does the patient have a history of rheumatic fever (RF)? RF is the most common cause of all diastolic murmurs (mitral → aortic → tricuspid → pulmonic) (2). Of patients with mitral stenosis, 50% will have a history of rheumatic fever (3).
      1. **Endocarditis.** Vegetations can lead to either AR/PR or MS/TS.
      2. **Pulmonary hypertension with PR** is classically associated with the Graham Steell murmur, heard in the left third interspace near the sternum and propagated down the sternum.
      3. **Connective tissue and collagen vascular diseases** predispose to aortic root dilatation and AR.
      4. **Congenital heart malformations** can be associated with multiple valvular lesions, left ventricular (LV) outflow tract abnormalities, or shunts (with resultant volume overload).
      5. **Atrial myxoma** is a rare cause of *variable* AV valve obstruction.
      6. **Syphilis** can cause aortitis and AR.

Table 7.3 Physical examination findings of diastolic murmurs

Timing	Murmur	Pitch	Location	Shape or quality	Maneuvers and other features
Early diastolic murmurs	Aortic regurgitation (AR)	High	Left lower sternal border (LLSB)	Decrescendo	Have patient lean slightly forward, hold breath in deep expiration, press diaphragm firmly against chest; increases with hand grip and squatting; listen for Austin-Flint murmur.
	Pulmonary regurgitation (PR) *with* pulmonary hypertension	High	LLSB	Decrescendo	Distinguish from AR by prominent jugular A-wave; right ventricular (RV) heave; RV S_4 that increases with inspiration
	PR *without* pulmonary hypertension	High	LLSB	Crescendo-decrescendo (short duration)	RV heave (sometimes); palpable thrill over pulmonic area may signify dilation of pulmonary artery; *follows silent gap after S_2* (unlike other PR murmur)
Middiastolic murmurs	Mitral stenosis	Low	Point of maximal impulse (PMI)	Rumbling; may have presystolic accentuation	Have patient on left side, hold bell lightly on chest; may be preceded by opening snap; increased with handgrip; decreased with inspiration.
	Tricuspid stenosis	Low	LLSB (near xyphoid)	Rumbling	Inspiratory augmentation.
	Nonstenotic rumbles	Low	PMI or LLSB	Rumbling	No presystolic component; preceded by low-pitched S_3 instead of high-pitched opening snap.
	Austin-Flint (mitral origin, associated with AR)	Low	PMI	Rumbling	Begins after S_3; increased with handgrip and squatting. In severe AR, this murmur may be absent.

III. Physical examination (PE)
  A. Table 7.3 lists characteristic PE findings of diastolic murmurs.
  B. **Fine points of the physical examination**
    1. Is the murmur of AR louder at the right sternal border? If so, consider aortic root dilation. Remember, whereas the duration of the *chronic* AR murmur is directly proportional to the severity of the regurgitation, the duration of the *acute* AR murmur may not predict its severity (3).
    2. Is the murmur of MS shorter, or does it extend closer to S_2? The length of this murmur, not its intensity, is directly proportional to the severity of the stenosis (3). In addition, the murmur may not be audible with increased heart rates because of shortening of diastole.
    3. Does the murmur of MS vary from examination to examination? If so, and especially if it is introduced by a "plop" sound, consider atrial myxoma.
IV. Testing. Echocardiogram is the essential test for confirming the anatomic location of the murmur and its severity. Transthoracic echocardiography (ECHO) is generally sufficient, unless endocarditis is suspected, in which case a transesophageal ECHO is preferred to evaluate for vegetations. If aortic root dilatation is present on ECHO, a computed tomography or magnetic resonance imaging scan may help to delineate the anatomy further. Additional laboratory testing may be warranted to further evaluate the underlying cause (e.g., serologic studies for collagen vascular disease, serologic test for syphilis, and so on).
V. Diagnostic assessment. With a careful examination and thorough history, the valve causing the murmur and the probable cause of the valvular lesion can be identified prior to ordering the definitive test (ECHO). The most common cause of all diastolic murmurs is still rheumatic heart disease, even though the incidence of acute rheumatic fever has decreased. Mitral stenosis is almost invariably caused by rheumatic heart disease (98% in one study of excised valves) (3,4), with the remainder caused by vegetations (from endocarditis) or congenital factors (4). Tricuspid stenosis is also predominantly rheumatic in origin and is rarely an isolated lesion. Other causes of TS include carcinoid and congenital malformations. Rheumatic heart disease is the leading cause of chronic AR, followed by congenital bicuspid valves and aortic root dilatation (Marfan's syndrome, Ehlers-Danlos syndrome, ankylosing spondylitis, and syphilitic aortitis). If chronic, AR can result in LV dilation and compensation; if acute, it can be associated with severe LV overload and significant symptoms. Acute AR is most often related to endocarditis, aortic dissection, and trauma. Pulmonary regurgitation without hypertension has multiple causes, including pulmonary trunk dilation, endocarditis, carcinoid, trauma (from balloon-tipped catheters), and rheumatic fever. The nonstenotic physiologic murmurs are related to high-flow states across an otherwise normal mitral or tricuspid valve. For a mitral flow murmur, the primary lesions are usually mitral regurgitation, ventricular septal defects, or patent ductus arteriosus. For a tricuspid flow murmur, an atrial septal defect or severe tricuspid regurgitation is the most common cause. The Austin–Flint murmur, caused by increasing left ventricular pressure pushing the anterior mitral leaflet into the flow of blood coming from the atrium, is the result of significant aortic regurgitation.

References

1. Chizner MA, ed. *Classical teachings in clinical cardiology.* Chatham, New Jersey: Laennec Publishing, 1996.
2. Coblyn JS, Weinblatt ME. Rheumatic disease and the heart. In: Braunwald E, ed. *Heart disease: a textbook of cardiovascular medicine*, 5th ed. Philadelphia: WB Saunders, 1997:1776–1785.
3. Abrams J, ed. *Synopsis of cardiac physical diagnosis.* Philadelphia: Lea & Febiger, 1989.
4. Olson LJ, Subramanian MB, Ackermann DM, Orszulak TA, Edwards WM. Surgical pathology of the mitral valve: a study of 712 cases spanning 21 years. *Mayo Clin Proc* 1987;62:22–34.

7.7 Heart Murmur, Systolic

Dale Bishop

Systolic murmurs can herald significant clinical deterioration and sudden death, or they can represent stable or clinically insignificant conditions. Although technologic advances in cardiac diagnostic testing continue, auscultation remains the mainstay of diagnosis and is the key to the cost-effective use of technology.

I. **Approach.** Systolic murmurs can develop in all age groups. Close attention should be given to the history [looking for associated symptoms (e.g., dyspnea)] and to the physical examination (looking for specific murmur characteristics described below).

II. **History**

A. **General issues in the history.** The history can provide important clues as to whether the murmur is clinically significant. Any history of rheumatic fever, previously known valvular disease, congenital heart disease, or intravenous drug abuse would be important to ascertain.

Murmurs of early adulthood suggest congenital or rheumatic disease, whereas murmurs with onset later in life are consistent with degenerative valvular changes.

B. **Patient symptoms.** Patients should be asked about shortness of breath, dyspnea on exertion, orthopnea, and paroxysmal nocturnal dyspnea. Patients with these symptoms warrant an expedited evaluation because these symptoms suggest cardiac decompensation. Advanced aortic stenosis specifically is associated with chest pain, syncope, and heart failure, although a gradient across the valve can exist for years prior to symptom onset. Chest discomfort is often present in advanced disease, but sudden death occurs in 15% of patients with no previous symptoms (1).

C. **Association of a murmur with a specific disease.** Recent myocardial infarction endocarditis could cause papillary muscle dysfunction resulting in mitral or tricuspid regurgitation. Mitral regurgitation can be seen in connective tissue disease, coronary artery disease, and congenital disease, but is commonly associated with conditions leading to left ventricular dilatation such as congestive heart failure (CHF) (Chapter 7.5). Endocarditis, myocardial infarction, trauma, prolapse, or congenital heart disease usually precede tricuspid regurgitation. Mitral valve prolapse, which is clinically characterized by palpitations, fatigue, and chest pain, is often associated with anxiety. Hypertrophic cardiomyopathy can be seen in patients with a family history and usually presents between the ages of 20 and 40 years. Presenting symptoms include dyspnea on exertion, chest pain, palpitations, or syncope. It is an important cause of sudden death in athletes. A history of anemia, thyroid disease, or fever should also be elicited from patients being evaluated for a systolic murmur as each of these conditions can cause a murmur from increased flow.

III. **Physical examination**

A. **Technique.** Auscultate the heart with the bell to best detect lower frequencies and the heart sounds (S_1-S_4). The quality of the murmur is best heard with the diaphragm. Inspiration increases the audibility of right ventricular sounds.

B. **Murmur characteristics.** Table 7.4 presents a summary of the characteristics of different causes of systolic murmurs (2,3). Etchell et al. (3) have prepared a comprehensive review on the usefulness of specific physical examination findings in the diagnosis of systolic murmurs.

IV. **Testing.** Testing of an undiagnosed cardiac murmur can include an electrocardiogram (ECG), a chest x-ray study (CXR), and an echocardiogram.

Table 7.4 Characteristics of systolic murmurs

Systolic murmurs	Murmur type	Maneuvers
Tricuspid regurgitation	Early systolic (low pressure) Holosystolic (high pressure)	Inspiration intensifies murmur
Aortic stenosis	Midsystolic crescendo, decrescendo with delayed and decreased peripheral pulses	Palpable thrill in aortic area on full expiration
Mitral valve prolapse	Late systolic	Squatting and prompt standing may augment murmur
Tricuspid insufficiency	Holosystolic on left sternal border	Large jugular waves; increased murmur with inspiration
Mitral regurgitation	Apical holosystolic radiating to axilla and left sternal border	If left ventricle dilatation present, grade II–IV murmur with S_3 mid to late or holosystolic with palpable thrill
Pulmonic stenosis	Midsystolic	Murmur increases with inspiration
Ventricular septal defect	Harsh, holosystolic murmur	Differentiated from mitral regurgitation by radiating to right of sternum rather than apex
Hypertrophic cardiomyopathy	Midsystolic; if murmur present, associated with S_4 and heard best at left lower sternal border	

Echocardiograms, although useful for quantification of stenotic valvular disease, can overestimate the degree of regurgitation.

A. Aortic stenosis. Specific ECG findings in aortic stenosis can include left ventricular hypertrophy (LVH), left axis deviation, conduction disturbances, and atrial hypertrophy. On CXR, cardiac size remains normal until stenosis is severe, then signs of CHF may be present. The echocardiogram may reveal thickened or calcified aortic leaflets, bicuspid valve, and LVH. The size of the valve can be estimated and the pressure gradient across the valve can be assessed. Cardiac catheterization can also be used to assess the size of the valve and the gradient. Even though echocardiography is accurate in measuring valve area and gradient, catheterization is usually indicated because 50% of patients above age 40 years have coronary artery disease.

B. Mitral regurgitation. In mitral regurgitation, the ECG may reveal LVH with left atrial enlargement and later in the course, atrial fibrillation. In severe disease, CXR usually reveals cardiomegaly without pulmonary venous congestion. The echocardiogram reveals valvular anatomy, but can overestimate the severity of the regurgitation. Exercise testing can be used to deter-

Table 7.5 Auscultation resources available on-line

The Auscultation Assistant: www.med.ucla.edu/wilkes/intro.html
Cardiac Auscultation: www.xs4all.n1/~medicine
Virtual Stethoscope: www.music.mcgill.ca/~tkatsia/auscultation.html

mine clinical deterioration in mitral regurgitation. Catheterization is used to assess the contractile state of the ventricle as well as the regurgitant and forward stroke volume.

C. **Other disease processes.** The ECG with tricuspid insufficiency often reveals atrial fibrillation. The CXR may show right atrial hypertrophy, and the echocardiogram shows valvular anatomy. Pulmonic stenosis will lead to ECG findings consistent with right ventricular hypertrophy. Hypertrophic cardiomyopathy is best diagnosed by echocardiography. ECG may reveal LVH and occasionally a shortened PR interval is seen. Cardiac catheterization can be used to quantify the gradient caused by the hypertrophic lesion.

V. **Diagnostic assessment.** The history and physical examination with special emphasis on auscultation are the keys to the diagnosis of systolic murmurs. Those with symptomatic murmurs or in whom valvular disease is suspected should have an ECG, CXR, and echocardiogram. Murmurs of unknown duration or new murmurs should be worked up promptly with consideration of acute infarction in mind. If aortic stenosis is suspected, the workup should be expedited because sudden death can be the first clinical presentation. Valvular disease must always be considered with new onset congestive heart failure. Table 7.5 lists some of the online resources available to assist in the evaluation of heart murmurs.

References
1. Rackley C. Valvular heart disease. In: Bennett JC, Plum F, eds. *Cecil textbook of medicine*, 20th ed. Philadelphia: WB Saunders, 1996.
2. O'Connor D. The art of auscultation. *Patient Care* 1998;38:56–60.
3. Etchells E, Bell C, Robb K. Does this patient have an abnormal systolic murmur? *JAMA* 1997;277:564–571.

7.8 Hypertension

Duane D. Bland and Jay S. Roitman

One of four American adults has hypertension (HTN) (1). Despite its well-recognized role in cardiovascular disease, close to one-third of those with HTN are still unaware of it. Further, of those diagnosed with HTN, less than one-third have their condition under adequate control. HTN is most often found when the patient presents for an unrelated problem or for healthcare screening. The unfortunate exception may be when the patient presents with end-organ damage or with an acute hypertensive emergency.

I. **Approach.** In the evaluation of HTN, the most important tasks are to determine the severity, assess for other cardiovascular risk factors, and look for evidence of secondary causes.

A. **Essential HTN.** Most patients will have essential HTN. Further, most patients who present with HTN have mildly elevated values. Therefore, usually ample opportunity exists to assess for variation in readings and to stage the patient's HTN, to assess for other cardiovascular risk factors and for comorbid disease, and to distinguish primary from secondary HTN.

B. **Special concerns.** A small percentage of patients will present with a hypertensive emergency. In general, these patients have severe HTN with symptoms and signs indicating end-organ involvement (e.g., encephalopathy, congestive heart failure, angina). These patients require immediate management of their blood pressure and associated medical problems.

II. History

A. **Assessment for comorbid conditions.** The patient's past medical history should include an assessment for previous blood pressure readings. Any history of secondary disease or comorbid conditions should be documented: age more than 60 years, obesity, ischemic heart disease (IHD), cerebrovascular disease, peripheral vascular disease, retinopathy, nephropathy, dyslipidemia, diabetes mellitus, and menopausal status in women. A family history of these problems should also be documented, with particular emphasis on premature IHD in women aged less than 65 years, and in men aged less than age 55 years.

B. **Medication history.** The medication history should document the use of prescription, over-the-counter, and herbal preparations that may have hypertensive side effects.

C. **Social history or habits.** In addition, determine the use of tobacco, alcohol, or street drugs. The social history should also address leisure time physical activity and relevant psychosocial factors, which could affect ongoing HTN management.

D. **Dietary history.** Explore the ingestion of salt and saturated fats. Note recent weight changes, which can have significant effects on blood pressure.

III. Physical examination

A. **Blood pressure measurement**. Use a standardized technique (2,3) when measuring blood pressure to avoid spuriously high or low values. Patients should be seated in a chair, upright with back support, feet flat on the floor, arms bared, and supported at heart level. The patient should be resting at least 5 minutes before blood pressure measurements are taken. Stimulants such as nicotine and caffeine should be avoided at least 30 minutes prior to measurement. Appropriate cuff size is very important; the bladder within the cuff should circle at least 80% of the arm. Initial blood pressure measurements should include both arms; the arm with the higher reading should be used thereafter. It is recommended that two or more readings, separated by 2 minutes, be averaged. If the first two readings differ by more than 5 mm Hg, then additional readings should be obtained and averaged.

B. **Additional physical examination.** Height and weight should be measured. In a focused physical examination, pay particular attention to the fundi (for hemorrhages or vascular changes), the carotid arteries (for bruits), the heart (for murmurs), the abdomen (for bruits), and the extremities (for pulses, bruits, edema).

IV. Testing

A. **Routine clinical laboratory tests.** These include a urinalysis, hemoglobin, serum electrolytes, blood urea nitrogen, creatinine, blood glucose, total cholesterol, and high density lipoprotein (HDL) cholesterol. Obtain a 12-lead electrocardiogram.

B. **Optional laboratory tests and studies.** Additional testing may be warranted given the findings on history, physical examination, or the initial laboratory screening. Specifically, for patients with diabetes, urine microalbumin and serum glycohemoglobin. For patients with an elevated screening cholesterol, low-density lipoprotein (LDL) cholesterol and triglycerides. For patients with proteinuria on initial screening, 24-hour urinary protein and creatinine clearance (Chapter 16.6).

C. **Blood pressure measurement outside the office.** Self-measurement and ambulatory blood pressure monitoring are generally unnecessary but may be useful in certain circumstances. Self-measurement can help identify patients with "white coat hypertension." Potentially, it may help assess response to antihypertensive medications and improve patient compliance. Ambulatory blood pressure monitoring is significantly more expensive and should not be used routinely; however, it can also be useful in evaluating suspected "white coat hypertension."

IV. Diagnostic assessment

    A. Table 7.6 provides a summary of the sixth report of the Joint National Committee on Detection, Evaluation, and Treatment of High Blood Pressure (JNC-VI).

    B. Important considerations in the assessment of high blood pressure:

        1. The patient should not be acutely ill or already on antihypertensive agents.

        2. Classification should be based on the average of two or more readings taken at each of two or more visits after an initial screening.

        3. When the systolic and diastolic blood pressures fall into different classifications, the higher classification should be used.

        4. For patients with renal insufficiency and greater than 1 g/d of proteinuria, a blood pressure of 125/75 is recommended.

        5. For blood pressures greater than 160–170 over 105–110, the diagnosis of HTN is probable even without additional measurements.

        6. Follow-up may need to be modified based on the patient's cardiovascular risk factors, history of prior blood pressure measurements, or evidence of target organ disease.

    C. Secondary HTN. Secondary causes of HTN should be considered in patients responding poorly to medications, (particularly those with previously well-controlled HTN); in patients with stage 3 HTN; and those with sudden onset HTN. Many potential causes are found for secondary HTN. Some of the relatively more common causes and possible findings found during screening include:

        1. Aortic coarctation

            a. Short, rough systolic murmur in the second left interspace (Chapter 7.7)

            b. Bruits heard over the back

            c. Marked decrease in femoral pulses or blood pressures in the legs

        2. Cushing's disease

            a. Central obesity with wasted extremities

            b. Atrophic skin with abdominal striae and poor wound healing

            c. Hyperglycemia (Chapter 14.1)

        3. Exogenous substances. History of prescription drug, illicit drug, or alcohol use.

        4. Primary hyperaldosteronism

            a. Muscle weakness and cramps

            b. Serum potassium less than 3.5 mEq/L off diuretics or less than 3.0 mEq/L on diuretics

Table 7.6 Classification of blood pressure for adults aged 18 years and older (2)

Category	Systolic (mm Hg)	Diastolic (mm Hg)	Follow-up
Optimal	<120	<80	Recheck in 2 years
Normal	<130	<85	Recheck in 2 years
High normal	130–139	85–89	Recheck in 1 year
Hypertension			
Stage 1	140–159	90–99	Confirm within 2 months
Stage 2	160–179	100–109	Evaluate within 1 month
Stage 3	≥180	≥110	Evaluate immediately or within 1 week, depending on clinical situation

From Joint National Committee on Prevention, Detection, Evaluation, and Treatment of High Blood Pressure. The sixth report of Joint National Committee on Prevention, Evaluation, and Treatment of High Blood Pressure. *Arch Intern Med* 1997;157:2413–2446, with permission.

     5. Renal disease
       a. Proteinuria
       b. Elevated creatinine
     6. Renal vascular hypertension
       a. New onset HTN over the age of 55 years (particularly with history of smoking) or HTN in a child aged less than 12 years
       b. Sudden increase in previously well-controlled blood pressure
       c. Failure of triple drug therapy
       d. Periumbilical bruit with radiation to the flanks
     7. Pheochromocytoma
       a. Anxiety, headaches, palpitations tremor, and excessive sweating
       b. Weight loss (Chapter 2.13)
       c. Orthostatic hypotension
       d. Rapid pulse (Chapter 7.12)

References
1. American Heart Association [Web Page]. http://www.amhrt.org
2. Joint National Committee on Prevention, Detection, Evaluation, and Treatment of High Blood Pressure. The sixth report of Joint National Committee on Prevention, Evaluation, and Treatment of High Blood Pressure. *Arch Intern Med* 1997;157: 2413–2446.
3. Izzo JL, Black HR. *Hypertension primer: the essentials of high blood pressure*, 2nd ed. Chicago: American Heart Association, 1997.

7.9 Palpitations

David M. Schneider

Palpitations (PPTs), defined as an uncomfortable or abnormal awareness of the heart beat, are common in primary care patients. In one study, recurrent symptoms occurred in 75% of patients and 33% reported lower quality of life, but the 1-year mortality rate was 1.6% (1).

   I. Approach. The initial task is to detect a life-threatening cause of the PPTs. Studies have shown a 7% to 40% incidence of potentially serious arrhythmias in these patients, although the cause in up to 31% is psychiatric (1–3). Because the heart is electrically paced, the mnemonic E-PACED [**E**lectrolytes, **P**sychiatric, **A**nemia, **C**ardiac, **E**ndocrine (hyperthyroidism, hypoglycemia, menopause, pheochromocytoma), **D**rugs] may bring to mind the major causes of PPTs. Not all patients with arrhythmias experience PPTs, and individual patients vary greatly in sensitivity to PPTs.

  II. History. The history alone may suggest the underlying diagnosis.
     A. Characteristics of the PPTs. Are the PPTs regular or irregular? Fast or slow? What descriptors does the patient use? Are the PPTs only in the chest? Ask patients to tap out the rhythm of their PPTs, and to check their pulse during an episode (3).
       1. Rapid, irregular PPTs imply atrial fibrillation, multifocal atrial tachycardia, or atrial flutter with variable conduction.
       2. Rapid, regular PPTs occur with supraventricular tachycardias (SVTs), including sinus tachycardia and ventricular tachycardia (VT).
       3. A "stop-start," "flip-flop," or "turning over" sensation in the chest (postectopic pause and subsequent accentuated beat) is usually caused by premature ventricular contractions (PVCs) or premature atrial contractions (PACs).

4. PPTs felt in the neck represent atria contracting against closed atrioventricular (AV) valves, with blood refluxing into the superior vena cava. The most common cause is AV nodal reentrant tachycardia (AVNRT), which generally causes rapid, regular, sustained pounding; it can also occur with PVCs (slower, less regular, less sustained) (3).

B. Situations in which PPTs occur. PPTs can be associated with anxiety or somatization disorders. Although overlap is seen among patients with PPTs and those with psychiatric disorders, true arrhythmias do occur in such patients. Arrhythmias (SVT, VT, torsades de pointes) can occur with catecholamine release (exercise, emotional stress); PPTs occurring at rest may indicate benign conditions. PPTs associated with position may result from SVT or PVCs.

C. Onset and termination. Although abrupt onset and termination of PPTs suggests PSVT, this finding is neither sensitive nor specific. Anxiety can lead to sinus tachycardia following an arrhythmia, precluding the patient from sensing an abrupt cessation.

D. Associated symptoms. When syncope, presyncope, or dizziness occurs with PPTs, sustained or nonsustained VT must be ruled out (Chapters 2.2 and 2.12).

E. Other information. Patients with structural heart disease are more likely to have arrhythmias. Age of onset in childhood or adolescence suggests SVT, especially preexcitation syndromes or long QT syndrome. Various substances can be associated with SVT (nicotine, caffeine, adrenergic or anticholinergic drugs, cocaine, amphetamines) or atrial fibrillation (alcohol). Findings consistent with hyperthyroidism or less common disorders causing PPTs (diabetes, Lyme disease, sarcoidosis, amyloidosis) should be pursued. Ask if the patient has found relief with beta-blockers (PVCs) or vagal maneuvers (SVT). Family history (arrhythmias, sudden death, other cardiovascular disease, syncope) can be helpful.

III. **Physical examination (PE).** If the patient is not seen during an episode, aim the PE at detecting abnormalities that are associated with PPTs. Midsystolic click and murmur (mitral valve prolapse), harsh holosystolic murmur (hypertrophic cardiomyopathy), diastolic murmur (aortic regurgitation), or signs of congestive heart failure may aid in diagnosis. Look for stigmata of hyperthyroidism and other conditions noted above **(II.E)** (Chapter 14.8).

IV. **Testing**

A. 12-lead electrocardiogram (ECG). All patients with PPTs should have an ECG. The presence of an arrhythmia may be diagnostic. Findings between episodes can include short PR interval and delta waves (preexcitation), Q waves (VT, PVCs), long QT interval (drugs, long QT syndrome), left ventricular hypertrophy with left atrial abnormality (AF), and complete heart block (PVCs, torsades de pointes) (3).

B. Laboratory testing. Initial laboratory testing consists of serum potassium, hemoglobin and hematocrit, and thyroid-stimulating hormone; serum glucose can be added with a suspicion of hypoglycemia.

C. Ambulatory ECG recording (AECG). For patients in whom a diagnosis has not been made with the initial evaluation, AECG monitoring is indicated. A Holter monitor (24- or 48-hour continuous ECG) should be the initial study for patients with daily symptoms. In those with less frequent episodes, a continuous-loop event recorder worn for a duration of 2 weeks is more cost-effective (4,5).

V. **Diagnostic assessment.** The history, PE, and ECG are important steps in the evaluation of PPTs, although many patients will require ambulatory ECG testing to reach a diagnosis. If symptoms correlate with arrhythmias on AECG monitoring, a diagnosis can be made and treatment begun, if appropriate. If no arrhythmia occurs and the patient has typical PPTs, a benign cause is likely. When no symptoms and no arrhythmias are found, the AECG is nondiagnostic and repeat testing or referral may be necessary, especially with underlying heart disease or poorly tolerated PPTs.

References
1. Weber BE, Kapoor WN. Evaluation and outcomes of patients with palpitations. *Am J Med* 1996;100:138–148.
2. Barsky AJ, Cleary PD, Coeytaux RR, Ruskin JN. The clinical course of palpitations in medical outpatients. *Arch Intern Med* 1995;155:1782–1788.
3. Zimetbaum P, Josephson ME. Evaluation of patients with palpitations. *N Engl J Med* 1998;338:1369–1373.
4. Kinlay S, Leitch JW, Neil A, Chapman BL, Hardy DB, Fletcher PJ. Cardiac event recorders yield more diagnoses and are more cost-effective than 48-hour Holter monitoring in patients with palpitations. *Ann Intern Med* 1996;124:16–20.
5. Zimetbaum PJ, Kim KY, Josephson ME, Goldberger AL, Cohen DJ. Diagnostic yield and optimal duration of continuous-loop event monitoring for the diagnosis of palpitations. *Ann Intern Med* 1998;128:890–895.

7.10 Pericardial Friction Rub

Mark A. Marinella

The pericardial friction rub is the characteristic physical finding of acute pericarditis (AP), the most common disease process involving the pericardium (1).

  I. **Approach.** When evaluating the patient with a friction rub, it is important to recognize potentially serious causes of AP (Table 7.7).
 II. **History.** This is a very important element in the evaluation of a friction rub.
    A. **Pain characteristics.** Where is the pain? What is the nature of the pain? Does the pain radiate? Does body position affect the pain? Are systemic symptoms present?
       1. The pain of AP is typically precordial and sharp; it can worsen with recumbency, movement, inspiration, coughing, or swallowing.
       2. Pain can radiate to the trapezius ridge, a symptom characteristic of AP (1,2).
       3. Fever, myalgias, and malaise may be present, especially with viral AP (Chapter 2.6).
    B. **Other symptoms.** AP can complicate several serious diseases. Examples of "red flags" in the history include substernal chest pressure (myocardial infarction), "tearing" pain (aortic dissection), weight loss (malignancy), productive cough (pneumonia with purulent pericarditis), or hemoptysis (tuberculosis).

Table 7.7 Selected causes of acute pericarditis (AP)

LIFE-THREATENING
Myocardial infarction, malignancy, uremia/dialysis, aortic dissection, chest trauma, purulent AP.

OTHER CAUSES
Viral, autoimmune disorders, drugs, myxedema, radiation, Dressler's syndrome, cardiac surgery, idiopathic.

SPECIAL CONCERNS
Is a pericardial effusion or tamponade present?
On occasion, AP may present with pericardial tamponade or a very large effusion (2). As such, the clinician must consider this when examining the patient and ordering diagnostic tests (section **IV**).

Patients with viral or idiopathic AP typically do not have the aforementioned symptoms.

C. **Past medical history.** Is there a history of recent pericardiotomy? Is there a history of renal failure or hemodialysis? Has there been a previous diagnosis of collagen vascular disease? Noting any prior illnesses associated with AP may assist in the diagnosis of a rub.

D. **Drug history.** Drugs associated with AP include hydralazine, procainamide, minoxidil, cromolyn, and isoniazid (2).

III. **Physical examination**

A. **Vital signs.** Fever may be present with viral AP. Hypotension or pulsus paradoxus can occur with a large pericardial effusion or pericardial tamponade. Tachycardia may be caused by fever or tamponade (Chapter 7.12).

B. **Cardiac auscultation.** A quiet room is essential. The pathognomonic physical finding of AP is the pericardial friction rub that has been likened to creaking leather or a scratching sound (1–3). The rub may be evanescent and vary in intensity; hence, multiple attempts should be made to elicit this finding. The rub is best heard with the stethoscope diaphragm firmly applied to the chest wall at the left-lower sternal border at end-inspiration (2). Having the patient lean forward may be helpful. The classic friction rub occurs in three phases: atrial systole, ventricular systole, and ventricular diastole. However, eliciting all three phases is uncommon. The presence of a rub does not exclude a large pericardial effusion or cardiac tamponade (2,3).

IV. **Testing**

A. **Laboratory tests.** AP is mainly a clinical diagnosis but many patients have an elevated erythrocyte sedimentation rate or leukocytosis. Patients with connective tissue disease may have a positive antinuclear antibody test. Creatine phosphokinase or troponin levels can be slightly elevated if the underlying myocardium is inflamed (3).

B. **Electrocardiogram.** The electrocardiogram (ECG) is the most useful clinical tool in the diagnosis of AP, as repolarization changes occur in up to 90% of patients (1,3). The most sensitive indicator of AP is diffuse, concave-upward ST-segment elevation. A less sensitive, but very specific, indicator of AP is PR-segment depression (2,4). In addition, the P wave and QRS complex are normal and reciprocal changes and Q waves are absent.

1. Later findings of AP include T-wave flattening and T-wave inversion, which typically occur several days after ST-segment elevation.

2. Early repolarization is limited to the precordial leads. Notching of the terminal component of the QRS complex is characteristic of early repolarization.

3. Low-voltage QRS complexes can be a clue to pericardial effusion.

C. **Diagnostic imaging.** Imaging studies are unnecessary in most patients with idiopathic or classic viral AP. However, if clinical signs of pericardial tamponade or a large effusion are present, echocardiography should be performed (3). Chest radiography may reveal a "water-bottle" heart if a large effusion is present.

V. **Diagnostic assessment.** The diagnosis of a pericardial friction rub depends largely on the patient's history. Chest pain that is sharp, pleuritic, worsened with recumbency, and relieved by leaning forward is very suggestive of pericardial inflammation. Radiation of pain to the trapezius ridge is very characteristic as well. Inquiring about conditions associated with pericarditis is paramount (e.g., autoimmune disease, drugs, recent heart surgery, renal failure). The friction rub is best heard at end-inspiration with the patient leaning forward. The ECG is the most useful diagnostic test, but if there is evidence of cardiac tamponade, an echocardiogram should be obtained.

References

1. Marinella MA. Electrocardiographic manifestations and differential diagnosis of acute pericarditis. *Am Fam Physician* 1998;57:699–704.
2. Shabeti R. Acute pericarditis. *Cardiol Clin* 1990;8:639–644.
3. Dehmer GJ, O'Meara JJ. Update on acute pericarditis. *Hosp Med* 1995;31:39–44.

4. Baljepally R, Spodick DH. PR-segment deviations as the initial electrocardiographic response in acute pericarditis. *Am J Cardiol* 1998;81:1505–1506.

7.11 Raynaud's Phenomenon

Brian V. Reamy and Douglas C. Warren

Raynaud's phenomenon (RP) is an episodic vascular disorder of varying severity that results in digital artery ischemia and manifests clinically as a sequence of color changes in the digits. It affects between 3% to 20% of the general population (1).

I. **Approach.** The important steps in the evaluation of suspected RP are to establish its presence, then to distinguish primary RP (idiopathic RP or Raynaud's disease) from secondary RP.
  A. **Classification.** Primary RP is distinguished by the lack of an associated illness. Secondary RP indicates that an underlying disease is responsible. The differentiation between primary and secondary RP is readily made on the basis of the history and physical examination.
  B. **Epidemiology.** RP occurs four times more commonly in women than men. Primary RP usually begins before the age of 30 and a familial history is sometimes present. The prevalence is influenced by geographic location, with more cases reported in colder climates.
  C. **Special concerns.** Although primary RP is a relatively benign disorder, secondary RP is associated with significant morbidity and mortality because of the underlying illness, as well as tissue necrosis from prolonged vasospasm.
II. **History**
  A. **Description of attack.** What is the sequence of color changes, including their location, frequency, and duration? Are there associated symptoms?
    1. The classic sequence of events is a symmetric, white, blanching, sharply demarcated discoloration, followed by cyanosis, and then redness with resolution of the attack after approximately 15 minutes. Two colors, most commonly white and blue, are sufficient for a firm diagnosis. The presence of only one color makes the diagnosis tenuous.
    2. Fingers are usually involved, whereas the thumb and toes are less commonly affected. Rarely, the earlobes, nose, and lips are involved.
    3. Associated symptoms can include clumsiness, paresthesias, or pain.
    4. Symmetric, mild attacks without tissue loss are typical of primary RP.
    5. Asymmetric, prolonged, or intensely painful attacks associated with tissue injury are characteristic of secondary RP.
  B. **Triggers**
    1. Cold exposure is by far the most common trigger.
    2. Other triggers include emotional stress and nicotine.
  C. **Underlying illnesses or causes.** Are there symptoms or a known underlying disease that suggest secondary RP is present? The most common disorders are connective tissue diseases, especially systemic sclerosis or CREST syndrome; atherosclerotic disease; hyperviscosity syndromes; occupational exposure to intense vibration or vinyl chloride; and medications such as beta-blockers, clonidine, ergot drugs, and some chemotherapeutic agents (vinblastine, bleomycin, and cisplatin).
  D. **Other information.** Does the patient take unopposed estrogen or have a history of migraine headaches, chest pain, or possible *Helicobacter pylori* infection?
    1. Unopposed estrogen therapy or the presence of *H. pylori* infection can be associated with an increased risk of RP (2,3).
    2. Patients with RP report a higher prevalence of migraine headache, and both variant angina and musculoskeletal chest pain (4) (Chapters 2.7 and 7.1).

III. **Physical examination**
- A. **Focused physical examination (PE).** The goal of the PE is to uncover sentinel markers for illnesses responsible for secondary RP. In primary RP, the physical examination should be normal. Evaluate for thoracic outlet syndrome, examine distal extremity pulses, and perform an Allen test. Signs of scleroderma, such as sclerodactyly or telangiectasia should be sought, and digital necrosis or ulceration should be identified.
- B. **Additional PE.** If the history suggests an underlying connective tissue disorder, examine the heart, lungs, joints, skin, and nervous system.

IV. **Testing**
- A. **Clinical laboratory tests.** No "gold standard" test for RP exists. Evaluation is aimed at uncovering secondary causes and should include a complete blood count, erythrocyte sedimentation rate, and antinuclear antibodies (1).
- B. **Other tests.** Angiography can be considered with evidence of vascular occlusive disease. Abnormal nailfold capillary microscopy is a reliable indicator of the presence of underlying connective tissue disorders or of the risk of developing such a disorder. It is a useful adjunctive test in cases where the distinction between primary and secondary RP is unclear. It is performed by placing a drop of immersion oil on the nailfold and observing the capillaries with an ophthalmoscope set at diopter 40. The absence of fine capillaries and the presence of markedly dilated or tortuous vessels are characteristic abnormal findings.

V. **Diagnostic assessment.** A history of typical color changes of the digits is essential in the diagnosis of RP. Characterization of the attack as primary or secondary RP is accomplished through history, PE, and basic screening laboratory tests. More than 85% of patients with RP have the primary form, but 10% of patients with apparent primary RP will manifest an underlying disorder an average of 10 years from the onset of their RP (5). Nailfold capillary microscopy and laboratory tests to confirm specific connective tissue diseases should be performed in those cases where a suspicion for secondary RP exists, such as RP onset after age 30, asymmetric digital involvement, prolonged attacks resulting in tissue injury, or abnormal screening laboratory test results. Periodic monitoring for transition to secondary RP in these patients is prudent.

References
1. Wigley FM, Flavahan NA. Raynaud's phenomenon. *Rheum Dis Clin North Am* 1996;22:765–781.
2. Fraenkel L, Zhang Y, Chaisson CE, Evans SR, Wilson PWF, Felson DT. The association of estrogen replacement therapy and the Raynaud phenomenon in postmenopausal women. *Ann Intern Med* 1998:129:208–211.
3. Gasbarrini A, Massari I, Serricchio M, et al. Helicobacter pylori eradication ameliorates primary Raynaud's phenomenon. *Dig Dis Sci* 1998:43:1641–1645.
4. O'Keeffe ST, Tsapatsaris NP, Beetham WP. Increased prevalence of migraine and chest pain in patients with primary Raynaud disease. *Ann Intern Med* 1992;116:985–989.
5. Spencer-Green G. Outcomes in primary Raynaud phenomenon: a meta-analysis of the frequency, rates, and predictors of transition to secondary diseases. *Arch Intern Med* 1998:158:595–600.

7.12 Tachycardia

Gehan Devendra

Tachycardia is commonly found in both hospitalized and ambulatory patients. It can be either physiologic or pathologic and is defined as a heart rate greater than

100 beats/ minute. Tachycardia can initiate in two main areas, either supraventricular or ventricular, and can be divided into wide complex or narrow complex tachycardia.

I. Approach. In the evaluation of tachycardia, the important tasks are to determine if an underlying cause exists and to determine precisely the specific dysrhythmia producing tachycardia (1).

II. History

  A. Determining the cause. The clinical history is directed toward determining the underlying cardiac disease. Symptoms associated with tachycardia are palpitations, lightheadedness or presyncope, syncope, or congestive heart failure (CHF) (Chapters 2.12, 7.5, and 7.9). Some patients will also complain of irregular heartbeat, whereas others can be asymptomatic even with a profoundly abnormal rhythm. Prior history of myocardial infarction, cardiomyopathy (both ischemic and nonischemic heart disease), arrhythmias, pulmonary hypertension, cardiac surgery, rheumatic heart disease, valvular disease, and family history of cardiac arrythmias are all important. Medications such as any of the class IA or III antiarrythmic agents or over-the-counter cold preparations can cause tachyarrhythmias. Even a combination of medicines (e.g., certain antibiotics and newer nonsedating antihistamines) can contribute to tachyarrythmias.

III. Physical examination. The physical examination should include vital signs; pulse rate and blood pressure are the most important. Decreased blood pressure suggests a need for immediate treatment. A general assessment of mental status and skin perfusion also provides clues to the stability of the patient. A good cardiovascular and pulmonary examination is essential. Palpation of the heart (point of maximal impulse, PMI) can discern left ventricular enlargement. Auscultate systematically. The rhythm should be assessed to whether it is regular or irregular. Determine the specific heart rate. Next, determine if an associated murmur, rub, or gallop exists. Include in the examination an assessment for evidence of ventricular failure (e.g., pulmonary crackles, jugular venous distension, and lower extremity edema). In the respiratory assessment, include respiratory rate and evidence of labored breathing.

IV. Testing

  A. Electrocardiogram (ECG). The main diagnostic test is the 12-lead ECG: a rhythm strip during a tachycardia event is ideal. The Holter or event monitor can also be used in diagnosis in an outpatient setting. Rhythm and the QRS width are important in distinguishing the major types of tachycardia.

  B. Laboratory tests. Electrolyte abnormalities, especially hypomagnasemia and hypokalemia, can precipitate tachycardia. Digitalis toxicity can be another cause and, therefore, levels should be monitored. Also consider tests for common problems such as anemia, hyperthyroidism, and hypoxemia.

V. Diagnostic assessment

  A. Narrow complex tachycardia (QRS < 120 msec)

    1. Sinus tachycardia. Sinus tachycardia is normal in infants and children aged less than 2 years. In adults, it is often secondary to physiologic factors (anxiety, fever), pharmacologic factors (β-agonist therapy), and pathologic factors (anemia, thyrotoxicosis, hypoxemia, hypotension, pulmonary embolism). ECG findings reveal a normal P wave and PR interval. Management of sinus tachycardia is directed at correcting the underlying cause; specific therapy is rarely indicated.

    2. Atrial fibrillation. Atrial fibrillation (AF) occurs in approximately 10% of patients aged more than 70 years. The hallmark on ECG is an irregularly irregular rhythm and rate with the absence of P waves. The rate in AF can vary from normal to fast (> 200 beats/min). The QRS morphology can vary a great deal as well. Usually, the impulse originates from the atrium and travels down the His or Purkinje system with depolarization of the ventricle. Occasionally, the impulse from the atrium travels down

to the ventricle abnormally, resulting in aberrant conduction, and it can mimic ventricular tachycardia (VT). The key to distinguishing the two is recognizing a regular rhythm for VT and irregular rhythm for AF with aberrant conduction. In addition, patients with a prior bundle branch block who go into rapid AF can also mimic VT (see below). AF can result from cardiac [coronary artery disease, Wolff-Parkinson-White (WPW) syndrome, congestive heart failure, valvular abnormalities] or noncardiac (thyrotoxicosis, pulmonary embolism) sources. The underlying cause of the AF must be elucidated.

3. Atrial flutter. As with AF, atrial flutter can also be caused by both cardiac and noncardiac sources. The ECG is classically a "sawtooth" pattern in leads II, III, and aVF. The rate of the flutter waves is usually between 280 and 320 beats/minute. Ventricular conduction varies and usually demonstrates blocked conduction. The usual block is 2:1 or 4:1, with a ventricular rate of 150 to 75 beats/minute, respectively. Occasionally, the rate is too fast to discern any flutter waves. Carotid massage slows the ventricular rate, allowing for diagnosis. If carotid massage fails, pharmacologic treatment with adenosine or digitalis can slow the ventricular rate.

4. Paroxysmal supraventricular tachycardia (PSVT). PSVT is precipitated by reentry of the atrial impulse at the level of the atrioventricular (AV) node. This is the most common mechanism in the initiation of PSVT. PSVT is characterized by sudden onset of a narrow, regular QRS complex without discernible P waves. The rate varies from 160 to 190 beats/minute but can be as slow as 120 to 130 beats/minute. If the patient has a prior bundle branch block, a wide QRS complex will also be seen with PSVT. A specific subset of PSVT caused by reentry is the WPW syndrome. Conduction in WPW can occur via an accessory pathway. In the resting ECG, this is usually manifested by an upsloping tracing on the ECG prior to the QRS complex, known as the "delta wave." PR interval is also shortened. The accessory tract can predispose to PSVT, atrial flutter, or AF.

5. Multifocal atrial tachycardia (MAT). This arrhythmia is usually seen in the setting of pulmonary disease, metabolic or electrolyte abnormalities, or, rarely, digitalis toxicity. ECG findings in MAT consists of an irregular rhythm combined with three different morphologies of P waves. The rate of this arrhythmia usually does not exceed 140 beats/minute. Removal of the inciting event can relieve the tachycardia, but patients may frequently have to tolerate a low-grade tachycardia (1,2).

B. **Wide complex tachycardia (QRS > 120 msec)**
1. Ventricular tachycardia versus SVT with aberrant conduction. This is probably the hardest to diagnose of the tachycardias. Brudaga (3) put forth a schema to diagnose VT from SVT with aberrant conduction. The criteria are as follows:
   a. Initially rule out right or left bundle branch block.
   b. Is there an absence of an RS complex in all precordial leads? If yes then VT, if no then proceed to c.
   c. Is the RS interval more than 100 msec in any one precordial lead? If yes then VT, if no then proceed to d.
   d. Is there AV dissociation? If yes then VT. If no is answered to all the above then the specificity or sensitivity that this is a SVT with aberrant conduction is 98% and 99%, respectively. Inexact features of VT are QRS more than 0.14 second, QRS concordance in all precordial leads, fusion or capture beats, and QRS negative in leads I and II.
2. Ventricular fibrillation (VF). VF is not really a tachycardia but represents abnormal ventricular depolarization. The ventricle has numerous areas of depolarization and, therefore, cannot have organized contraction. This type of unorganized contraction produces no cardiac output. On ECG, it

often appears as a "bag of worms" with coarse or fine waves varying in amplitude and duration. Coarse VF indicates the recent onset of VF and is usually correctable with defibrillation, whereas fine VF is indicative of prolonged VF that approaches asystole.

References

1. Scheinman M. Tachyarrythmias in primary cardiology. In: Goldman L, Braunwald E, ed. *Heart disease: a textbook of cardiovascular medcicine.* Philadelphia: WB Saunders, 1998:330–352.
2. Ganz LI, Friedman PL. Supraventricular tachycardia. *N Engl J Med* 1995; 332:162–173.
3. Brugada P. A new approach to the differential diagnosis of a regular tachycardia with a wide QRS complex. *Circulation* 1991;83:1649–1659.

8. RESPIRATORY PROBLEMS

JOSEPH E. SCHERGER

8.1 Cough

Désirée A. Lie

Cough is among the top 10 reasons for visits to family physicians in the United States. It accounts for 200 to 400 million episodes of illness per year. Three causal conditions increasing in frequency over the past two decades are asthma, gastroesophageal reflux disease (GERD), and chronic obstructive airways disease (COPD) (1,2). Bronchitis is one of the most common causes of cough in the primary care setting (3).

I. **Approach**
   A. **Cough characteristics.** In evaluating cough as a symptom (4), a distinction has to be made among the following:
      1. Normal versus pathologic cough
      2. Acute (<3 weeks) versus chronic (>3 weeks) cough
      3. Respiratory versus nonrespiratory causes
      4. Pediatric versus adult conditions
   B. **Special concerns.** Failure to improve with appropriate management over 4 weeks signals a need for more extensive workup to exclude tuberculosis (TB), adult-onset asthma, penicillin-resistant pneumococcus, lung cancer, and immunosuppression.

II. **History**
   A. **Characteristics of the cough**. What is the type of cough (barking, brassy, wheezy, nocturnal, paroxysmal)? What are the duration, timing, and triggers? Are there associated symptoms of fever, sputum production, dypsnea, hemoptysis, and weight loss? Are there clear relieving factors? Ask specifically about postnasal drip as patients often do not volunteer this information. A good history is the key to diagnosis.
      1. Upper respiratory causes most commonly relate to postnasal drip. In adults, sinusitis, pharyngitis, and allergic rhinitis should be considered. In children, concomitant otitis media should be excluded.
      2. Lower respiratory causes include lung (bronchitis, asthma, pneumonia, bronchiectasis, and in children, foreign body aspiration) and cardiac [congestive heart failure (CHF) and mitral stenosis].
      3. Nonrespiratory causes include GERD, drug effects [e.g., angiotensin converting enzyme (ACE)-inhibitors], and psychogenic.
   B. **Smoking patients** should be identified early as bronchitis and lung cancer are possibilities. Passive smoking is also a risk factor, especially in children. Office visits for cough represent teachable moments for smoking cessation education. Smoking cessation has been shown to reduce respiratory symptoms by 50%.
   C. **Psychosocial impact** of the cough reflects severity and the need for further workup. Has the patient missed school or work? Is the sleeping partner disturbed? Is there avoidance of exercise because it triggers cough? In chronic, episodic cough, a correct diagnosis of asthma can considerably improve quality of life. A psychogenic cause for cough and behavioral problems in children may be unmasked here.
   D. **Other information**. Associated chest pain should direct the history toward pleurisy or rib fracture secondary to chronic cough. Occupational exposures (toxic fumes, chemicals, birds and animals), systemic diseases [rheumatoid arthritis, breast and prostate cancer metastases, human immunodeficiency virus disease (HIV)] and drug exposure (ACE-inhibitors, cyclophosphamide, and methotrexate) are important factors to consider in the cause. Cough with significant weight loss should trigger a workup for TB, HIV, or lung cancer in the smoker.

III. **Physical examination**
   A. **Focused physical examination (PE)** should include vital signs (temperature, pulse, respiratory rate, and blood pressure), ear, nose, sinuses, throat (ENST), and a full lung examination with the chest uncovered. Normal lung examination often excludes pneumonia but not asthma, bronchitis, COPD, GERD, or lung cancer. It is more effective to examine the lung before the ENST in young children because the ENST examination is more traumatic and can induce crying. In the older patient, especially the postmenopausal woman, rib palpation may be included to isolate fracture secondary to osteoporosis.
   B. **Additional PE.** The cardiovascular examination is directed at a diagnosis of CHF. Associated lymphadenopathy suggests infection or neoplasm. Wasting can be ominous (cancer or HIV). Abdominal examination may reveal a tender enlarged liver in CHF, or epigastric tenderness in GERD (Chapters 7.5 and 9.6).

IV. **Testing**
   A. **Clinical laboratory tests.** Most acute presentations of cough do not require blood, urine, or other laboratory tests. White blood count with differential and blood cultures are indicated for pneumonia. Gram's stain and culture of sputum are rarely practical in the office. A purified protein derivative (PPD) test should be placed early if TB is suspected, unless the patient is known to be anergic or thought to have overwhelming active TB disease. Systemic causes require testing specific to the disease in question.
   B. **Radiologic tests.** A chest x-ray study is not indicated for upper respiratory causes or bronchitis. It is only useful when pneumonia, TB, COPD, CHF, or cancer (primary or metastatic) are being considered. Computed tomography of the sinuses is more sensitive and specific than PE to differentiate sinusitis from other causes of cough.
   C. **Pulmonary function tests.** The simple peak flow meter used with a therapeutic trial of bronchodilators will identify most cases of asthma. This important test should be supervised by the physician or an experienced nurse. Additional testing is suggested for COPD and pulmonary fibrosis.
   D. **Invasive tests.** Bronchoscopy is useful for foreign body aspiration, cancer, or chronic interstitial lung disease. Esophageal pH monitoring will most likely confirm suspected GERD.

V. **Diagnostic assessment.** A thorough history is vital to accurate diagnosis. *Acute cough* is likely to be infectious. A pertinent observation is that physicians overtreat acute bronchitis with antibiotics. The literature suggests that most cases are viral in origin and antibiotics are ineffective. *Chronic cough* has a longer list of differential diagnoses. Asthma tends to be underdiagnosed in adults and children. Smoking-related causes should prompt educational intervention and workup, especially in older patients. GERD is a diagnosis often missed because it is not considered. Often, more than one office visit is needed to unravel the cause of chronic cough. Up to 80% of cases have multiple causes (5). Making an accurate diagnosis is essential to successful treatment. Of cough presentation, 90% can be adequately managed in the family physician's office, although it can take 3 to 5 months to arrive at a correct diagnosis in some cases (2). Referral to a pulmonary specialist is needed only in complicated cases (e.g., cancer, occupational and connective tissue diseases, and failed therapy).

References
1. Weiss BD. *20 common problems in primary care*. New York: McGraw-Hill, 1999.
2. Lawler WR. An office approach to the diagnosis of chronic cough. *Am Fam Physician* 1998;58(9):2015–2022.
3. Heath JM. Chronic bronchitis: primary care management. *Am Fam Physician* 1998;57(10):2365–2372, 2376–2378.
4. Irwin RS. Managing cough as a defense mechanism and as a symptom. A consensus report of the American College of Chest Physicians. *Chest* 1998;114:133S–181S.
5. Irwin RS. Silencing chronic cough. *Hosp Pract* 1999;34:53–60.

8.2 Cyanosis

Janis F. Neuman

Cyanosis is a bluish discoloration of the skin and mucous membranes caused by increased amounts of unsaturated hemoglobin in the blood. For cyanosis to appear, 5 g/100 ml of reduced blood hemoglobin is required. An oxygen saturation (O_2 sat) less than 75% or a PaO_2 of 40 mm Hg will result in cyanosis (1). Cyanosis can be considered central or peripheral, based on the underlying abnormality. Central cyanosis includes conditions that lead to arterial desaturation such as decreased inspired oxygen tension, pulmonary disease, and conditions causing right to left shunts (e.g., congenital heart disease and intrapulmonary shunts). Abnormal hemoglobins are also considered central. Peripheral cyanosis is caused by reduced cardiac output, cold exposure, and arterial or venous obstruction.

I. **Approach.** When the patient is cyanotic, the objective is to determine the underlying cause and correct it. Oxygen delivery to the tissues depends on an intact respiratory system to provide oxygen for hemoglobin saturation, the concentration of hemoglobin, the cardiac output and regional microvasculature, and an oxyhemoglobin unloading mechanism (2).

A. **Decreased blood oxygenation (central cyanosis) is usually caused by one of the following:**
1. Obstruction to the intake of oxygen (epiglottitis and acute laryngotracheobronchitis, asthma, chronic bronchitis or emphysema, and foreign body aspiration).
2. Decreased absorption of oxygen as occurs with an alveolar-capillary block (sarcoid, pulmonary fibrosis, pneumonia, pulmonary edema, or alveolar proteinosis). Ventilation-perfusion defects from emphysema, pneumoconioses, and sarcoid will also decrease O_2 absorption.
3. Decreased perfusion of the lung with blood (shock, septic or cardiogenic; pulmonary embolus; pulmonary vascular shunts from pulmonary hemangioma; or congenital heart disease).
4. Reduced intake of oxygen from an atmosphere with a decreased oxygen concentration.
5. A defective hemoglobin unable to attach to oxygen (methemoglobinemia, sulfhemoglobinemia, carbon monoxide poisoning, and other hemoglobinopathies).

B. **Peripheral cyanosis will occur with:**
1. Reduced cardiac output from acute myocardial infarction or other causes of pump failure.
2. Local or regional phenomenon from cold exposure, arterial obstruction from embolus or thrombosis, and venous stasis or obstruction.
3. Cold exposure (Raynauds' phenomenon) (Chapter 7.11).

II. **History**
A. **When did the cyanosis appear?** Is cyanosis of recent onset or has it been present since birth? A history of "squatting" episodes in childhood and congenital cyanosis suggest congenital heart disease. Chronic cyanosis caused by methemoglobinemia can be congenital or acquired. Other causes of chronic cyanosis include chronic obstructive pulmonary disease (COPD), pulmonary fibrosis, and pulmonary atrioventricular fistula. Acute and subacute cyanosis is caused by acute myocardial infarct, pneumothorax, pulmonary embolus, pneumonia, or upper airway obstruction.
B. **Is the patient symptomatic or asymptomatic?** Asymptomatic patients may have methemoglobinemia (congenital or drug-induced), or sulfhemoglobinemia. Exposure to drugs (prescribed and illicit) or environmental factors are important in these patients. Intermittent cyanosis, skin color changes, and pain with cold exposure suggests Raynaud's phenomenon. Symptomatic

patients, especially with chest pain and respiratory distress, are more likely to have a cardiac or pulmonary cause of cyanosis.

C. **Does the patient have known risk factors for cardiac or pulmonary disease, including smoking, hyperlipidemia, asthma, drug abuse (especially methamphetamines), severe obesity (sleep apnea), neuromuscular disease, or autoimmune disease?** Does the patient have chest pain or intermittent cyanosis with exercise, suggesting angina? Chest pain can be present with acute pulmonary emboli or pneumothorax. Is there a cough and fever suggesting pneumonia? Has the patient had any occupational or environmental exposures that might cause pulmonary problems?

D. **Other.** Is there a family history of abnormal hemoglobins or pulmonary disease? Has the patient suffered an episode of hypotension that could produce adult respiratory distress syndrome (ARDS), such as sepsis or heart failure?

III. **Physical examination**

A. **Initial assessment.** Vital signs are very important: tachycardia suggests cardiac arrhythmia, shock, volume depletion, anemia, or fever (Chapter 7.12). An increased or decreased respiratory rate and use of accessory musculature suggests hypoxia from any cause. Hypotension can signal vascular collapse from myocardial infarction, septic shock, or pulmonary embolus.

B. **Additional physical examination.** Stridor suggests upper airway obstruction. Examine the pharynx for evidence of obstruction. If epiglottitis or foreign body is suspected, be prepared to intubate the patient. Check the neck for evidence of jugular venous distention (JVD). Auscultate the chest for rales, suggesting pulmonary edema; wheezing and rhonchi consistent with reactive airway disease; or absence of breath sounds, suggesting pneumonia or pneumothorax. Auscultate the heart for murmurs, arrhythmias, and abnormal heart sounds. Feel the pulses in the extremities to assess for arterial embolus or venous thrombosis, especially if cyanosis is localized to one extremity. Examine the abdomen for evidence of intraabdominal catastrophe or aneurysm. Examine the nails for evidence of clubbing, suggesting chronic pulmonary disease.

IV. **Testing**

A. **Pulse oximetry** estimates oxygen saturation, but does not measure it directly. Direct measurements using arterial blood gases (ABGs) are necessary to assess a cyanotic patient. Patients with abnormal hemoglobins will have a normal PaO_2 but a decreased hemoglobin oxygen saturation. Cyanotic patients will have an O_2 sat. less than 75% and a PaO_2 less than 40 mm Hg if they have a normal hemoglobin concentration. A low PaO_2 is caused by respiratory or cardiac problems in most circumstances.

B. **A chest radiograph** helps assess heart size and lung parenchyma. Infiltrates suggest pneumonia, ARDS, or pulmonary edema. Exclude pneumothorax. Look for evidence of interstitial lung disease. Pleural effusion can represent infection, malignancy, or pulmonary edema (Chapter 8.4).

C. **An electrocardiogram** may demonstrate acute myocardial infarction, arrhythmia, or pericardial process. P-pulmonale, right ventricular hypertrophy (RVH), and R axis suggest chronic pulmonary disease.

D. **Other tests.** Ventilation-perfusion scans may demonstrate pulmonary embolus. Pulmonary artery catheterization and pressure measurements help distinguish cardiac from pulmonary causes of cyanosis. Pulmonary function testing can help in the diagnosis of various pulmonary diseases.

V. **Diagnostic assessment.** A focused history, physical examination, and diagnostic testing will elucidate the cause of cyanosis in affected patients. Response to supplemental O_2 can also help pinpoint the cause of cyanosis (2). Decreased oxygenation secondary to mild to moderate $\dot{V}/\dot{Q}$ mismatches caused by pneumonia, pulmonary embolus, and asthma may be reversible with supplemental oxygen. Severe $\dot{V}/\dot{Q}$ mismatch caused by intrapulmonary shunting from severe pulmonary edema or ARDS may be refractory to supplemental O_2. Moderate $\dot{V}/\dot{Q}$ mismatch associated with ventilatory failure (COPD) may respond to supplemental O_2, but be aware of increasing CO_2 levels. ABGs directly measure PaO_2

and O_2 saturation. Abnormal hemoglobins will also be measured and help guide therapy. Hypoxia with an elevated CO_2 suggests COPD or asthma, whereas hypoxia with a normal or decreased CO_2 suggests pneumonia, ARDS, pulmonary edema, pulmonary emboli, or interstitial lung disease (1). Once the cause of the cyanosis is determined, the objective is to treat the underlying process. Causes of pseudocyanosis include argyria or bismuth poisoning (slate blue-gray color), hemochromatosis (brownish color), or polycythemia (ruddy red color). For peripheral cyanosis caused by decreased cardiac output, correct the causes of hypovolemia (e.g., dehydration, shock, heart failure from whatever cause). Surgical consultation may be required for acute embolization of an extremity, and anticoagulation for venous thrombosis.

References

1. Khan MG. *Cardiac and pulmonary management*. Philadelphia: Lee & Febiger, 1993:818–825.
2. Woodley M, Whelan A. *Manual of medical therapeutics*. Boston: Little, Brown and Company, 1993:179–181.
3. Hurst JW. *Medicine for the practicing physician*. Boston: Butterworth–Heineman, 1983:973–975.
4. Collins RD. *Dynamic differential diagnosis*. Philadelphia: JB Lippincott, 1981: 386–388.

8.3 Hemoptysis

Kathryn M. Larsen and Mary Knudtson

Hemoptysis is defined as the coughing up or expectoration of blood from the tracheobronchial tree, which can be from the trachea, major airways, or the lung parenchyma. It is an alarming symptom that usually prompts the patient to seek immediate medical attention. Hemoptysis can range in severity from trivial to life-threatening and has numerous causes.

   I. **Approach.** The clinician must determine the anatomic bleeding site and the underlying cause for the bleeding (1). Bleeding originating from the nasopharynx or bleeding from the gastrointestinal tract, can mimic hemoptysis (Chapter 9.7). A thorough evaluation is necessary because the amount of blood expectorated does not correlate with the seriousness of the cause. After extensive evaluation, up to 30% of patients have no identifiable cause for their hemoptysis; these patients are classified as having cryptogenic hemoptysis.

   The pathogenesis of hemoptysis generally results from inflammation or injury to the tracheobronchial mucosa (e.g., bronchitis, bronchiectasis, tuberculosis, sarcoidosis, and bronchogenic carcinoma); injury to the pulmonary vasculature (e.g., lung abscess, necrotizing pneumonia, and pulmonary infarction secondary to embolization); or elevation of the pulmonary capillary pressure (e.g., pulmonary edema, Wegener's granulomatosis, and Goodpasture's syndrome). The most common causes are acute and chronic bronchitis, followed by bronchogenic carcinoma and pneumonia (2). Lung tumors account for 20% of the cases of hemoptysis; they are usually associated with smokers aged more than 40 years who have had a change in cough pattern with an ache or pain in the chest. A bleeding diathesis or the use of anticoagulant medicine may present with hemoptysis but underlying pulmonary disease must always be excluded. Chest trauma is a less common cause of hemoptysis.

  II. **History**
      A. **Identification of the site of bleeding.** What is the source of the bleeding? Is the problem truly hemoptysis or could the bleeding originate in a nonpulmonary location such as the nose and oropharynx or the gastrointestinal

tract? Blood that is coughed from the respiratory tract is bright red in color and may be frothy or mixed with sputum. Hemoptysis is more likely with a history of underlying pulmonary disease, smoking, or mitral valve disease. Hematemesis is associated with blood that is dark red, brown, or coffee ground in appearance and that may be mixed with food particles. Hematemesis is favored in the presence of preexisting gastrointestinal condition, especially with a history of liver disease, alcohol use, or peptic ulcer disease. Sputum that is blood-streaked often arises from the nasal mucosa and oropharynx.

B. **Characteristics of the sputum.** What are the characteristics of the sputum in terms of color, odor, and consistency? A description of the sputum can assist in defining the disease process causing the hemoptysis: (a) frothy, pink sputum is suggestive of pulmonary edema fluid; (b) putrid or foul-smelling sputum suggests a lung abscess; (c) currant jelly sputum may suggest a necrotizing pneumonia; (d) the sputum of pneumococcal pneumonia is typically rust-colored and can be confused with true hemoptysis; (e) large amounts of blood-streaked sputum often suggest bronchiectasis.

C. **Other information.** Does the patient have other associated symptoms? Cough, dyspnea, and sputum production over several years may suggest chronic bronchitis or bronchiectasis. Weight loss and fatigue may suggest an underlying malignancy, and fever and night sweats might indicate tuberculosis. Does the patient have a history of known pulmonary, cardiac, or hematologic problems? Does the patient have hematuria, which might suggest a pulmonary-renal syndrome (Chapter 10.2)? Is the patient a smoker or have specific environmental exposures? Is the patient taking medications, especially anticoagulants, that might contribute to the bleeding?

III. **Physical examination.** A focused physical examination should include vital signs and examinations of the nose, sinuses, oropharynx, neck, lungs, and heart. The neck should be palpated for the presence of lymphadenopathy and inspected for jugular venous distension. The lower extremities should be checked for edema. Examination of the skin may reveal lesions associated with systemic lupus erythematosus; Kaposi's sarcoma; clubbing (consistent with neoplasm, bronchiectasis, or lung abscess); or ecchymosis related to a coagulopathy.

IV. **Testing.** The evaluation should begin with a chest x-ray study to look for possible clues to the diagnosis: a mass lesion, focal or diffuse parenchymal disease, pneumonitis, abscess, infiltrate, hilar adenopathy, enlarged heart, pulmonary edema, coin lesion of aspergilloma, or the peribronchial cuffing suggestive of bronchiectasis. A computed tomography scan may be necessary to define a lesion seen on chest x-ray film (3). Additional basic testing should include a complete blood count with differential and a coagulation profile. For patients in whom infection is suspected, skin testing, a Gram's stain, acid fast stain, or sputum cultures may be appropriate. Cytologic examination of the sputum is indicated in cases of suspected malignancy.

A. **Other special tests.** Fiberoptic bronchoscopy is used to localize the bleeding site of specific lesions noted on x-ray film. It is also used in cases of persistent or recurrent bleeding and for smokers aged more than 40 years with a negative chest x-ray study. Ventilation-perfusion scanning is indicated if pulmonary embolism is suspected.

V. **Diagnostic assessment.** Determining the site of bleeding is the first step. If the bleeding is from the nasopharynx or gastrointestinal tract then it is not classified as hemoptysis. The basic approach depends on the severity of the bleeding. Most cases of blood-tinged sputum are upper respiratory in nature and do not require extensive workup. Bronchitis is the most common cause. However, bronchogenic carcinoma and bronchiectasis are also common causes that do require further evaluation (4). Mild hemoptysis can be evaluated with elective bronchoscopy of the respiratory tract. Massive hemoptysis (definitions in the literature range from 100 ml/24 hours to 1,000 ml over several days) requires an emergent diagnostic approach, typically with rigid bronchoscopy (5). If hemoptysis persists despite treatment of a presumed infection, bronchial arteriography with embolization or resection of the involved segment may be necessary.

References
1. Colice GL. Hemoptysis: three questions that can direct management. *Postgrad Med* 1996;100(1):227–236.
2. DiLeo MD, Amedee RG, Butcher RB. Hemoptysis and Pseudohemoptysis: the patient expectorating blood. *Ear Nose Throat J* 1995;74(12):822–824, 826, 828.
3. Marshall TJ, Flower CD, Jackson JE. The role of radiology in the investigation and management of patients with hemoptysis. *Clin Radiol* 1996;51(6):391–400.
4. Marwah OS, Sharma OP. Bronchiectasis: how to identify, treat, and prevent. *Postgrad Med* 1995;97(2):149–150, 153–156, 159.
5. Cahill BC, Ingbar DH. Massive hemoptysis: assessment and management. *Clin Chest Med* 1994;15(1):147–167.

8.4 Pleural Effusion

Mark F. Giglio

Pleural effusions occur in a variety of illnesses. The underlying causes range from benign atelectasis to malignancy. Pleural effusions develop in 1 million patients each year in the United States (1). Although effusions occur within the lungs and pleura, the source is often from outside the pulmonary system.

I. **Approach.** Two main tasks are involved in approaching the patient with pleural effusion. First, document the presence and size of the effusion, using history, physical examination, and radiologic studies. Second, determine the cause of the effusion. Thoracentesis helps by differentiating the two main types of effusions: transudative and exudative.

   A. **Transudative effusions** result from an elevated net hydrostatic pressure gradient. Common causes include congestive heart failure (CHF), nephrotic syndrome, and cirrhosis. Generally, they require no further workup when identified and respond to treatment of the primary problem.

   B. **Exudative effusions** result from increased permeability of the pleural vessels. The differential diagnosis encompasses a broader range of conditions, including malignancy and infections.

II. **History.** The patient's history can often suggest that a pleural effusion is present. Small effusions, however, may cause no symptoms. Frequently, an underlying disease causes the patient's initial symptoms.

   A. **Pulmonary.** Dyspnea is the most common symptom. Did it develop acutely or gradually? Is there a dry cough present? Does the patient experience chest pain, especially pleuritic pain? Does the pain vary in quality (Chapter 8.5)?

   B. **Associated symptoms.** The main goal here is to think about underlying illnesses that might produce a pleural effusion. Orthopnea, paroxysmal nocturnal dyspnea, dyspnea on exertion, and pedal edema suggest CHF. Does the patient have exertional chest pain that may be angina? Hemoptysis, weight loss, and anorexia point to malignancy. Has the patient been acutely ill? Productive cough, fever, chills, and night sweats suggest pneumonia. Does the patient have risks for deep venous thrombosis (e.g., recent travel, prolonged immobilization or fracture)? Symptoms of pulmonary embolism include tachycardia, hemoptysis, and dyspnea.

   C. **Past medical history.** Has the patient had prior pulmonary diseases? Are cardiac risk factors present? Is there a history of hepatic or renal disease? Has the patient had cancer before?

   D. **Family history.** Are there family members with premature coronary artery disease, tuberculosis, or malignancy?

   E. **Social history.** Does the patient smoke? Does the patient use alcohol to excess? Where does the patient work? Is there solvent or asbestos exposure at work?

III. Physical examination (PE)

A. **Focused PE.** Observe the patient's appearance and respiratory effort. Is the patient splinting or showing signs of respiratory distress? Vital signs should include respiratory rate. Is there tachycardia present (Chapter 7.12)? Typical findings on pulmonary examination include decreased or absent breath sounds over the affected side, dullness to percussion, decreased tactile fremitus, and possibly splinting of the affected side. Findings can be bilateral (e.g., CHF) or unilateral. The examination can also vary with the severity of the effusion. Findings are usually normal when less than 300 ml of fluid is present. A pleural rub may be noted. With a large effusion (>1,500 ml), the affected hemithorax is often larger with bulging interspaces (2).

B. **Additional physical examination.** Think in terms of differential diagnosis to look for signs of underlying causes. Cardiac examination should look for signs of congestive heart failure, including cardiomegaly, displaced point of maximal impulse, and an S_3 gallop. Is a heart murmur present? Abdominal examination may reveal hepatomegaly, liver tenderness, a fluid wave, and other signs of ascites. Are there signs of malignancy, including generalized or regional lymphadenopathy (Chapters 15.1 and 15.2)?

IV. Testing

A. **Radiographic study.** Initial testing focuses on confirming that a pleural effusion is present. A chest x-ray study is the typical starting point. On the upright anteroposterior view, a small effusion may show up as blunting of the costophrenic angle. Larger effusions will show a meniscus sign at the air fluid border. Lateral decubitus views help estimate the size of the effusion.

B. **Ultrasound and other modalities.** Unfortunately, the chest x-ray study can fail to show small effusions, even with decubitus views. Ultrasound can detect as little as 5 to 50 ml of fluid. It is also helpful in locating pockets of fluid and guiding thoracentesis for small effusions. Computed tomography scan, which is very sensitive, can differentiate pleural fluid from pleural thickening and focal masses.

C. **Thoracentesis.** Thoracentesis allows evaluation of any undiagnosed pleural effusion. Note that not all effusions require diagnostic thoracentesis. If the cause is apparent from the clinical presentation (e.g., CHF), observation may be appropriate (3). In general, parapneumonic effusions require thoracentesis to confirm diagnosis and assess the need for chest tube placement.

1. Relative contraindications include bleeding diathesis, systemic anticoagulation, small volume of pleural fluid, mechanical ventilation, inability of patient to cooperate, and cutaneous disease at the needle entry site.

2. Transudate or exudate? Based on a revision of the "modified" Light criteria, pleural fluid is an exudate if it meets one or more of the following parameters (5):

   a. Pleural fluid serum lactate dehydrogenase (LDH) more than 0.45 the upper limit of normal LDH

   b. Pleural:serum LDH more than 0.6

   c. Pleural:serum protein more than 0.5

3. Other measures used to test for an exudate include pleural fluid cholesterol, fluid:serum albumin gradient and fluid:serum bilirubin ratio. Cell count, pH, glucose, Gram's stain and culture help assess for infection.

V. Diagnostic assessment.
In developing a diagnostic assessment for the patient with pleural effusion, it is important to consider that pleural fluid analysis does not establish a specific diagnosis, but supports a clinical impression. Ordering and interpreting tests must be guided by pretest clinical impressions (4). Initially, it may be appropriate to order only pleural fluid LDH and protein levels to determine the presence or absence of an exudate. Additional fluid can be reserved for further testing if an exudate is found.

If the pleural fluid analysis shows a transudate, the most likely diagnosis is CHF. Additional possibilities include cirrhosis with ascites, nephrotic syndrome, hypoalbuminemia, and acute atelectasis. Further diagnostic evaluation of the pleural fluid would not be necessary.

If the pleural fluid is exudative, the most likely diagnostic possibilities are malignancy, infection, or tuberculosis, but the differential diagnosis is quite broad. In one study, malignancy accounted for 25% of all pleural effusions seen in the general hospital setting. Cytology is helpful in looking for malignancy. In 54% to 63% of patients with malignant effusions, pleural fluid cytology will be positive (4). Glucose level, cell count, and pH will help guide management in the setting of parapneumonic effusions and aid in determining the need for chest tube placement. Tuberculous effusions may require pleural biopsy to confirm the diagnosis. Amylase can be elevated in pancreatitis, pancreatic pseudocyst, malignancy, and esophageal rupture. Triglycerides would be elevated in the setting of chylothorax.

Studies on pleural fluid will yield a definitive or presumptive diagnosis in 74% of cases (4). Those that are undiagnosed may require repeat thoracentesis, pleural biopsy, bronchoscopy, or thoracoscopy to ascertain the cause.

References
1. Stagner SW, Campbell GD. Pleural effusion: What can you learn from the results of the a "tap"? *Postgrad Med* 1992;91:439–454.
2. Jay SJ. Diagnostic procedures for pleural disease. *Clin Chest Med* 1985;6:33–48.
3. Burgher LW, Jones FL, Patterson JR, Selecky PA. Guidelines for thoracentesis and needle biopsy of the pleura. *Am Rev Respir Dis* 1989;140:257–258.
4. Bartter T, Santarelli R, Akers S, Pratter M. The evaluation of pleural effusion. *Chest* 1994;106:1209–1214.
5. Heffner JE, Brown LK, Barbier C. Diagnostic value of tests that discriminate between exudative and transudative pleural effusions. *Chest* 1997;111:970–980.

8.5 Pleuritic Pain

Hal S. Shimazu

Pleuritic pain is the characteristic pain of inflamed pleura (i.e., pleurisy—a term often used synonymously with pleuritic pain). Pleuritic pain arises from parietal pleura and is typically sharp, stabbing, unilateral, and aggravated by deep inspiration and coughing. The visceral pleura is insensitive.

  I. **Approach**. Pleuritic pain is a frequent presenting complaint in an urgent or emergent care setting.
   A. **Etiology.** It is important to distinguish true pleuritic pain (Table 8.1) from conditions that mimic this pain (Table 8.2).

Table 8.1 Causes of pleuritic pain

Pleuritis/pleurisy: infectious (viral, especially Coxsackie B; primary or reactivated tuberculosis, fungal), autoimmune (e.g., systemic lupus, rheumatoid arthritis, Dressler's syndrome—pleuropericarditis), uremic, radiation, drug reaction, and idiopathic

Pulmonary embolism

Pneumonia

Spontaneous pneumothorax

Trauma (hemothorax, pneumothorax)

Neoplasia

Asbestosis

Table 8.2 Pleuritic pain mimics

Chest wall: costochondritis, rib fracture, muscle strain/spasm, herpes zoster
Abdominal: pancreatitis, abscess (hepatic, splenic, subphrenic), splenic infarction
Cardiac: pericarditis

    B. Special concerns. In acute pleuritic pain, urgent exclusion of pulmonary embolism (PE) is paramount with less than 10% mortality in treated patients and 30% mortality in untreated patients (1). Because of the low specificity of the presenting signs and symptoms of PE, in the absence of an obvious cause for acute pleuritic pain, suspicion for PE must remain high; further evaluation is required, typically with a ventilation-perfusion ($\dot{V}/\dot{Q}$) lung scan (2,3).

II. History

    A. Characteristics of the pleuritic pain. What is the acuity of the pain, its location, and exacerbating features?

        1. Acute onset suggests sudden development as viral or idiopathic pleurisy, PE, pneumonia, or pneumothorax.
        Insidious onset suggests a slower inflammatory or irritative process usually resulting in a pleural effusion with the pain generally diminishing as fluid accumulates (Chapter 8.4).

        2. Pleuritic chest pain localizes above the underlying pleural pathology through intercostal innervation.

        3. Through phrenic innervation, shoulder pain can indicate ipsilateral diaphragmatic involvement, usually by abdominal pathology (Table 8.1).

        4. Substernal pain improved by leaning forward suggests pericarditis (Chapter 7.1).

        5. Provocation of pain by shoulder movement indicates a musculoskeletal cause.

    B. Focused review of systems. What symptoms or history accompany the pain that might suggest a respiratory infection, PE, or malignancy? A nonproductive cough is nonspecific, and a productive cough suggests infection. Hemoptysis suggests malignancy, tuberculosis, or pulmonary embolism. A fever suggests infection but can occur with PE. Recent surgery or lower extremity trauma or swelling increase the risk for PE. Unexplained weight loss suggests malignancy or tuberculosis (TB).

    C. Past medical history. Past history can provide clues to the cause including malignancy, recent myocardial infarction, uremia, lupus, and rheumatoid arthritis.

    D. Other history. Inquire about oral contraceptives (PE risk), TB, or asbestos exposure.

III. Physical examination

    A. Focused physical examination. This should include vital signs with attention to temperature and respiratory rate and examination of the chest. Tenderness to palpation indicates a musculoskeletal cause. Dullness to percussion suggests pleural effusion or parenchymal pathology and hyperresonant percussion indicates pneumothorax. On auscultation, a pleural friction rub is the only sign of pleurisy; crackles suggest pneumonia; and decreased breath sounds indicate pneumothorax or effusion. The examination result is frequently normal.

    B. Additional physical examination. Abdominal tenderness can suggest a subdiaphragmatic process (Table 8.2, *Abdominal*). Lower extremity edema, tenderness, or Homans' sign can imply deep vein thrombosis (DVT) and PE. Lymphadenopathy can represent lymphoma or metastatic disease.

IV. Testing

A. Clinical laboratory tests. Routine studies (e.g., complete blood count and metabolic panels) are of limited usefulness; leukocytosis in pneumonia, uremia, or hepatic abnormalities may suggest the cause.

B. Diagnostic imaging. The chest x-ray (CXR) study is essential, potentially revealing pneumonia, neoplasm, pneumothorax, or pleural effusion; the decubitus view is sensitive at 100 ml effusion. Nonspecific findings of atelectasis, pulmonary parenchymal abnormalities, or both are seen in 68% of PE; pleural effusion is found in 48% of PE (3). The CXR study is commonly normal. Notably, PE and viral pleurisy frequently have a normal CXR study. Ultrasound has diagnostic and therapeutic adjunctive roles with pleural effusions and computed tomography has a role with both effusions and parenchymal abnormalities.

C. Pleural effusion analysis. Diagnostic thoracentesis is indicated if the cause of the effusion and pain is not apparent (Diagnostic assessment of pleural effusion is discussed in Chapter 8.4.) Effusion associated with pleuritic pain is nearly always an exudate with a notable exception of PE which can be a transudate (4).

D. Additional studies. $\dot{V}/\dot{Q}$ lung scan is typically obtained for any suspicion of PE. If the $\dot{V}/\dot{Q}$ scan is intermediate or has low probability for PE, then evaluating for possible DVT with leg impedance plethysomography or ultrasound is useful. If the DVT studies are negative and strong clinical suspicion for PE exists, then either a pulmonary angiogram or serial leg venous study can be obtained (3). Obtain an electrocardiogram and echocardiogram if pericarditis is suspected.

V. Diagnostic assessment.

After performing a focused history and physical examination and excluding chest wall pain and other mimics (Table 8.2), order a CXR study, which may reveal an obvious cause (e.g., neoplasm, pneumonia, or pneumothorax). The CXR film may nonspecifically reveal a PE or, commonly, it may be normal. Causes of pleuritic pain with a normal CXR result are PE, viral or idiopathic pleurisy, and serositis, especially from systemic lupus (5). Viral pleurisy, usually Coxsackie virus B, is characterized by unilateral acute pleuritic pain, variable low-grade fever, and nonproductive cough with typically a normal CXR film, which is an indistinguishable presentation from PE—20% presenting with acute pleuritic pain to the emergency room have PE and approximately 50% have viral or idiopathic pleurisy (1,2). Hence, acute pleuritic pain without an obvious cause on history and physical examination and CXR film requires exclusion of PE. A possible exception to this tenet is the young adult (aged <40 years) who is highly unlikely to have a PE if all three of the following clinical features are absent: (a) risk factors for or past history of venous thromboembolic disease, (b) physical findings of phlebitis, and (c) pleural effusion on CXR film (2). In the presence of an effusion without a clear cause of the pleuritic pain and PE either ruled out or clinically highly unlikely, a diagnostic thoracentesis is indicated. The effusion associated with pleuritic pain is nearly always an exudate. The most common causes of exudate in descending order of frequency are malignancy (most commonly lung cancer, breast cancer, lymphoma), pneumonia, PE, and viral, which together constitute 95% of these effusions (4).

References

1. Palevsky HI, Kelley MA, Fishman AP. Pulmonary thromboembolic disease. In: Fishman AP, ed. *Fishman's pulmonary diseases and disorders*. New York: McGraw-Hill, 1997:1297–1329.
2. Hull RD, Raskob GE. Pulmonary embolism in outpatients with pleuritic chest pain. *Arch Intern Med* 1988;148:838–844.
3. Stein PD. Acute pulmonary embolism. *Dis Mon* 1994;XL(9):467–515.
4. Light RW. *Pleural diseases*, 3rd ed. Baltimore: Williams & Wilkins, 1995:75–82, 187–191.
5. Staton Jr GW, Ingram Jr RH. Disorders of the pleura, hila, and mediastinum. In: Dale DC, ed. Sci Am Med St. Louis: Mosby, 1997; 14RespIX:1–19.

8.6 Pneumothorax

Kathleen E. Gallagher

Pneumothorax occurs when air enters the pleural space, the area between the visceral and parietal pleura. It is a common problem with a variety of different causes. In all cases, air enters the space because of a disruption or break in either the visceral or parietal pleura.

I. **Approach.** Pneumothorax can be classified into two major categories, spontaneous and traumatic.
   A. **Spontaneous pneumothorax**
      1. Primary spontaneous pneumothorax occurs in previously healthy individuals. It is seen generally in tall, slender persons, and in males approximately six times more often than in females (1). It is most common in persons in their early twenties, and is uncommon in those older than 40 years. Primary spontaneous pneumothorax is caused by a rupture of apical blebs or bullae. Cigarette smoking increases the possibility of primary spontaneous pneumothorax (1,4). The incidence in the United States is estimated at 10,000 cases per year (2).
      2. Secondary spontaneous pneumothorax occurs as a complication in individuals with underlying pulmonary disease. It is most common in persons with chronic obstructive pulmonary disease (COPD). Secondary spontaneous pneumothorax is also seen in persons with interstitial lung disease; infections, particularly *Pneumocystis carinii* pneumonia and tuberculosis; and neoplasms, either primary lung or metastatic tumors. The incidence is the same as that of primary spontaneous pneumothorax, an estimated 10,000 cases per year in the United States (2).
   B. **Traumatic pneumothorax**
      1. Iatrogenic pneumothorax occurs as a complication of medical procedures such as transthoracic needle biopsy, central venous catheter placement, thoracentesis, and bronchoscopy, or as a complication of mechanical ventilation.
      2. Penetrating and blunt trauma. Penetrating trauma, such as a stab wound, as the causative factor of pneumothorax is obvious: the wound allows air to enter through the chest wall. Pneumothorax can also be a result of blunt trauma, as sometimes occurs when a rib fracture pierces the visceral pleura. More often, however, decelerating forces of blunt chest trauma can lead to chest compression that can directly cause pneumothorax.
   C. **Special consideration—tension pneumothorax.** Tension pneumothorax occurs when a one-way valve allows air into, but not out of the pleural space. As pressure in the pleural space exceeds the atmospheric pressure, the ipsilateral lung, mediastinum, and contralateral lung are compressed. This is a medical emergency.
II. **History**
   A. **Spontaneous pneumothorax.** Chest pain, most often pleuritic and localized to the side of the pneumothorax, and dyspnea are the major symptoms. Onset is generally sudden. In primary spontaneous pneumothorax, symptoms are often mild, onset is usually at rest, and patients often do not immediately seek medical attention (2). Symptoms are generally more severe in patients with underlying lung disease who have impaired pulmonary reserve (3).
   B. **Traumatic pneumothorax.** Symptoms are the same as in spontaneous pneumothorax; although, in iatrogenic pneumothorax, they may not occur for 24 hours or more after the diagnostic or therapeutic procedure (3). Clin-

ical deterioration of patients on ventilators should raise suspicion of pneumothorax. This is more likely in patients with acute respiratory distress syndrome, necrotizing or aspiration pneumonia, COPD, or interstitial lung disease (3).

III. **Physical examination.** Vital signs can be normal, except for mild tachycardia, in healthy patients with spontaneous pneumothorax. Significant tachypnea can occur in patients with large pneumothoraces, or in patients with underlying pulmonary disease. Hypotension and severe tachycardia can be present in patients with tension pneumothorax. On chest and lung examination may be found unilateral enlargement of the chest cavity, loss of tactile fremitus, hyperresonance to percussion, and decreased, or absent, breath sounds on the affected side. Tracheal deviation may be seen, especially with tension pneumothorax.

IV. **Testing.** Arterial blood gas typically shows hypoxia and, occasionally, hypocarbia secondary to hyperventilation. Electrocardiographic changes may be seen, especially with left-sided pneumothorax, including axis deviation, nonspecific ST- and T-wave changes, ST depression, and T-wave inversion (3).

Chest x-ray study is generally paramount in the diagnosis, with visualization of the visceral pleural line and the absence of lung markings distal to this line. This is best seen on an upright film and can be enhanced by expiratory films, especially with small pneumothoraces. Lateral decubitus films may be helpful in critically ill patients who cannot sit upright (5). Computed tomography scans can also be useful when the chest x-ray study is not diagnostic.

V. **Diagnostic assessment.** In tall, slender, young men who have had acute onset of chest pain and dyspnea, the diagnosis of pneumothorax can be made by the history and physical examination, and confirmed with a chest radiograph visualizing the visceral pleural line. Patients who have had primary spontaneous pneumothorax are at risk for recurrence.

Secondary spontaneous pneumothorax can be a bit more difficult to diagnose. Although symptoms are more prominent, signs on physical examination are often subtle, especially in patients with COPD who tend to have decreased breath sounds and decreased tactile fremitus because of their underlying disease. Radiographic evaluation can be more difficult as well. Because of the lack of interstitial markings in the emphysematous lung, little difference is seen in the appearance proximal and distal to the visceral line. Also, an emphysematous bleb might be mistaken for a visceral line.

It is common to obtain a chest x-ray film after procedures that might lead to pneumothorax. Pleuritic chest pain and dyspnea, after associated diagnostic or therapeutic procedures, should alert practitioners, even if these symptoms occur many hours after the procedure. All patients with significant blunt trauma to the chest should be evaluated for pneumothorax, including all patients with rib or scapula fractures.

The diagnosis of tension pneumothorax must be made clinically, because there is not enough time for imaging studies. The diagnosis is confirmed by treatment: place a large bore needle through the second intercostal space approximately 2 to 3 cm from the edge of the sternum. A rush of air and relief of symptoms confirm the diagnosis.

References

1. Baum GL, Wolinsky E. *Textbook of pulmonary diseases*, 5th ed. Volume II. Boston: Little, Brown and Company, 1994;1871–1875.
2. Light RW. *Pleural diseases*, 3rd ed. Baltimore: Williams & Wilkins, 1995:242–277.
3. Jantz MA, Pierson DJ. Pneumothorax and barotrauma. *Clin Chest Med* 1994; 15(1):75–91.
4. Schramel FMNH, Postmus PE, Vanderschueren RGJRA. Current aspects of spontaneous pneumothorax. *Eur Respir J* 1997;10:1372–1379.
5. Spillane RM, Shepard JO, Deluca SA. Radiographic aspects of pneumothorax. *Am Fam Physician* 1995;51(2):459–464.

8.7 Shortness of Breath

Robert M. Theal

Shortness of breath, or dyspnea, accounts for 3.7% of all visits to medical clinics (1).

I. **Approach.** The initial history, physical examination, and chest x-ray (CXR) study are diagnostic in 66% to 92% of the patients (1). This symptom is present in many different illnesses. Fortunately, only a handful of disorders cause most of the cases; therefore, the most economical approach is to exclude acute life-threatening problems during the initial clinical examination. These include pneumonia, pulmonary embolus, acute heart failure, toxic exposure or ingestion, myocardial infarction, pneumothorax, life-threatening neuromuscular disease, or airway obstruction. If these are unlikely, then the next step is to systematically evaluate the patient for the most frequent disorders using common tests.

Shortness of breath has a long differential diagnosis, but respiratory and cardiac diseases account for 85% of the cases; in the remaining 15%, only a few illnesses are usually found (3). Of all the final diagnoses in dyspneic patients, the frequency of asthma is 18% to 33% and chronic obstructive pulmonary disease is 9% to 19% (1–4). Congestive heart failure (CHF) or pulmonary edema represents 11% to 63% of the cases (1–4). Other important diagnoses are deconditioning or obesity in 3% to 5% (1–4). Final diagnoses ranging between 0% and 10% include interstitial lung disease and ischemic heart disease (1–4). Table 8.3 lists less common diagnoses.

II. **History.** Are historical features helpful? Historical findings are neither sensitive nor specific; however, some symptoms are associated with specific diseases. Regardless of the cause, people associate shortness of breath with words that describe a sense of "work" or "effort" to breathe. Asthma is associated with words that denote a sense of "tightness." Patients with interstitial lung disease choose terms emphasizing the sense of "rapid" breathing. Did the patient select terms indicating difficulty with both inhalation and exhalation? This is often reported by patients with CHF (Chapter 7.5). Patients who are deconditioned select rapid, breathing more, or heavy to describe their dyspnea. Patients suffering from neuromuscular disorders select terms denoting rapid breathing or difficulty with inhalation. Is the patient aged less than 40 years? Are the patient's symptoms episodic? Reactive airway disease and hyperventilation are associated with these terms (2).

III. **Physical examination.** In the physical examination, focus on signs of respiratory or cardiac disease. For the respiratory system, this means a careful exami-

Table 8.3 Less common diagnoses of shortness of breath[a]

Anemia	Acute myocardial infarction
Acidosis	Atrial septal defect
Thyroid disease	Ventricular septal defect
Neuromuscular disease	Mitral stenosis
Pulmonary infection	Pericardial disease
Pulmonary embolus	Chest wall deformity
Pulmonary hypertension	Gastroesophageal reflux disease
Pulmonary effusion	Postnasal drip
Neoplasia	Sleep apnea
Airway obstruction	Hyperventilation
Arrhythmia	

[a] Frequencies between 0% and 5%.

nation starting at the nose. Specifically, on head, eyes, ear, nose, and throat examination look for evidence of obstruction, infection, or postnasal drip. Exclude obstruction, subcutaneous emphysema, or tracheal deviation. On cardiac examination, look for evidence of cardiomegaly, S_3 gallop, or hepatojugular reflux (HJR). In this setting, HJR is very specific for CHF (1). Assess the lungs for abnormal breath sound intensity, rales, wheezing, rhonchi, or tachypnea. Examine the chest for abnormal movements or deformities. Exclude abdominal masses, ascites, pregnancy, or abdominal distention. Evaluate the extremities for edema, tenderness, or asymmetry. Do a complete neurologic examination, and screen for weakness atrophy, sensory loss, and fasciculations.

IV. Testing. Most patients require a CXR study and pulse oximetry to screen for cardiac and pulmonary diseases. Use an arterial blood gas (ABG) analysis to confirm hypoxia, hypercapnia, hypocapnia, and acidosis. Complete blood count (CBC), electrolytes, thyroid-stimulating hormone (TSH), and drug screens are useful for suspected cases of anemia, acidosis, hyperthyroidism, hypothyroidism, or drug ingestions.

Pulmonary function studies (PFTs) are important to document the presence of obstructive or restrictive lung diseases. A methacholine challenge test is used if the symptoms are intermittent, the patient is aged less than 40 years, or if lung disease is suspected and the PFTs are normal. In this setting, the results will confirm or exclude asthma (3). In dyspneic patients, a lung diffusion capacity (DLCO) has a high positive predictive value and a high negative predictive value for interstitial lung disease (3). Low maximal inspiratory and expiratory pressures suggest neuromuscular disease.

The cardiac causes of dyspnea are CHF, intracardiac shunts, valvular heart disease, pulmonary hypertension, and pericardial disease. They have abnormal or characteristic findings on echocardiography and Doppler echocardiography. An electrocardiogram (ECG) or exercise stress test (EST) screens for arrhythmias and ischemic heart disease. **Warning:** A negative EST does not exclude ischemia in dyspneic patients (3) (Chapter 7.1).

Other tests are used in selected patients. High resolution computerized tomography (CT) of the chest detects early interstitial lung disease in patients with normal CXR films. Electromyogram (EMG) and nerve conduction studies are useful for confirming and differentiating the most common neuromuscular problems: myasthenia gravis and Guillain-Barré syndrome. A therapeutic response to H_2 blockers confirms gastroesophageal reflux disease (GERD) in most dyspneic patients (2). Screen for acute or chronic pulmonary embolism with a nuclear medicine ventilation and perfusion ($\dot{V}/\dot{Q}$) scan.

V. Diagnostic assessment. The initial assessment usually requires a clinical evaluation, CXR study, and pulse oximetry. This identifies about 70% of the underlying diseases (1). For the remainder, a systematic evaluation for the most common diseases will correctly identify the cause. If appropriate, consider obtaining an ECG, CBC, TSH, and electrolytes. If theses are nondiagnostic, then further testing is indicated.

Exclude pulmonary diseases if the initial evaluation is nondiagnostic, or if pulmonary diseases are suspected, which account for 75% of the cases (3). Start with PFTs and an ABG. If the PFTs are normal, then order a methacholine challenge test to rule out asthma. If interstitial lung disease is suspected or if the PFTs show a restrictive pattern, then order a DLCO. Abnormally low maximal inspiratory and expiratory pressures suggest neuromuscular disease. Confirm the diagnosis with an EMG.

When pulmonary disease has been excluded, or if cardiac disease is suspected, the next step should be a cardiac evaluation. An echocardiogram will suggest or identify most of the cardiac causes. If the echocardiogram is normal, consider exercise stress testing or a Holter monitor. If these are normal, then most patients will have either GERD, deconditioning, or psychogenic disorders. Other low frequency causes of shortness of breath that need further evaluation include neuromuscular diseases, pulmonary emboli, postnasal drip, and sleep apnea. With a clinical suspicion of these disorders, obtain an EMG, $\dot{V}/\dot{Q}$ scan, or polysomnogram. Otherwise, they are not indicated.

References

1. Mulrow CD, Lucey CR, Farnett LE. Discriminating causes of dyspnea through clinical examination. *J Gen Intern Med* 1993;8:383–392.
2. DePaso WJ, Winterbauer RH, Lusk JA, Dreis DF, Springmeyer SC. Chronic dyspnea unexplained by history, physical examination, chest roentgenogram, and spirometry. *Chest* 1991;100:1293–1299.
3. Pratter MR, Curley FJ, Dubois J, Irwin RS. Cause and evaluation of chronic dyspnea in a pulmonary disease clinic. *Arch Intern Med* 1989;149:2277–2282.
4. Schmitt BP, Kushner MS, Wiener SL. The diagnostic usefulness of the history of the patient with dyspnea. *J Gen Intern Med* 1986;1:386–393.
5. Mahler DA, Harver A, Lentine T, Scott JA, Beck K, Schwartzstein M. Descriptors of breathlessness in cardiorespiratory diseases. *Am J Respir Crit Care Med* 1996;154:1357–1363.

8.8 Stridor

Alexandra Duke and Tahany Maurice-Habashy

Stridor is a common type of wheezing (Chapter 8.9). It is characterized by a harsh, raspy, medium-pitched sound produced as air flows through a partially blocked airway. It is usually seen in early childhood.

  I. **Approach.** Stridor can be inspiratory, indicating obstruction at or above the larynx; or expiratory, indicating obstruction below the larynx. Biphasic stridor is an obstruction in the trachea; it is heard with inspiration and expiration. When hoarseness or aphonia accompanies stridor, the vocal cords are involved (Table 8.4) (1–5).
 II. **History**
     A. **Characteristics of stridor.** When confronted with stridor, check the age of the patient and the duration of the symptoms.
        1. A child aged less than 6 months with stridor of a few weeks to months has a congenital cause of stridor.
        2. Patients aged more than 6 months with stridor lasting hours to days usually have an acquired cause of stridor, most commonly viral croup, epiglottitis, or aspiration of a foreign body.
        3. A typical history is a child aged less than 6 years with a 2- to 3-day history of upper respiratory infection (URI) and gradually worsening cough,

Table 8.4 Common causes of stridor

CONGENITAL[a]	INFLAMMATORY
Laryngomalacia	Laryngotracheobronchitis (croup)
Laryngeal cysts and webs	Epiglottitis, bacterial tracheitis
Laryngeal hemangiomas	Retropharyngeal abscess
Tumors	Allergic edema
Subglottic stenosis	Diphtheria, tetanus
Vocal cord dysfunction	
Micrognathia	NONINFLAMMATORY
Vascular ring	Foreign body
Ectopic thyroid	Gastroesophageal reflux disease
Cri du chat	Hysterical stridor
Macroglossia	

[a] More common under 6 months of age.

especially at night. A barking cough with the inspiratory stridor heralds the diagnosis of croup, which accounts for 90% of all cases of stridor. This condition will classically improve with moist air (1,3).

4. A history of choking, coughing, or gagging points to aspiration or ingestion of a foreign body.

5. In older children and adults, a concomitant sore throat and fever may indicate acute supraglottitis, which constitutes an emergency.

B. Other information

1. Whether stridor is acute, recurrent, or chronic.

2. Personal or family history of atopy, would suggest spasmodic croup, which presents with stridor at night, not necessarily associated with a URI.

III. Physical examination

A. Focused physical examination (PE)

1. The PE should include vital signs, notably temperature and respiratory rate, and pulse, with emphasis on general appearance and examination of the head and neck, including ears, nose, and throat.

2. Signs of respiratory distress may be present, including dyspnea, tachypnea, chest retractions, nasal flaring, and stridor. If cyanosis is present, this is an ominous sign (2,4) (Chapter 8.2).

B. Additional physical examination may reveal:

1. A toxic-appearing child with high fever, drooling, severe respiratory distress, and preference for a sitting and forward-leaning position (1,4)

2. Varying degrees of anxiety, which will increase during examination, cause a worsening of stridor (1,4)

IV. Testing

A. The best test is a lateral neck x-ray study to assist with a diagnosis that is mostly made on clinical grounds. Films of the larynx and trachea in anteroposterior and lateral neck views may show narrowing of the trachea or extrinsic pressure on the tracheobronchial airway. Acutely, lateral neck radiographs showing the classic swollen glottis described by some as a thumbprint, assist with the diagnosis of acute supraglottitis and eminent respiratory collapse. Chest x-ray studies are of little value. Films showing hyperinflation or bronchial thickening may help to make a diagnosis of asthma rather than stridor. Additionally, foreign body aspiration or mass will be elucidated in x-ray studies (2).

B. Tomograms or computed tomography (CT) of the neck may provide additional information, especially in chronic stridor (2).

C. Blood tests (e.g., complete blood count) can be useful in the acutely ill patient, especially if viral or bacterial infection is suspected.

D. With suspicion that the stridor is a result of a laryngomalacia or laryngeal lesions such as papilloma, direct laryngoscopy is the test of choice for accurate diagnosis. Direct observation via fiberoptic bronchoscope positioned in the pharynx would provide diagnostic views of the larynx (2,4).

V. Diagnostic assessment.
In making the diagnosis of stridor, two key elements exist: acute onset in a toxic-appearing patient, versus chronic stridor in a relatively stable patient.

A. Acute stridor

1. The most likely cause of acute stridor in the febrile child with the additional features of barking cough and antecedent coryza is laryngotracheobronchitis or croup. Acute stridor is a non–life-threatening condition accounting for 90% of stridor cases. Classically, it improves with exposure to moist air. It has a viral cause, usually from one of the following: respiratory syncytial virus, rhinovirus, adenovirus, parainfluenza virus, and influenza virus. Generally, this diagnosis is made on clinical grounds (1). The child is less ill and, although often febrile, not toxic appearing. The entire illness usually abates in 5 days. Hospitalization, unlike with epiglottitis, is rarely needed (2).

2. In the toxic patient with fever, respiratory distress, sore throat, or drooling, especially in the younger age group, consider epiglottitis—a medical

emergency. As use of the *Haemophilus influenzae* vaccine has increased in recent years, acute epiglottis is becoming increasingly rare. *H. influenzae* is the most common bacterial cause of stridor, although streptococcus, staphylococcus and viral agents are also possible causes.

3. The patient with a history of suspected foreign body aspiration will have similar symptoms without fever. Foreign body aspiration is common in the 1- to 2-year age groups, although it does occur in adults. It can be a cause of chronic stridor (3).

4. Additionally, an acute allergic reaction can cause stridor. The history should herald a possible offending agent and, although respiratory collapse may be eminent, the patient will not be toxic, as no infectious agent is involved.

5. Trauma can also cause laryngeal damage; however, the history will assist with this diagnosis.

B. **Chronic stridor.** For the most part, these causes of stridor occur in early childhood. With the exception of laryngeal papillomas, tumors, and subglottic stenosis after instrumentation as in intubation (there is a congenital form also), foreign body aspiration with partial obstruction and hysterical stridor can occur at any age. Laryngomalacia and laryngeal lesions are caused by webs, hemangiomas, and cysts; they are usually identified early in life (1–3).

References

1. Pryor MP. Noisy breathing in children. *Postgrad Med* 1997;101:103–112.
2. Behrman RE, Kliegman RM, Arvin AM. *Nelson textbook of pediatrics*. Philadelphia: WB Saunders, 1996:241, 1173, 1198, 1238.
3. Behrman RE, Vaughan VC. *Nelson textbook of pediatrics*. Philadelphia: WB Saunders, 1983:1031–1032, 1076–1077.
4. Tintinalli JE, Ruiz E, Krome RL. *Emergency medicine: a comprehensive study guide*. New York: McGraw-Hill, 1996:247–251.
5. Campbell AGM, MacIntosh N. *Textbook of pediatrics*. London: Pearson Ltd., 1998: 508–513, 563.

8.9 Wheezing

Thomas C. Bent

Wheezing is one of the most common respiratory complaints to present to primary care physicians. Although most often caused by asthma or chronic obstructive pulmonary disease, there are multiple causes. The correct diagnosis can usually be made with a careful history and physical examination and simple diagnostic testing.

I. **Approach.** Although asthma is the first consideration in the wheezing patient—and most often the correct diagnosis—careful consideration of less common but potentially more dangerous causes must be considered.

A. **Wheezing in infants, children, and adults.** The reasons patients wheeze vary dramatically, depending on age. For example, whereas asthma is the most common chronic pediatric disease in industrialized nations (1), inhalant allergens appear to be unimportant precipitants of wheezing in infancy (2). (Table 8.5).

B. **Wheezing versus stridor.** Stridor, discussed in Chapter 8.8, is characterized as an inspiratory wheeze that implies major obstruction of the upper airway. Wheezing, in contrast, is defined as high-pitched, continuous (or of long duration) adventitious lung sounds that are superimposed on the normal breath sounds (3). The inspiratory phase of respiration is usually normal and the expiratory phase is prolonged. Unfortunately, the difference is

Table 8.5   Etiology of wheezing by age group

INFANTS

bronchiolitis, pertussis, recurrent aspiration during feeding, gastroesophageal reflux disease, foreign body inhalation, bronchopulmonary dysplasia, cystic fibrosis, tracheoesophageal fistula, congenital malformations

CHILDREN

asthma, bronchiolitis, tracheomalacia, gastroesophageal reflux, sinusitis, foreign bodies, cystic fibrosis, and pulmonary hemosiderosis

ADULTS

asthma, chronic obstructive pulmonary disease, acute infections, foreign body inhalation, intra-airway tumor, extrinsic tumor with airway compression, interstitial lung disease

---

not always obvious to the clinician. Vocal cord dysfunction, which is a psychosomatic disorder, can be difficult to differentiate from asthma. The episodes can include both inspiratory and expiratory wheezing and an upper airway cause is not clear (4).

C. **Special concerns: the emergency assessment.** The immediate assessment of the acutely wheezing patient is essential. Regardless of whether the patient presents with an initial episode or a chronic condition, determine the degree of airway obstruction and the potential deterioration of the patient quickly. The reduction in intensity of wheezing can indicate acute decompensation, as air obstruction becomes too severe to allow the mechanical sounds of wheezing.

II. **History**

A. **Onset.** Is this the first episode? If so, were there problems with wheezing or asthma in childhood?

B. **Exposures.** Are there any precipitating factors? Have there been any recent exposures? Is there an exposure to cigarette smoke? What is the patient's occupation?

  1. Cigarette smoke is one of the most potent and ubiquitous avoidable allergens.

  2. Occupational exposures can frequently be identified, especially among agricultural and industrial workers.

  3. Family or household exposure to tuberculosis or pertussis can indicate an infectious cause.

C. **Concurrent illnesses.** Has the patient recently suffered an upper respiratory infection or sinusitis? Is there a history of gastroesophageal reflux disease?

D. **Family history.** A history of asthma, allergies, or atopic disease in family members can support the diagnosis of asthma.

E. **Past history.** A childhood history of atopic disease or allergies suggests adult onset asthma. Past history of exercise-induced wheezing also supports this diagnosis.

F. **Psychosocial aspects.** Emotional stress can lead to exacerbation of chronic asthma. Psychogenic wheezing is a conversion disorder, which can coexist with other psychopathology.

III. **Physical examination**

A. **Vital signs.** A full set of vital signs is essential to the assessment of the wheezing patient. The respiratory rate and the pulse are a more objective, and often more accurate, assessment of the severity of wheezing than the auditory volume of the wheezing itself. Fever suggests a concurrent respiratory infection. Hypotension is an ominous sign that points to a decompensating patient.

B. **Lung examination.** During auscultation, note the location, intensity, and duration of wheezing. Wheezing caused by asthma, chronic obstructive pulmonary disease (COPD), or interstitial disease should be diffuse and symmetric and present during expiration. The expiratory phase will be prolonged. Focal obstruction (e.g., tumors and foreign bodies) can give asymmetric findings and inspiratory wheezing. Mucus plugging will change with cough. Rhonchi and crackles suggest a concurrent infectious process. Percussion and egophony can be present with consolidation.

IV. Testing

   A. Pulmonary function. A peak flow meter is a valuable initial assessment of airway obstruction and can be done quickly and cheaply in the office. It is also an excellent measure of progression of disease or success of treatment. Pulse oximeter is another quick, noninvasive office technique to assess the severity of both chronic disease and acute respiratory distress. Full spirometry, although not available in all primary care offices, gives additional diagnostic information that can differentiate among asthma, COPD, and fixed airway obstruction.

   B. Chest x-ray study. Plain chest films will identify consolidation, masses, mediastinal shifts, and hyperaeration.

   C. Clinical laboratory tests. A complete blood count may demonstrate signs of an acute bacterial infection. Polycythemia is a sign of chronic hypoxia (Chapter 16.5). Eosinophilia can indicate asthma or allergic disease (Chapter 16.2). Angiotensin-converting enzyme levels are elevated in sarcoidosis. A tuberculin skin test should be considered in all patients with wheezing or chronic cough.

V. Diagnostic assessment. The history and physical examination are the key elements to an acute diagnosis. A consistent exposure or reaction history, coupled with an elevated serum IgE or eosinophilia, indicates allergic disease. Wheezing in the setting of acute bronchitis or sinusitis is not true asthma and the patient can be reassured that this is not the beginning of a chronic disease. Inspiratory wheezing, or stridor, indicates upper airway obstruction or psychogenic wheezing. A normal, or nearly normal, peak flow is reassurance that good air exchange is occurring, regardless of the loudness of the wheezing. The pulse oximetry will differentiate between severe obstruction and poor cooperation with the peak flow testing. When confusion still exists, spirometry will clarify the diagnosis in most cases. The diagnosis and treatment of most cases of wheezing is within the scope of practice of the primary care physician.

References

1. Pryor MP. Noisy breathing in children. *Postgrad Med* 1997;101:103–111.
2. Martinati LC, Boner AL. Clinical diagnosis of wheezing in early childhood. *Allergy* 1995;50:701–710.
3. Meslier N, Charbonneau G, Racineux JL. Wheezes. *Eur Respir J* 1995;8:1942–1948.
4. Goldman J. All that wheezes is not asthma. *Practitioner* 1997;241:35–38.

9. GASTROINTESTINAL PROBLEMS

MICHAEL R. SPIEKER

9.1 Abdominal Pain

Richard W. Emerine

Abdominal pain of varying causes, ranging from the functional to the organic, is one of the top ten outpatient complaints; it is the chief complaint for 5% to 10% of patients presenting to emergency departments (1).

I. **Approach.** Rapid assessment is aimed at determining whether the abdominal pain is emergent or nonemergent. This assessment should be tempered with the understanding that in certain populations (the elderly, the young, the immune compromised) signs and symptoms of ominous disease can be blunted or absent.
   A. **Emergent abdominal pain.** Did the patient experience sudden or severe pain or demonstrate hemodynamic changes—hypotension or tachycardia? Is the patient pregnant? (Up to 13% of women with a positive pregnancy test and abdominal pain have an ectopic pregnancy.) Emergent intervention is required for abdominal aortic aneurysm (AAA), bowel obstruction, ruptured spleen, and ruptured ectopic pregnancy.
   B. **Nonemergent abdominal pain.** When emergent causes are reasonably excluded, nonemergent causes can be considered. Common nonurgent conditions include functional bowel syndrome, urinary tract infections (UTI), constipation, renal stones, cholelithiasis, gastroenteritis, and dysmenorrhea.
II. **History**
   A. **History of present illness.** Medication use, alcohol and tobacco history, and menstrual history in women are vital. When did the pain begin and what are the characteristics of the pain? Use the "OPQRST" approach outlined below to question the patient about pain characteristics.
      1. **O:** Onset of pain. Pain of sudden onset or that awakens a patient from sleep can represent appendicitis, leaking abdominal aortic aneurysm, ectopic pregnancy, pancreatitis, or perforating ulcer. Gradual onset of pain can represent cholecystitis, diverticulitis, inflammatory bowel disorders, or pancreatitis. Longstanding pain without debility that is worsened by emotional stress is suggestive of irritable bowel syndrome.
      2. **P:** Palliative or Provocative factors (diet, exercise, sleep, bowel movement, and so on).
      3. **Q:** Quality of pain—pain descriptors are often associated with specific causes:
         a. "Burning" pain—ulcer
         b. "Agony"—pancreatitis
         c. "Shearing" or "tearing"—abdominal aortic aneurysm
         d. "Colicky" or "cramping"—cholecystitis, bowel obstruction, urolithiasis, irritable bowel syndrome
         e. "Constant ache"—appendicitis, peritonitis, herpes zoster
      4. **R:** Radiation or Referred—pain from appendicitis, simple colic, and bowel obstruction from strangulation or volvulus is often first felt in the epigastrium. Abdominal causes may result in referred or radiating pain to extraabdominal sites:
         a. Abdominal aortic aneurysm—to the midback
         b. Biliary colic—to the right scapula
         c. Renal colic—to the costovertebral angles, testicle, or thigh
         d. Hernias—to the genitalia
      5. Extraabdominal pathology can cause referred pain to the abdomen.
         a. Cardiac ischemia—to the epigastrium
         b. Scrotal pathology—to the abdomen

6. **S:** Severity—level of intensity (some use a 1–10 scale)
7. **T:** Time or Temporal relationships—with meals, after bowel movement, menses, and so on

B. **Past medical history.** Is there a history of previous abdominal or pelvic surgery? Prior abdominal surgery increases the risk for bowel incarceration, obstruction, and strangulation. Fallopian tube surgery and prior pelvic inflammatory disease (PID) increase a woman's risk for ectopic pregnancy (Chapter 11.3).

C. **Review of systems.** Are there associated symptoms that point to a specific etiology? Chills and fever suggest infectious causes (UTI, PID, prostatitis, and pneumonia). Emesis occurring before the onset of pain is associated with appendicitis; with the onset of pain, cholecystitis or urolithiasis; after onset of pain, gastroenteritis. Late onset or feculent emesis suggests bowel obstruction; bilious emesis occurs in cholecystitis. Postprandial right upper quadrant pain is common in cholecystitis. Diarrhea with a recent travel history suggests dysentery or parasitic infections. Genitourinary complaints (dysuria, frequency, hematuria, vaginal discharge, and dypareunia) should prompt evaluation for UTI, sexually transmitted disease, and PID.

III. **Physical examination.** A thorough, targeted physical examination, directed by a complete history, leads to a correct diagnosis in most cases (2).

Complete vital signs are essential. Tachycardia or hypotension can indicate hypovolemia and the need for urgent intervention (Chapter 7.12). Rapid, shallow breaths occur with peritoneal irritation. Inspect the abdomen for distention (obstruction), pulsations (AAA), or scars from past surgery. High-pitched hyperactive bowel sounds occur with bowel obstruction. Palpation and percussion help localize tenderness, organomegaly, and masses. Pain with movement, rebound tenderness, or rigidity are indicative of peritonitis and should prompt surgical consultation.

Cardiovascular, pulmonary, and digital rectal and genitourinary examinations should be included in all evaluations of significant abdominal pain. The pelvic examination must be done to exclude ectopic pregnancy and PID. Among patients in whom pregnancy is a possibility, the presence of peritoneal signs, cervical motion tenderness, or lateral (or bilateral) abdominal or pelvic tenderness should raise concern about possible ectopic pregnancy (3).

IV. **Testing**
A. **Clinical laboratory tests.** Human chorionic gonadotrophin should be obtained if the patient has any potential for pregnancy. If appendicitis is suspected, sensitivity approaches 96% when both the total white blood cell count and neutrophil counts are elevated. Overall, however, hemograms do not by themselves often result in a change of disposition. Serum electrolytes are generally of little diagnostic value, except for the anesthesia provider if surgery is contemplated.

Urinalysis may identify urinary infection or calculi. Liver function tests in patients with right upper quadrant pain may help differentiate hepatitis and hepatobiliary disease (Chapter 9.8). Serum amylase is not a specific test for pancreatitis; it can be elevated in many other conditions that cause abdominal pain. Serum lipase has a higher sensitivity and specificity for pancreatitis than total amylase (4).

B. **Diagnostic imaging**
1. **Plain films.** Plain radiographs have utility primarily when attempting to identify specific abdominal pathology such as renal stones, perforated viscus, or bowel obstruction. They can detect as little as 5 ml of free air. Up to five air-fluid levels of less than 2.5 cm in length may be normal; however, dilation of the small bowel beyond 2.5 cm suggests obstruction.
2. **Ultrasonography.** Abdominal and pelvic sonograms are rapid, inexpensive, and noninvasive. They are especially accurate in detecting hepatobiliary, pancreatic, aortic, pelvic, and renal pathology.
3. **Computed tomography (CT).** Consider for patients with challenging presentations. CT is valuable in identifying abscesses, hematomas, and

pancreatitis, and in evaluating solid organs and the abdominal vascular system; it is remarkably useful in evaluating patients with trauma. Magnetic resonance imaging has not proved particularly beneficial in the evaluation of acute abdominal pain.

V. **Diagnostic assessment.** The critical key is to identify the patient with an acute surgical abdomen. Physical examination coupled with a careful history narrows the differential diagnosis so that confirmation can be made by appropriately selected laboratory and imaging studies. In most cases, a good clinical history augmented by a focused physical examination leads to a correct diagnosis with limited need for further testing. Extremes of age, an impaired immune system, use of pain medications, and obesity can complicate the evaluation. Surgical consultation should be obtained immediately for patients with abdominal pain accompanied by peritoneal signs or shock.

References

1. Powers RD, Guertler AT. Abdominal pain in the ED: stability and change over 20 years. *Am J Emerg Med* 1995;13:301–303.
2. Silen W, ed. *Cope's early diagnosis of the acute abdomen*, 19th ed. New York: Oxford University Press, 1996.
3. Dart RG. Predictive value of history and physical examination in patients with suspected ectopic pregnancy. *Ann Emerg Med* 1999;33:283–290.
4. Gwozdz GP, Steinberg WM, Werner M, Henry JP, Pauley C. Comparative evaluation of the diagnosis of acute pancreatitis based on serum and urine enzyme assays. *Clin Chim Acta* 1990;187:243–254.

9.2 Ascites

C. Randall Clinch

Ascites, the accumulation of fluid within the abdominal cavity, is the most common major complication of cirrhosis; it is present in 50% of patients with cirrhosis of 10 years' duration (1). Ascites has important prognostic implications, carrying a 50% 2-year mortality rate (1). Once identified, an investigation should follow to determine its cause and plan appropriate management.

In the United States, most (80%) adult patients with ascites have cirrhosis caused by alcoholic hepatitis (Laennec's cirrhosis), hemochromatosis, Wilson's disease, autoimmune cirrhosis, or an idiopathic cause (1). Heart failure, constrictive pericarditis, peritoneal infection and inflammation (e.g., tuberculosis, viral hepatitis, chlamydia), nephrotic syndrome, malignancy, pancreatitis, marked hypoalbuminemia (<2 g/dl), trauma, or fulminant hepatic failure are the cause of ascites in approximately 20% of patients. Of patients, 5% have "mixed ascites," or ascites from two causes (e.g., hemochromatosis and heart failure; Laennec's cirrhosis and pancreatitis).

I. **Approach**
   A. **Urgent need for diagnosis.** An urgent approach to diagnosis may arise in patients with an extremely distended abdomen and respiratory compromise. Patients with a large umbilical herniation, which can rupture, or patients with encephalopathy, fever, and decreased urine output also warrant immediate diagnosis.
   B. **Nonurgent need for diagnosis.** Nonurgent scenarios are more common. The approach to diagnosis is the same, based on a thorough history, physical examination, and ascitic fluid analysis.
II. **History**
   A. **Does the patient use alcohol or drugs?** Alcoholic hepatitis is the most common cause of cirrhosis and ascites. Intravenous drug use places the patient at risk for ascites from either acute or chronic viral hepatitis (hepatitis B and C).

B. **Is the patient at risk for sexually transmitted diseases?** Hepatitis B is commonly acquired sexually, therefore a complete sexual history is mandatory.

C. **Is the patient otherwise at risk for acquiring hepatitis?** Other individuals at risk include hemodialysis patients, recipients of organ transplantations, close contacts of persons with hepatitis, members of high-risk populations (Asia, the South Pacific, sub-Saharan Africa), recipients of blood or blood products, individuals with tattoos, prior acupuncture or ear piercing, and needlestick victims.

D. **Does the patient have signs of fluid retention?** Ask about increased abdominal girth, weight gain, leg edema, penile or scrotal edema, and umbilical herniation (Chapter 2.3).

E. **Are there any secondary symptoms to suggest fluid retention?** Increased abdominal fluid leads to vague complaints of nausea, anorexia, early satiety, heartburn, abdominal pain, shortness of breath, or orthopnea.

F. **Is there a suspicion of infection?** Of patients admitted with ascites, 10% to 27% have spontaneous bacterial peritonitis (SBP); 48% to 57% of these patients will die (4). Ask about fever, abdominal pain, or mental status changes (encephalopathy) (Chapters 2.6, 3.2, and 9.1).

G. **Is there a past history of heart failure, cancer, or tuberculosis?** These are included in the 20% of nonhepatic causes of ascites.

III. **Physical examination.** Obtain vital signs (temperature, respiratory rate, blood pressure, and weight). Ascites is rarely the sole physical finding. Examine for evidence of liver disease (jaundice, spider angiomata, Dupuytren's contracture, caput medusae); hepatomegaly may be absent if chronic cirrhosis exists. Examine the skin for evidence of intravenous (IV) drug use, tattoos, and pigment changes (hemochromatosis). Jugular venous distention, a third heart sound, pulmonary crackles, and peripheral edema suggest heart failure. Abdominal tenderness can reflect pancreatitis or infection. Tests for ascites include shifting dullness, bulging flanks, flank dullness, fluid wave, and the "puddle" sign (i.e., percussing the abdomen with the patient on hands and knees). The reliability of these tests are unpredictable (2). These techniques are not helpful when a small volume (<1,000 ml) of ascites exists; 1,500 ml of fluid must be present before shifting dullness is detected. The "puddle" sign is no longer considered valuable because of its low sensitivity and patient discomfort (2,5).

IV. **Testing**

A. **Diagnostic paracentesis** should be performed to determine the nature of the ascitic fluid and to evaluate for the presence of SBP.

B. **An ascitic fluid polymorphonuclear leukocyte count** of more than 250 cells/mm^3 indicates infection (SBP) and the patient should be empirically treated as such.

C. **If a culture** is obtained, 10 ml of ascitic fluid should be injected into blood culture bottles at the bedside to increase sensitivity (1,4).

D. **The serum-ascites albumin gradient (SAAG)** is the difference between the serum albumin concentration and the ascitic fluid albumin concentration. This gradient is 97% accurate in determining the underlying mechanism of ascites and replaces the former classification of ascitic fluid as either a transudate or an exudate (1). An SAAG of more than 1.1 g/dl indicates the patient has portal hypertension (seen with diagnoses such as cirrhosis, heart failure, alcoholic hepatitis, massive metastatic liver disease, or Budd-Chiari syndrome) (4). An SAAG of less than 1.1 g/dl indicates the patient does not have portal hypertension and a process such as peritoneal carcinomatosis, tuberculous peritonitis, pancreatic ascites, serositis from connective tissue diseases, nephrotic syndrome, or biliary ascites may be present (1,4).

E. **Cytology, smear, and culture for mycobacteria** are expensive and have very low yields. They should only be ordered if there is a very high pretest probability.

F. **Other tests** that can be ordered include amylase (pancreatic ascites), triglycerides (chylous ascites), and lactate dehydrogenase and glucose (secondary peritonitis) (4).

G. Ultrasonography can detect as little as 100 ml of fluid in the abdomen (3). It is useful both for confirming the presence of ascites and in guiding diagnostic paracentesis.

V. Diagnostic assessment. If ascites is suspected on history and physical examination, a diagnostic paracentesis should be performed. Basic orders include a cell count and differential and albumin concentration (ascitic and serum). The SAAG should be calculated. Culture and other optional tests should be performed, based on clinical suspicion. If the diagnosis is uncertain because of a low volume of ascites, an ultrasound should be performed to guide a diagnostic paracentesis. If the patient is having significant symptoms or tense ascites, a therapeutic large-volume paracentesis should be performed and the fluid analyzed as above. Complications of paracentesis have been reported in approximately 1% of patients (i.e., abdominal wall hematomas), including those with an underlying coagulopathy (1).

A. Indications for hospitalization (5) or referral include:
1. Worsening ascites despite initial management attempts
2. Tense ascites
3. Systemic signs or symptoms (liver failure, renal failure, encephalopathy, pancreatitis, gastrointestinal bleeding)
4. Suspicion of infection (SBP)
5. Patient noncompliant with medical management

References

1. Runyon BA. Management of adult patients with ascites caused by cirrhosis. AASLD practice guidelines. *Hepatology* 1998;27(1):264–272.
2. Cattau EL, Benjamin SB, Knuff TE, Castell DO. The accuracy of the physical examination in the diagnosis of suspected ascites. *JAMA* 1982;247:1164.
3. Goldberg BB, Goodman GA, Clearfield HR. Evaluation of ascites by ultrasound. *Radiology* 1970;96:15–22.
4. Habeeb KS, Herrera JL. Management of ascites. Paracentesis as a guide. *Postgrad Med* 1997;101(1):191–200.
5. Lipsky MS, Sternbach MR. Evaluation and initial management of patients with ascites. *Am Fam Physician* 1996;54(4):1327–1333.

9.3 Constipation

W. Robert Kiser

I. Approach. Constipation, defined as the passage of two or fewer stools per week (1), is the most frequently reported gastrointestinal (GI) complaint in primary care, responsible for as many as 1.25 million patient visits annually (2).

A. The potential causes are legion, but can be generally classified by the acrostic **MADE-O-FUN:**
1. **M:** medications (anticholinergics, antispasmotics, antacids containing aluminum or calcium, diuretics, clonidine, calcium channel blockers, overuse of laxatives, narcotics, and others)
2. **A:** activity—general inactivity or debility
3. **D:** dietary—inadequate fluid and food intake
4. **E:** electrolytes and endocrine—hypokalemia, hypercalcemia, hypothyroidism, uremia, diabetes mellitus
5. **O:** obstruction—tumor, stricture, rectocoele, foreign body
6. **F:** functional—depression or irritable bowel syndrome
7. **U:** unusual things—thankfully, rare!
8. **N:** neurologic disorders—parkinsonism, multiple sclerosis, autonomic insufficiency associated with diabetes mellitus

II. History. The assessment and evaluation of the constipated patient begins with the history.

    A. What is the patient's description of the onset, duration, and frequency of constipation? Constipation of recent onset is suggestive of tumor.

    B. Is rectal bleeding, melena, or narrowing of the stool caliber (all suggesting neoplasia) present (Chapter 9.11)?

    C. What over-the-counter (OTC) medications are being used? (Is this patient potentially abusing OTC laxatives or taking OTC "cold" medicine containing an antihistamine?) Does the onset of constipation coincide with the taking of any of the medications listed in the MADE-O-FUN acrostic?

    D. Does the past medical history, past surgical history, systems review, or chart review suggest any of the associated systemic illness listed in MADE-O-FUN? Is the patient known to have parkinsonism, renal failure, diabetes mellitus, hypertension (possibly treated with medications such as clonidine, calcium channel blockers, or potassium depleting diuretics, or other medications potentially causing decreased colonic tone), or hypothyroidism? Is there a history of cancer (potentially associated with hypercalcemia)?

III. Physical examination. Undertake a general physical examination looking for the stigmata of the associated constitutional illnesses mentioned in the MADE-O-FUN acrostic. Target the abdominal examination specifically for masses or abdominal tenderness and the rectal examination for fecal occult blood, rectal tone, rectal masses, rectal foreign body, impaction, anal fissure, hemorrhoids, or rectocoele—essential parts of the evaluation.

IV. Diagnostic testing. Laboratory evaluation should consist of fecal occult blood testing (FOBT) looking for rectal bleeding; serum potassium and calcium to rule out hypokalemia and hypercalcemia (both associated with decreased colonic tone); serum glucose to evaluate possible diabetes; complete blood count looking for anemia (possibly related to chronic GI blood loss from tumor); blood urea nitrogen, serum creatinine, or both to rule out renal failure; and thyroid stimulating hormone to evaluate for hypothyroidism.

    Visualize the lower colon via flexible sigmoidoscopy in patients aged more than 40 years whose constipation is of recent origin. Flexible sigmoidoscopy alone is insufficient for patients whose findings could suggest colonic neoplasia (melena, positive FOBT, hematochezia, abdominal mass, unexplained weight loss, or unexplained anemia). These patients should be offered either (a) colonoscopy or (b) barium enema plus flexible sigmoidoscopy.

V. Diagnostic assessment. The key diagnostic task in adults presenting with constipation is identifying those occasional patients whose constipation is caused by colorectal cancer. Because survival from colon cancer is directly related to the stage of the disease at time of diagnosis (3), patients whose history, examination, or laboratory findings are more suggestive of this diagnosis merit prompt investigation, including referral if necessary.

    For patients whose constipation can be related to a particular systemic disease (e.g., hypercalcemia or hypothyroidism) or the use of particular medications (e.g., clonidine or an aluminum-containing antacid), identifying that link can be instrumental in ensuring that inciting issues are appropriately addressed in the management of the patient as a whole entity and not just as "a colon."

    In that greater host of patients whose initial evaluation suggests a more benign cause of constipation, or for whom constipation seems to be an incidental feature in an otherwise well individual, the decision to proceed with colonic visualization, or to begin a search for more unusual causes (the "U" in the MADE-O-FUN acrostic) will depend on the degree to which the constipation subjectively has an impact on the patient's ability to live a fulfilling, happy, and rewarding life.

References
1. Drossman DA, McKee DC, Sandler RS, et al. Bowel patterns among subjects not seeking health care. Use of a questionnaire to identify a population with bowel dysfunction. *Gastroenterology* 1982;83:529–534.

2. Sonnenberg A, Koch TR. Physician visits in the United States for constipation: 1958–1986. *Dig Dis Sci* 1989;34:606–611.
3. Steele G. Colorectal cancer. In: Murphy GP, Lawrence W, Lenhad RE, eds. *American Cancer Society textbook of clinical oncology*, 2nd ed. Atlanta: The American Cancer Society, 1995:Chap 14.

9.4 Diarrhea

Francis G. O'Connor

Diarrhea is one of the most common clinical complaints encountered by primary care providers. Although diarrhea infrequently requires a significant diagnostic evaluation and no more than symptomatic oral rehydration and reassurance, in selected clinical settings (e.g., impoverished, immunocompromised), this ailment can be life-threatening.

I. **Approach.** Identify those individuals with diarrhea who need urgent treatment or an acute diagnostic workup. In more than 90% of patients with acute diarrhea, the illness is mild and self-limited and no laboratory evaluation is necessary. The goal of the initial evaluation of the adult with diarrhea, therefore, is to distinguish these patients from those with more serious disorders.

   A. **Definition.** Diarrhea is best defined as an increase in the fluidity, frequency, and volume of daily stool output, where stool weight is greater than 200 g. Chronic diarrhea is distinguished from acute in that it lasts more than 3 weeks. Infection is the leading cause of acute diarrhea, whereas irritable bowel syndrome is the leading cause of chronic diarrhea.

   B. **Pathophysiology.** Four major mechanisms of diarrhea are seen (1):

   1. Osmotic diarrhea: increased amounts of poorly absorbable, osmotically active solutes in the gut lumen; stool volume decreases with fasting (e.g., laxative abuse, fat malabsorption, Norwalk virus, rotavirus).

   2. Secretory diarrhea: increased chloride and water secretion with or without inhibition of normal active sodium and water absorption; large volume stools with little change with fasting (e.g., toxigenic *Escherichia coli*, gastrinoma, phenolphthalein).

   3. Exudative diarrhea: exudation of mucus, blood, and protein from sites of active inflammation into the bowel lumen; fever, abdominal pain, or both may be present (e.g., Crohn's disease, psuedomembranous colitis).

   4. Abnormal intestinal motility: increased or decreased motility and contact between luminal contents and mucosal surface (e.g., irritable bowel syndrome, thyrotoxicosis).

II. **History**

   A. **General.** How long has the diarrhea been present? Most cases of acute diarrhea are secondary to infection (Table 9.1) (2). The overwhelming majority of cases of acute diarrhea are benign and self-limited. Diarrheal illnesses lasting longer than 3 weeks are classified as chronic and should be clinically investigated (Table 9.2) (3,4). Other symptoms to inquire about include associated nausea, vomiting, chills, fever, or abdominal pain. Bloody or melanotic stools and weight loss are red flags that should prompt further diagnostic testing (Chapters 2.13 and 9.11).

   B. **Acute diarrhea.** Has the patient recently traveled, tried new foods, used any medications, or had recent illness? Traveler's diarrhea commonly begins 3 to 7 days after arrival in a foreign location after exposure to foods or water contaminated with enterotoxigenic *Escherichia coli*, *Salmonella* spp., or *Giardia* spp. Diarrhea that develops within 12 hours of food ingestion is most likely caused by a bacterial preformed toxin. If diarrhea occurs in the setting of a recent course of antibiotic therapy, pseudomembranous colitis

Table 9.1 Common causes of acute diarrhea

VIRAL INFECTIONS Rotavirus Norwalk virus	FOOD POISONING *Staphylococcus aureus* *Clostridium botulinum*
BACTERIAL INFECTIONS *Campylobacter* species *Escherichia coli* *Salmonella* species *Shigella* species *Clostridium difficile* *Vibrio cholera*	DRUGS Laxatives Antacids Lactulose MISCELLANEOUS Fecal impaction Diverticulitis
PARASITIC INFECTIONS *Giardia lamblia* *Cryptosporidium* species *Entamoeba histolytica*	Ischemic bowel disease

caused by *Clostridium difficile* toxin should be suspected. A thorough medication history includes all products, including over-the-counter agents, alcohol, and caffeine.

C. **Chronic diarrhea.** In patients with chronic diarrhea, the history should focus on the characterization of the stools and the pattern of the diarrhea. Diarrhea at night favors an organic cause. Associated periods of constipation can be a clue to irritable bowel syndrome (Chapter 9.3). Is there a family history of diarrhea? Family history can provide clues to a diagnosis of irritable bowel syndrome, inflammatory bowel disease, or a multiple endocrine neoplastic disorder. Concurrent diarrheal illness among family members suggests the possibility of shared pathogens (e.g., *Giardia*) with a contaminated water source. The history should also detail other medical problems, prior surgeries, and allergies. A sexual history should be sought. Homosexual individuals are at higher risk for exposure to infectious agents, including amebiasis, giardiasis, and shigellosis. In patients with acquired immune deficiency

Table 9.2 Common causes of chronic diarrhea

INFECTION *Giardia lamblia* *Entamoeba histolytica* *Clostridium difficile*	MALABSORPTION Disaccharidase deficiency Pancreatic insufficiency Short bowel syndrome Celiac sprue Whipple's disease
INFLAMMATION Ulcerative colitis Crohn's disease Collagenous colitis Diverticulitis Ischemic colitis	ENDOCRINE DISORDERS Zollinger–Ellison syndrome Hyperthyroidism Villous adenoma Adrenal insufficiency Diabetes mellitus
DRUGS Laxatives Antibiotics Antacids Diuretics Ethanol, caffeine Nonsteroidal antiinflammatory drugs	MOTILITY DISORDERS Irritable bowel syndrome Postvagotomy syndrome

syndrome, infectious agents may include *Candida* spp., cytomegalovirus, and *Cryptosporidium* spp. A careful medication history should also screen for laxative abuse.

III. **Physical examination**

A. **Focused physical examination.** Obtain vital signs (notably temperature) and include orthostatic blood pressure measurements. Assess the patient's weight and general nutritional status. The abdomen should be examined for bowel sounds, localized tenderness, and organomegaly. A rectal examination may demonstrate a fistula or abscess that can be a clue to Crohn's disease. Occult or gross blood can indicate an invasive inflammatory diarrheal illness, diverticular disease, or an ischemic bowel.

B. **Additional physical examination.** The history may lead to a more specific examination (e.g., thyroid for thyrotoxicosis) or a search for lymphadenopathy in an immunocompromised patient.

IV. **Testing (5)**

A. **Acute diarrhea.** Laboratory testing should be reserved for those patients with severe symptoms (e.g., fever, bloody diarrhea, abdominal pain, and dehydration, or symptoms not improving after 5 days) or a comorbid condition. Examination of the stool sample is the most important laboratory test. A single specimen should be submitted for a Wright's stain for leukocytes, occult blood, Sudan stain for fat, and selected bacterial cultures (*Salmonella*, *Shigella*, *Campylobacter*, and *Yersinia* organisms). Large numbers of white cells are consistent with inflammatory causes, whereas isolated occult or gross blood may suggest amebiasis, neoplastic disease, vascular disease, or intestinal ischemia. If excess fat is present, malabsorption should be considered (e.g., celiac sprue). *Clostridium difficile* toxin should be obtained in the elderly and in those with a recent antibiotic history. Tests for ova and parasites on three consecutive specimens should be done in patients with diarrhea that persists for more than 7 to 10 days. In patients where ova and parasite testing is negative and clinical suspicion is high, an enzyme-linked immunosorbent assay test for the *Giardia* antigen should be considered as well as a wet mount examination of the stool for amebiasis. Sigmoidoscopy is warranted acutely in patients with symptoms of severe proctitis and in patients with suspected *C. difficile* colitis who appear ill. Rectal swabs for *Chlamydia*, herpes simplex virus, and gonorrhea may additionally be warranted in sexually active patients with severe proctitis.

B. **Chronic diarrhea.** Additional tests to be considered include complete blood count, serum electrolytes, liver function tests, calcium, phosphate, albumin, B_{12}, folate, and iron studies to rule out significant abnormalities secondary to the diarrhea, nutritional abnormalities, or hepatobiliary disease. Thyroid studies, serum gastrin, and vasoactive intestinal peptide should be ordered if clinically indicated. Sigmoidoscopy, which allows direct visualization for biopsy and culture, may be helpful in detecting inflammatory bowel disease. Barium studies of the small and large bowel can identify Crohn's disease, blind loops, celiac sprue, fistulae, and tumors. The stool specimen can be alkalinized for phenolphthalein, consistent with laxative abuse. The presence of steatorrhea warrants a 72-hour collection of stool fat (Chapter 9.12). A gastroenterologist can pursue additional specialized testing, including upper endoscopy with biopsy, breath testing for malabsorption, and pancreatic function testing.

V. **Diagnostic assessment.** A careful history helps to classify the diarrhea, provides clinical clues for selected diagnostic testing, and aids in risk stratifying the patient. Comorbid diseases and associated symptoms increase the urgency for diagnostic workup and management (e.g., fever, symptoms > 5 days, bloody diarrhea, known exposures, weight loss). Abnormal vital signs or bloody diarrhea identify patients at higher risk who require early therapeutic intervention. Although most diarrhea is benign and self-limited, a thorough history, focused physical examination, and directed laboratory testing will identify those cases requiring early diagnostic evaluation, aggressive management, or referral.

References
1. Kroser JA, Metz DC. Evaluation of the adult patient with diarrhea. *Primary Care* 1996;23(3):629–647.
2. Blacklow NR, Greenberg HB. Viral gastroenteritis. *N Engl J Med* 1991;325(4): 252–264.
3. Donowitz M, Kokke FT, Saidi R. Evaluation of patients with chronic diarrhea. *N Engl J Med* 1995;332(11):725–729.
4. Norris TE. *Lower gastrointestinal problems.* Monograph, edition No. 198. Home Study Self-Assessment program. Kansas City, Mo: American Academy of Family Physicians, November 1995.
5. Kearney DJ, McQuaid KR. Approach to the patient with gastrointestinal disorders. In: Grendell JH, ed. *Current diagnosis and treatment in gastroenterology.* Norwalk, CT: Appleton & Lange, 1996.

9.5 Dysphagia

Michael R. Spieker

Dysphagia (difficult swallowing) is a common diagnosis, ranking in frequency alongside other complaints such as pneumonia, bronchitis, and otitis media (1). At least 7% to 10% of adults aged more than 50 years experience dysphagia and up to 25% of hospitalized patients and 30% to 40% of nursing home patients experience swallowing problems (2). Aspiration is the most serious potential complication.

I. **Approach.** Initially, categorize complaints as due to obstructive or neuromuscular causes (Table 9.3). Further categorize the dysphagia as occurring in the oropharyngeal or esophageal stages of swallowing (3).
    A. **Differential diagnosis of dysphagia.** Stroke and neuromuscular disease affect older patients. Drug-induced esophagitis is most common with patients taking alendronate (Fosamax), nonsteroidal antiinflammatory drugs, and slow release potassium chloride. α-Adrenergic blockers can cause xerostomia (dry mouth). Younger patients can have strictures secondary to gastric reflux associated with tobacco and alcohol use. Rapid progression of dysphagia associated with weight loss is considered a malignancy until proved otherwise (Chapter 2.13).
    B. **Other considerations.** True dysphagia must be distinguished from other esophageal complaints that do not cause difficulty with the swallowing mechanism. Odynophagia (painful swallowing) and globus (the sensation of a lump in the throat without organic defect) are separate symptoms from dysphagia. Up to 28% of patients with noncardiac chest pain can have abnormal esophageal motility disorders (Chapter 7.1).
II. **History.** More than 80% of the causes of dysphagia can be identified by history alone. Is there difficulty initiating the swallow or a sensation of the food bolus getting stuck in the chest? Oropharyngeal dysphagias cause difficulty initiating a swallow and have associated coughing, choking, or nasal regurgitation. The patient's speech quality may have a nasal tone. Esophageal dysphagias cause patients to complain of food sticking in their throat or chest.
    A. **Chronology and progression of the dysphagia.** Has the dysphagia acutely progressed or has it gradually worsened over a long time? A progressively rapid course can represent mechanical obstruction secondary to tumors, other mediastinal masses, and esophageal webs or rings. Gradual dysphagias requiring progressive, forceful swallows and the Valsalva maneuver are indicative of neuromuscular motor disease. Acute dysphagia suggests infection, irritation, or food bolus impaction.

Table 9.3 Causes of dysphagia

	Neuromuscular	Obstructive
Oropharyngeal	Central nervous system diseases	Tumors
	Cerebrovascular accident	Inflammatory masses
	Parkinson's disease	Trauma/surgical resection
	Brainstem tumors	Zenker's diverticulum
	Degenerative diseases	Esophageal webs
	Amyotrophic lateral sclerosis	Extrinsic structural lesions
	Multiple sclerosis	Anterior mediastinal masses
	Huntington's disease	Cervical spondylosis
	Postinfectious (poliomyelitis, syphilis)	
	Peripheral nervous system—peripheral neuropathy	
	Motor end plate dysfunction—myasthenia gravis	
	Skeletal muscle disease (myopathies)	
	Polymyositis	
	Dermatomyositis	
	Muscular dystrophy	
	Cricopharyngeal (UES) achalasia	
Esophageal	Achalasia	Intrinsic structural lesions
	Spastic motor disorders	Tumors
	Diffuse esophageal spasm	Strictures
	Hypertensive lower esophageal sphincter	Peptic
	Nutcracker esophagus	Radiation-induced
	Scleroderma	Chemical-induced
		Medication-induced
		Lower esophageal rings (Schatzki's ring)
		Esophageal webs
		Foreign bodies
		Extrinsic structural lesions
		Vascular compression
		Enlarged aorta or left atrium
		Aberrant vessels
		Mediastinal masses
		Lymphadenopathy
		Substernal thyroid

UES, upper esophageal sphincter.

B. Solid or liquid dysphagia. Does the patient have dysphagia for solids, liquids, or both? Solid food dysphagia and weight loss indicate mechanical obstruction; difficulty with both liquids and solids suggests neuromuscular disease. Cold foods and beverages can exacerbate neuromuscular dysphagia.

C. Social history. Does the patient use tobacco, alcohol, or any over-the-counter (OTC) or prescription medications? Smoking causes chest malignancies, including esophageal carcinoma. Alcohol and many OTC and prescription medications decrease esophageal motility, relax the lower esophageal sphincter, or induce esophagitis directly (4).

D. Associated symptoms. Pain with swallowing can be associated with achalasia or spasm. Pain on swallowing saliva alone suggests mucosal inflammation from infection. Heartburn and dysphagia for solids indicate distal esophageal stricture from reflux. Are there associated neurologic symptoms consistent with a stroke (Chapter 4.8)?

E. Evidence of aspiration. Does the patient cough when swallowing? Does the cough occur in the oropharyngeal stage or esophageal stage of swallowing? Pneumonia or other chest infection without a cough can indicate silent aspiration.

III. Physical examination. A general physical examination and focused organ- or symptom-specific examinations based on the history often confirm the cause of the patient's dysphagia.

A. Focused examination. Assess mental status, motor and sensory functioning, deep tendon reflexes, cerebellar function, and cranial nerves. Focus special attention on the cranial nerves (CN) associated with swallowing (CN IX, X). A decreased gag reflex is associated with an increased risk of aspiration. Inspect the oropharynx and note the patients' speech. A widened anteroposterior chest diameter and distant breath sounds are signs of chronic obstructive lung disease and may indicate chronic aspiration.

B. The swallow. Observe the patient swallowing a variety of liquids and solids. Can the patient chew, mix, and propel a food bolus to the posterior pharynx without choking or coughing? When in the swallowing sequence does the patient complain of difficulty?

IV. Testing

A. Clinical laboratory tests. Limit initial laboratory evaluations to specific studies based on the differential diagnosis generated after a complete history and physical examination. These can include thyroid function studies, erythrocyte sedimentation rate, and a complete blood count to screen for infectious or inflammatory conditions.

B. Special studies and diagnostic imaging. Additional diagnostic testing is indicated to confirm a diagnosis, to obtain biopsy specimens, or to establish the risk for aspiration. Specialists in radiology, otolaryngology, and gastroenterology will most often complete these tests.

1. **Nasopharyngoscopy.** Nasopharyngoscopy assesses patients with oropharyngeal dysphagia and those at risk for aspiration. It quickly identifies structural masses and lesions and assesses laryngeal sensitivity to contact. Patients demonstrating aspiration without cough are at high risk for pulmonary complications.

2. **Barium studies.** Barium swallow detects obstructive lesions and assesses motility better than endoscopy, but lacks precision in identifying the nature of some obstructive lesions. It is relatively inexpensive with few complications, but can be difficult to perform on sick or uncooperative patients. Double contrast studies provide better visualization of esophageal mucosa.

3. **Upper gastrointestinal (GI) endoscopy.** Patients with food impactions, esophageal mucosal symptoms, or masses identified by barium studies should undergo upper endoscopy. A consensus panel found endoscopy more sensitive (92% vs. 54%) and more specific (100% vs. 91%) than double contrast UGI in patients with dysphagia of all causes (5). Patients prefer endoscopy to UGI studies, and the higher initial cost of endoscopy may be offset by lower subsequent medical costs because of its improved diagnostic accuracy.

4. **Videoradiographic studies.** Patients at risk for silent aspiration (stroke, neurologic impairment) may benefit from videoradiographic studies performed by a team composed of a radiologist, otolaryngologist, and speech pathologist with expertise in swallowing disorders. The studies are expensive and require special equipment and facilities.

5. **Other studies.** Manometry detects abnormalities in only 25% of those with nonobstructive lesions. Esophageal pH monitoring is the gold standard for suspected reflux. Plain films of the chest or neck and ultrasound of the pharynx offer limited information. Computed tomography and magnetic resonance imaging scans provide excellent definition for suspected structural central nervous system abnormalities. Radionuclide studies can be used to evaluate transit function through the esophagus.

V. **Diagnostic assessment.** A thorough history and physical examination readily identify the cause of dysphagia in most patients. Confirmatory studies are predicated on the differential diagnoses generated. Referral to other specialists is warranted when the cause is not clear or if further diagnostic or therapeutic expertise is required. Elderly patients are at highest risk for dysphagia and complications, especially silent aspiration. Aggressive early evaluation and management of stroke victims reduce symptoms and risk of aspiration.

References

1. *National ambulatory medical care survey: 1993 summary.* Vital and Health Statistics, series 13. Hyattsville, Maryland: US Department of Health and Human Services, 1998;136:74.
2. Lindgren S, Janzon L. Prevalence of swallowing complaints and clinical findings among 50–79-year-old men and women in an urban population. *Dysphagia* 1991;6: 187–192.
3. Castell DO. Approach to the patient with dysphagia. In: Yamada T, ed. *Textbook of gastroenterology*, 2nd ed. Philadelphia: Lippincott-Raven, 1995:638–648.
4. Boyce HW. Drug induced esophageal damage: diseases of medical progress. *Gastrointest Endosc* 1998;6:547–550.
5. Dooley CP, Larson AW, Stace NH, et al. Double contrast barium meal and upper gastrointestinal endoscopy: a comparative study. *Ann Intern Med* 1984;101:538–545.

9.6 Epigastric Distress

Cindy Barter

Epigastric distress is a very common presenting complaint in both the emergency room setting and the outpatient setting. Of the multitude of diseases or diagnoses that can present with epigastric distress, gastroesophageal reflux disease (GERD) is commonly encountered; it affects approximately 25% to 35% of Americans during their lifetime (1).

I. **Approach.** The complaint of epigastric distress creates a very long differential diagnosis that involves many organ systems. A careful, thorough history will narrow, if not define, the diagnosis in most cases. It is important to differentiate between urgent and nonurgent causes of epigastric distress. Immediate evaluation is indicated when patients present with acute onset of pain. Possible diagnoses in such cases include, but are not limited to, the following: appendicitis, cardiac disease (acute myocardial infarction), cholecystitis, gastrointestinal (GI) bleed, ischemic bowel, pancreatitis, small bowel obstruction, and ruptured abdominal aortic aneurysm. Diagnoses made more often in patients who present with chronic epigastric distress and who can be evaluated and monitored over longer period of time include, but are not limited to, the following: GERD, nonulcer dyspepsia, peptic ulcer disease (PUD), gastritis, cholecystitis or cholelithiasis, hepatitis, gastroenteritis, constipation, pneumonia, pyelonephritis, neoplasms, inflammatory bowel disease, and irritable bowel syndrome (2).

II. **History**
   A. **Pain** is the usual presentation of epigastric distress. First priority is to ask questions about the onset, intensity, frequency, pattern, and location of the pain. Onset: When did the pain start? Is there any prior history of similar pain?

B. Intensity and quality. Can you describe the pain? (sharp, dull, burning, radiating, pressure). Burning pain is often used to describe GERD. Pressure sensation "like an elephant sitting on me" suggests cardiac ischemia (Chapter 7.1).

C. Frequency and pattern. Does the pain occur at any particular time of day? Is there anything that makes the pain better or worse? Pain that is worse at night when lying down suggests GERD. Pain that occurs after a high fat meal increases the likelihood of gallbladder disease (Chapter 9.1).

D. Location. Where is the pain? Does the pain radiate anywhere? Radiation to the back suggests pancreatitis. Pain radiating to the scapula can indicate gallbladder disease.

E. Associated symptoms. Has there been any nausea, vomiting, or hematemesis? The previous symptoms can indicate a Mallory-Weiss tear or PUD. If diarrhea is present, is there bright red blood or melena in the stool? The presence of blood or melena in the stool requires further workup for GI bleed.

F. Past medical history. Has the patient had any prior GI problems? Obtain a drug history, including the use of aspirin, nonsteroidal antiinflammatory drugs, alendronate sodium (Fosamax), steroids, antibiotics. Is there a history of tobacco or alcohol use? Both tobacco and alcohol use are associated with an increased incidence of GERD and PUD. Multiparity and obesity increase the risk of gallbladder disease. Are there risk factors for sexually transmitted diseases? Hepatitis B and human immunodeficiency virus can be transmitted sexually and can be causative factors in epigastric distress.

III. Physical examination

A. General assessment. Obtain vital signs. Is the patient febrile—indicating an infectious cause? Tachycardia and hypotension can indicate dehydration or GI bleed. Is the patient in acute distress? Jaundiced?

B. Cardiopulmonary assessment. Evaluate the heart and lungs to rule out any cardiac or pulmonic process that could present with epigastric distress. Is there evidence of an arrhythmia, myocardial infarction, or congestive heart failure? Are there crackles or rales suggesting a pneumonia?

C. Abdominal examination. Are bowel sounds present? Decreased or absent bowel sounds can indicate a small bowel obstruction, acute surgical abdomen (appendicitis, perforated ulcer), or pancreatitis. Rebound tenderness should prompt consideration of an acute surgical abdomen. The right upper quadrant (RUQ) should be palpated. A palpable liver warrants evaluation for other signs of liver disease—jaundice, ascites, skin changes. Murphy's sign—sudden cessation of the patient's inspiratory effort during deep palpation of the RUQ—is suggestive of acute cholecystitis (3). Tenderness to palpation of the left upper quadrant can indicate splenic infarct such as seen with sickle cell disease. Tenderness of the midepigastric area can represent peptic ulcer disease, dyspepsia, "nonclassical" presentation of acute appendicitis, or any other of the above-mentioned conditions. A rectal examination with testing for occult blood should be a part of the examination, particularly with any concern about GI bleeding (Chapter 9.7).

IV. Testing

A. Clinical laboratory tests. Laboratory tests should be directed by the history and physical examination. A complete blood count is indicated if signs are seen of infection or bleeding. An elevated white blood cell count is consistent with appendicitis or pneumonia. A decreased hemoglobin or hematocrit warrants further evaluation for GI bleed. Other laboratory tests that might be indicated by the history and physical examination include liver function tests (hepatitis, gallbladder disease), amylase and lipase (pancreatitis—although no single laboratory test is diagnostic for pancreatitis), creatine kinase-MB (CK-MB), and/or troponin (cardiac pathology). Laboratory testing for *Helicobacter pylori* is controversial except for those with documented PUD. Keep in mind that of patients who have PUD, 90% are infected with *H. pylori* and only 10% to 20% of patients infected with *H. pylori* develop PUD (4).

B. Diagnostic imaging. Plain film x-ray studies are helpful only if bowel obstruction or perforation is suspected. RUQ ultrasound is warranted if gallbladder disease or pancreatitis is suspected. Computed tomography scan of the abdomen could be considered in cases of difficulty in differentiating acute abdominal pain or when needed to evaluate for possible complications. Barium studies are not indicated in the acute setting, but can be helpful in the diagnostic workup for gastric ulcer, GERD, and esophagitis.

C. Endoscopy. Esophagogastrodoudenoscopy in the setting of an upper GI bleed may help to identify the source of the bleeding, assuming the patient is sufficiently stable to tolerate the procedure (Chapter 9.7). The diagnoses of PUD, gastritis, and esophagitis are best made using endoscopy, which also allows evaluation for the presence of *H. pylori* (5).

D. Other tests. Other tests useful in the evaluation of epigastric distress include an electrocardiogram to assess for possible cardiac disease and chest radiographs and a pulmonary function test to evaluate for possible pulmonary disease.

V. Diagnostic assessment. The key to the successful approach to a patient presenting with epigastric distress begins with a careful history. If the distress is of acute onset, a more urgent and directed evaluation is needed. Vital signs and physical examination should be directed to evaluate for fever (infection), hypotension (GI bleed), and non-GI causes (MI, ruptured aneurysm). Epigastric distress of a chronic nature can be evaluated using history, directed laboratory testing, and diagnostic imaging.

References

1. Scott M, Gelhot AR. Gastroesophageal reflux disease: diagnosis and management. *Am Fam Physician* 1999;59(5):1161–1169.
2. Isselbacher KJ, Podolsky DK. Approach to the patient with gastrointestinal disease. In: Fauci AS, ed. *Harrison's principles of internal medicine.* New York: McGraw-Hill, 1998:1579–1583.
3. Swartz MH. *Textbook of physical diagnosis, history and examination.* Philadelphia: WB Saunders, 1994:324.
4. NIH Consensus Conference. *Helicobacter pylori* in peptic ulcer disease. *JAMA* 1994; 272(1):65–69.
5. Rank JM, Vennes JA. Gastrointestinal endoscopy. In: Bennet JC, Plum F, eds. *Cecil textbook of medicine.* Philadelphia: WB Saunders, 1996:636–642.

9.7 Gastrointestinal Bleeding

Mark B. Stephens

Gastrointestinal (GI) bleeding is responsible for 1% to 2% of all hospital admissions in the United States (1). Bleeding can be either acute or chronic. The source can be upper or lower, overt or occult. The patient can be either hemodynamically stable or unstable on presentation. A systematic approach to the patient with GI bleeding is critical to an accurate diagnosis.

I. Approach. The key to successful evaluation of GI bleeding revolves around the following principles (2): (a) determine the hemodynamic stability of the patient; (b) determine the source of bleeding (Table 9.4); (c) stop the bleeding; (d) prevent recurrence.

II. History. Clinical history accurately points to the source of bleeding in only 40% of cases (3).

Table 9.4 Common sources of gastrointestinal (GI) bleeding

UPPER GASTROINTESTINAL BLEED (PROXIMAL TO THE LIGAMENT OF TREITZ)

Esophageal	Gastric	Duodenal	Miscellaneous
Varices	Peptic ulcer disease	Peptic ulcer disease	Iatrogenic
Mallory-Weiss	Varices	Cancer	Coagulopathy
Cancer	Gastritis	Arteriovenous fistula	Ischemia
Esophagitis	Cancer		Angiodysplasia
	Dieulafoy's lesion		Hemobilia

LOWER GASTROINTESTINAL BLEED (DISTAL TO THE LIGAMENT OF TREITZ)[a]

Small intestine	Large intestine	Rectum	Miscellaneous
Angiodysplasia	Diverticulosis	Hemorrhoids	Iatrogenic
Cancer	Angiodysplasia	Fissures	Coagulopathy
Ischemia	Cancer	Cancer	
Trauma	Inflammatory bowel disease	Ulceration	
Aortoenteric fistula	Trauma	Varices	
Meckel's diverticulum	Ischemia	Trauma	
	Radiation enteritis		
	Infection		
	Aortoenteric fistula		

[a] Bleeding from an upper GI source is another common cause of lower GI bleeding and must always be considered in patients presenting with rectal bleeding.

A. **Upper GI bleeding**. Hematemesis and melena are the most common presentations of acute upper GI bleeding. Important questions to ask: Is there a prior history of bleeding (60% rebleed from the same site) (3)? Is there any family history? Does the patient have any comorbid diseases (peptic ulcer disease, pancreatitis, cirrhosis, cancer)? Is the patient taking any medications (especially nonsteroidal antiinflammatory agents)? Does the patient use recreational drugs, cigarettes, or alcohol? What is the character of the pain? Peptic ulcer pain is epigastric, gnawing, rhythmic, and dull. GI cancers are associated with vague epigastric pain, dysphagia, or weight loss. Was there any retching (Mallory–Weiss tear)? Does the patient have a history of prior surgeries? Patients with a history of vascular grafting are at risk for aortoenteric fistulae, which is often associated with a "herald bleed."

B. **Lower GI bleeding**. How old is the patient? Age is an important feature in discriminating the source of lower GI bleeding. Patients aged less than 50 years usually bleed from infectious causes, anorectal disease, or inflammatory bowel disease. For patients aged more than 50 years, diverticulosis, angiodysplasia, cancer, and ischemia are most common (4). Are there any associated symptoms? Diverticular disease presents as painless, high volume bleeding. Angiodysplasia and cancer present with symptoms of chronic blood loss (fatigue, dyspnea on exertion). Inflammatory bowel disease presents with bloody diarrhea, cramping, weight loss, and fever. A prior history of inflammatory bowel disease, cancer, or radiation to the abdomen is also important.

III. **Physical examination**

A. **Vital signs**. The single most important aspect of the initial physical examination is determining the patient's hemodynamic stability. Unstable patients should be managed as trauma patients. Placement of a nasogastric (NG) tube is considered the "fifth vital sign" in patients with acute GI bleeding (2).

B. **Focused physical examination**. After ensuring hemodynamic stability, the initial physical examination should eliminate a nasal or oropharyngeal source of bleeding. Examine the skin and abdomen carefully for clues to an underlying cause. A rectal examination is mandatory.

1. Skin examination. Ecchymoses, petechiae, and varices should be noted. Conjunctival pallor is a sign of chronic anemia. Numerous mucosal telangiectasias can point to an underlying vascular abnormality.

2. Abdominal examination. Look for stigmata of chronic liver disease (hepatosplenomegaly, spider angiomata, ascites, palmar erythema, caput medusae, gynecomastia, and testicular atrophy) (Chapter 9.9).

3. Rectal examination. Rectal varices, hemorrhoids, and fissures should be noted.

IV. **Laboratory evaluation**

A. **Basic laboratory studies** should include a complete blood count with particular attention to the hematocrit, coagulation studies [prothrombin time (PT) and partial thromboplastin time (PTT)], liver function tests (LFTs), serum chemistries (blood urea nitrogen is elevated disproportionately to creatinine in patients with GI blood loss), electrocardiogram (ECG), and NG aspirate analysis. Acutely, the hematocrit is a poor indicator of blood loss; however, serial hematocrits can be useful in assessing ongoing blood loss. A prolonged PT or PTT suggests an underlying coagulopathy. Elevated LFTs suggest underlying liver disease. An ECG is important, especially in elderly patients, to search for evidence of cardiac ischemia. Finally, the NG aspirate is essential. If the aspirate is bright red, or "coffee grounds" in appearance, an upper GI source is likely.

B. **Endoscopy** plays a central role in the diagnosis and management of GI bleeding. Fiberoptic endoscopy is 90% accurate in pinpointing the source of upper GI bleeding. In addition, the endoscope can also be used to deliver therapy directly.

C. **Anoscopy** can be used to identify the source of lower GI bleeding; however, the yield is poor (5). Often the site of bleeding cannot be directly visualized or the volume of bleeding is sufficiently heavy to obscure clear visualization.

D. **Nuclear medicine** studies are useful in grossly localizing bleeding sources to the small intestine, right colon, or left colon. Nuclear scanning is also useful in detecting Meckel's diverticulae. These images can detect ongoing GI bleeding with a sensitivity of blood loss at 0.05 to 0.1 ml/minute.

E. **Angiography** can also identify the source of lower GI bleeding. It is not as sensitive as nuclear scanning, requiring a blood loss of more than 0.5 ml/minute.

V. **Diagnostic assessment.** The key to the successful approach to GI bleeding is ensuring the hemodynamic stability of the patient. Once done, a systematic search for the source of the bleeding should be undertaken. Although often unreliable, a careful patient history can provide valuable clues to factors that may predispose the patient to hemorrhage from a particular site within the GI tract. Physical examination (including placement of a NG tube) can further delineate whether an upper source or a lower source is most likely. The key diagnostic modality in GI bleeding is fiberoptic endoscopy. Following the clues provided by a careful history and physical examination, targeted endoscopy is then used to definitively identify the source of bleeding. In the rare cases where endoscopy is unable to adequately identify the source of GI bleeding, specialized nuclear medicine and angiographic studies can be used.

References
1. Zimmerman HM, Curfman K. Acute gastrointestinal bleeding. *AACN Clin Issues* 1997;8(3):449–458.
2. Laine L. Acute and chronic gastrointestinal bleeding. In: Feldman M, Sleisinger MH, Scharschmidt BF, eds: *Gastrointestinal and liver disease: pathophysiology, diagnosis, and management.* Philadelphia: WB Saunders, 1998:198–218.
3. McGuirk TD, Coyle WJ. Upper gastrointestinal tract bleeding. *Emer Med Clin N Am* 1996;14(3):523–545.
4. Zuccaro G. Management of the adult patient with acute lower gastrointestinal bleeding. *Am J Gastroenterol* 1998;93(8):1202–1208.
5. Bono MJ. Lower gastrointestinal bleeding. *Emer Med Clin N Am* 1996;14(3):547–556.

9.8 Hepatitis

Susan C. Cullom

Viral hepatitis is the most common cause of liver disease in the world. In the United States, more than 300,000 cases of acute viral hepatitis occur annually. Hepatitis B and C give rise to chronic hepatitis, with 5 million cases worldwide (1). In addition to the six hepatitis viruses (A,B,C,D,E,G) identified to date (2), multiple other causes of hepatitis exist: viruses (e.g., cytomegalovirus, Epstein-Barr, coxsackie virus), alcohol, drugs, and biliary tract disease. Drug-induced disease accounts for approximately 10% of hepatitis cases among all adult patients and for more than 40% of cases among patients aged more than 50 years (3).

I. **Approach.** The important tasks in the diagnosis are to identify infectious causes, so as to limit infectivity through appropriate precautions, and to identify those patients with fulminant hepatitis from noninfectious causes in an attempt to limit their morbidity (4). Hepatitis can be classified into five broad categories:
   A. Viral
   B. Drug-induced
   C. Alcoholic
   D. Chronic
   E. Autoimmune
II. **History.** Patients may complain of anorexia, fever, arthralgia, malaise, vomiting, diarrhea, or chills. Complaints of dark urine or jaundice are highly suggestive of hepatitis. As these symptoms are seen in many types of hepatitis, specific questions help categorize the cause.
   A. **Viral hepatitis.** Does the patient have exposure to blood (transfusions before 1990, tattoos, body piercing, shared razor, needlestick, sharing needles, intranasal cocaine use)? Hepatitis B is most commonly transmitted via contaminated blood or sexually via risky sexual behaviors (anal intercourse, prostitution, multiple sexual partners). Hepatitis A and E are transmitted via the fecal-oral route. Does the patient have a history of travel to developing countries, raw shellfish ingestion, or work in an institution or daycare?
   B. **Drug-induced hepatitis.** Does the patient use prescription or over-the-counter medication? The drugs most often associated with hepatitis are anesthetics (halothane), neuropsychotropics (chlorpromazine, haloperidol, tricyclics), anticonvulsants (phenytoin), analgesics (acetaminophen, ibuprofen), antigout (allopurinol), hormonal derivatives and drugs used in endocrine disease (glipizide, tamoxifen, anabolic steroids, oral contraceptives), antimicrobials (tetracyclines), cardiovascular drugs (amiodarone, procainamide), antineoplastic (cisplatin), vitamin A, propoxyphene, cimetidine, and ferrous sulfate.
   C. **Alcoholic hepatitis.** Could the patient be an alcoholic? Inquire about quantitative alcohol intake and obtain a history from both patient and

family members. Use the CAGE questionnaire to help identify individuals at high risk. Inquire about alcohol-associated illnesses (pancreatitis) and motor vehicle citations.

D. Chronic hepatitis. Has the patient ever been jaundiced or diagnosed with hepatitis before (Chapter 9.10)? Has the patient had elevated liver enzymes for at least 6 months? The most common cause of chronic hepatitis and cirrhosis is alcohol. Viral hepatitis B and C often cause chronic hepatitis, cirrhosis, or hepatocellular carcinoma. Other causes of chronic hepatitis are drug-induced, Wilson's disease, and α_1-antitrypsin deficiency.

E. Autoimmune hepatitis. Is there a history of arthritis, amenorrhea, or rash? Mediated by the deposition of circulating immune complexes, this disease is also referred to as "chronic active hepatitis." It is more common in female patients and adolescents; prior hepatitis B virus (HBV) or hepatitis C virus (HCV) infection is a triggering factor.

III. Physical examination

A. General examination. Common findings in viral, alcoholic, or drug-induced hepatitis include fever, jaundice, scleral icterus, weight loss, muscle tenderness or weakness, and a palpable tender liver. Ecchymosis or petechiae indicates significant clotting factor abnormalities and, coupled with a small liver which diminishes in size, is suggestive of severe hepatitis or impending hepatic failure.

B. Chronic liver disease results in progressive liver dysfunction, fluid retention, and portal hypertension. The liver plays a key role in the detoxification of endogenous hormones, drugs, and ingested substances. Abnormalities in estrogen metabolism have often been considered the cause of peripheral stigmata such as spider angiomata, palmar erythema, gynecomastia, parotid enlargement, and testicular atrophy.

C. Does the abdominal examination reveal hepatosplenomegaly? Modest enlargement of the liver occurs in acute viral and chronic hepatitis, whereas marked enlargement (>10 cm below the costal margin) is seen in alcoholic hepatitis. Ascites, prominent abdominal collateral veins, bruits, rubs, abdominal masses, or a palpable gallbladder can also indicate hepatitis, whereas a small liver can indicate cirrhosis.

IV. Testing. Laboratory tests differentiate between hepatocellular disorders (e.g., viral hepatitis) and cholestatic syndromes (e.g., primary biliary cirrhosis and bile duct obstruction).

A. Liver function tests (LFTs)

  1. Elevated alanine aminotransferase (ALT) and aspartate aminotransferase (AST) are nonspecific indicators of hepatocellular damage and do not distinguish viral from drug-induced hepatitis. Alcoholic liver disease is suggested when the AST:ALT ratio is greater than 2:1.

  2. Total serum bilirubin is not a sensitive indicator of hepatic dysfunction. Hepatitis impairs the excretion phase of bilirubin metabolism, resulting in an elevated direct (conjugated) bilirubin greater than 0.1 mg/dl.

  3. γ-Glutamyl transpeptidase (GGT) is a very sensitive indicator for minimal hepatocellular damage. Elevations are seen in alcoholic liver disease before other LFTs are abnormal.

  4. Alkaline phosphatase indicates cholestasis or obstruction. Approximately 75% of patients with prolonged cholestasis have alkaline phosphatase values increased fourfold or greater.

  5. Immunoglobulins (IgA, IgG, IgM) in acute hepatitis are normal or minimally increased. A moderate increase is seen in chronic active or autoimmune hepatitis. Indices are useful in monitoring response to immunotherapy.

  6. Circulating autoantibodies (e.g., antinuclear, smooth muscle, liver-kidney microsomal) may be seen in autoimmune hepatitis.

B. Hepatitis serology. Serologic testing (anti-HDV, anti-HCV) is now available for each type, except hepatitis E virus (HEV) (5) (Fig. 9.1). Hepatitis G virus (HGV) and GB virus C (GBV-C) are the most recently discovered

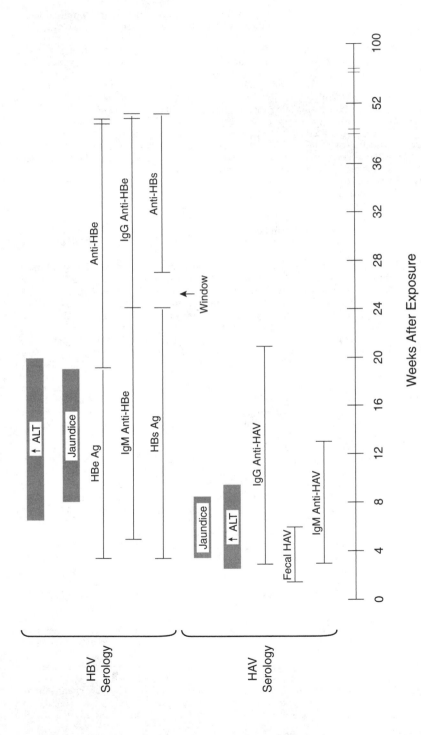

FIG. 9.1 Laboratory markers of hepatitis B and hepatitis A infection.

hepatitis viruses (2). HGV is present in asymptomatic blood donors and, although it is thought to cause chronic hepatitis, no causal relationship between HGV and hepatitis has been convincingly established (3).

C. **Radiologic and diagnostic procedures**
   1. Abdominal films are useful in detecting splenomegaly.
   2. Ultrasound is helpful in detecting gallstones in patients with jaundice and in detecting mass lesions (tumors or liver abscesses).
   3. Abdominal computerized tomography aids in the diagnosis of mass lesions of the liver and abnormalities of the gallbladder.
   4. Percutaneous needle biopsy of the liver permits an accurate diagnosis of diffuse parenchymal disorders such as hepatitis, drug reaction, cirrhosis, and liver tumors.

V. **Diagnostic assessment.** Viral hepatitis can be diagnosed by a thorough history and serology used in tandem. Individual susceptibility to hepatic injury in drug-induced hepatitis can be affected by genetic factors, age, gender, nutritional status, exposure to other drugs and chemicals, systemic disease, and other factors (4). Liver injury produced by drugs is either cytotoxic (hepatocellular), cholestatic, or a combination of the two. Knowledge of these mechanisms is extremely important in diagnosing the inciting agent. Alcoholic hepatitis is identified by the history coupled with the typical laboratory abnormalities. Chronic hepatitis requires elevated LFTs for at least 6 months and can result from infection with HBV or HCV, alcoholic liver disease, drug toxicity, or autoimmune causes. Liver biopsy is required for accurate assessment and classification of chronic hepatitis. Although effective vaccines are available for HAV and HBV and have yielded protection for decades, vaccines for HCV and HEV are only in early development and no vaccine exists for HDV.

References
1. Schiff ER, Sorrell MF, Maddrey WC. *Diseases of the liver*, 8th ed. Philadelphia: Lippincott Williams & Wilkins, 1999:234–235, 919–921.
2. Blum HE. Update hepatitis A-G. *Digestion* 1997;58(Suppl 1):33–36.
3. Zimmerman HJ. General aspects of drug-induced liver disease. *Gastroenterol Clin North Am* 1995;24:739–757.
4. Kools AM. Hepatitis A,B,C,D, and E. Update on testing and treatment. *Postgrad Med* 1992;91:109–114.
5. Schiff ER. Update in hepatology. *Ann Intern Med* 1999;130:52–59.

9.9 Hepatomegaly

Darryl G. White and Bruce A. Leibert

I. **Approach.** Hepatomegaly is a physical sign noted on abdominal examination that is present in hepatobiliary disease but is not specific or sensitive to one cause. Defining hepatomegaly can be enigmatic because of the highly variable liver size, which makes establishment of what constitutes normal somewhat difficult. The normal adult liver spans 8 to 12 cm for men and 6 to 10 cm for women, in the midclavicular line. Calculation methods for estimating liver size have been developed but they do not correlate well with percussion or ultrasound (1,2). Physical examination estimation of liver size and the clinical ability to suspect hepatomegaly are necessary to proceed with an appropriate workup.

II. **History**
   A. **Does the patient have known risk factors for liver disease** (Table 9.5)?
   B. **Does the patient have symptoms associated with liver disease** (Table 9.6)?

Table 9.5 Risk factors for liver disease

Acupuncture	Alcoholism	Bisexuality
Blood product transfusions	Dietary supplements	Family history of liver
Gallstones	Gastrointestinal	disease
Intravenous drug use	bleeding	Irritable bowel disease
Sexually transmitted	Male homosexuality	International travel
diseases	Tattoos	

III. Physical examination
A. How does a clinician diagnose hepatomegaly?
1. **Palpation and percussion.** Evaluation of the liver is difficult given its irregular shape and its location within the abdomen. Approach palpation of the right upper quadrant from one of two directions: palpate from below using the fingertips to palpate superiorly or from above with the fingertips hooked over the lower rib. Either method is facilitated by the patient's deep inspiration. Palpation must include the midline to identify an enlarged left lobe of the liver. On palpation, note the liver position, the extent of its palpation below the costal margin, and its texture and consistency. Palpate for the lower edge and percuss for the upper margin. These two points give the highest accuracy in estimating liver size. If the margin is not palpated but hepatomegaly is suspected, then attempt direct percussion of both margins.
2. **Auscultation.** The "scratch method" (gently stroking or scratching the skin surface in a parallel plane while listening with the stethoscope for change in sound and intensity of frequency) has been used to identify margins; however, a recent study by Tucker comparing ultrasound to the results of the scratch test found that this test was unreliable and inaccurate (3). Auscultation of the right upper quadrant has been described and several findings can be noted: friction rubs, bruits, and abnormal pulsations.
3. **Other associated signs.** Associated physical examination findings include jaundice, vascular spiders, palmar erythema, gynecomastia, ascites, splenomegaly, testicular atrophy, peripheral edema, Dupuytren's contracture, parotid enlargement, and encephalopathy. Although none of these physical examination signs are pathognomonic for hepatobiliary disease, their presence in the setting of hepatomegaly support further diagnostic testing.

B. How accurate is the physical assessment?
Palpation of the liver 2 cm below the costal margin correlates with a 50% chance of having hepatomegaly on further diagnostic workup. A 63% chance exists that a palpable liver relates to liver disease (4). The converse is also true: A nonpalpable liver could also be enlarged, therefore, the need for further assessment should be based

Table 9.6 Symptoms of liver disease

Abdominal pain	Arthralgias	Chills
Confusion	Diarrhea	Easy bruisability
Fatigue	Fever	Frequent epistaxis
Gastric bleeding	Heavy, irregular menses	Loss of appetite
Myalgia	Nausea	Night sweats
Pruritus	Rashes	Sleep disturbance
Vomiting		

on clinical context and associated signs. The liver span has classically been measured in the midclavicular line, although some have suggested that the use of the midclavicular line is too inaccurate. Several studies have attempted to establish a new reference point but no consensus has developed. Direct percussion (lightly tapping with index finger) is more accurate in identifying the extent of the margins than indirect percussion. Indirect percussion (heavy tapping of one finger against another finger held against the body firmly) often will not illicit a change over the thin lower margin or detect a change at the upper margin, depending on the contour of the diaphragm and the volume of the lower lungs (2). Nuclear medicine scintigraphy or ultrasound study defines hepatomegaly as greater than 15.5 cm. Studies comparing physical examination to these modalities have not shown physical examination to be accurate or consistent, with high interexaminer differences. Skrainka et al. evaluated liver size estimation by direct percussion, indirect percussion, palpation, and ultrasound. His results demonstrated that experienced clinicians (medicine consultants) accurately assessed liver size compared with ultrasound and that direct percussion measurements correlated the best with liver size in all groups (5).

IV. **Testing**
  A. **What are appropriate diagnostic tests in the setting of hepatomegaly?** An ultrasound of the right upper quadrant should be obtained, as well as a chest x-ray, and kidney, urinary tract, and bladder studies. Initial laboratory evaluation should include a complete blood count, electrolytes, creatinine, glucose, liver enzyme testing (alanine aminotransferase, aspartame transferase, γ-glutamyl transpeptidase, alkaline phospatase), and true liver function tests (albumin, prothrombin time, partial thromboplastin time and bilirubin). If liver enzymes are elevated, a hepatitis serology panel is added. Nondiagnostic ultrasound or hepatic masses should prompt computed tomography scan. Further differential testing is shown in Table 9.7.
  B. **Liver biopsy** is indicated for unexplained hepatomegaly or jaundice, persistent abnormal liver tests, chronic viral hepatitis, suspected cirrhosis or portal hypertension, primary or secondary malignancy, suspected hemochromatosis, suspected Wilson's disease, and hepatic dysfunction following liver transplantation.
V. **Diagnostic assessment.** How are the physical examination findings used to form a differential diagnosis?
  A. **Smooth nontender liver:** suspect fatty infiltration, congestive heart failure (CHF), portal cirrhosis, primary biliary cirrhosis, lymphoma, portal obstruction, hepatic venous thrombosis, hepatic vein thrombosis, lymphocytic leukemia, amyloidosis, schistosomiasis, or kala-azar.
  B. **Smooth tender liver:** suspect early CHF, acute hepatitis, amoebic abscess, or hepatic abscess.
  C. **Nodular liver:** suspect late portal cirrhosis, tertiary syphilis, hydatid cyst, or metastatic carcinoma.
  D. **Very hard nodular liver:** nearly always indicates metastatic carcinoma.

Table 9.7 Specific tests to evaluate hepatomegaly

Suggested Diagnosis	Test
Autoimmune hepatitis	Smooth muscle antibody, anti-LKM
Biliary cirrhosis	Antimitochondrial antibody
Hemochromatosis	Ferritin
Wilson's disease	Ceruloplasmin
Hepatocellular cancer	α-fetoprotein
α₁-antitrypsin deficiency	Enzyme assay of same

LKM, liver and kidney microsomal (antibodies).

VI. Summary. The combination of history, physical examination, and appropriate laboratory studies should yield a quick and accurate diagnosis. New therapies for chronic liver disease, specifically chronic viral liver diseases, make the early diagnosis and accurate identification of hepatobiliary disease highly beneficial to patients. Any suspected liver disease should be pursued completely.

References

1. Castell DO, O'Brien KD, Muench H, Chalmers TC. Estimation of liver size by percussion in normal individuals. *Ann Intern Med* 1969;70:1183–1189.
2. Naylor CD. Physical examination of the liver. *JAMA* 1994;27:1859–1865.
3. Tucker WN, Saab S, Leland SR, Matthews WC. The scratch test is unreliable for determining the liver edge. *J Clin Gastroenterol* 1997;25:410–414.
4. Rosenfield AT, Laufer I, Schneider PB. The significance of a palpable liver: a correlation of clinical and radioisotope studies. *Am J Roentgenol Radium Ther Nucl Med* 1974;122:313–317.
5. Skrainka B, Stahlhut J, Knight F, Holmes RA, Butt JH. Measuring liver span: bedside examination versus ultrasound and scintiscan. *J Clin Gastroenterol* 1986;8: 267–270.

9.10 Jaundice

James M. Brian and Cara K. Fox

The hepatobiliary system removes bilirubin, a byproduct of hemoglobin metabolism, from the blood stream. Jaundice, a yellowing of the skin and sclera, results from tissue build-up of bilirubin when the hepatobiliary system does not function properly.

I. **Approach**. The most important task in evaluating jaundice is to determine whether the jaundice is caused by the overproduction of bilirubin, by the inability of the hepatocyte and biliary drainage system to adequately clear the blood of bilirubin, or by a combination of both. Possible causes are then established based on the mechanism (1).

  A. **Increased bilirubin production** results from hemolysis, ineffective erythropoiesis, reabsorption of hematoma, or transfusion.

  B. **Impaired bilirubin elimination** can be a result of either decreased hepatobiliary excretion, cholestasis, or a combination of both. Decreased hepatobiliary excretion usually results from a hereditary defect or hepatocyte damage. Poor excretion occurs because of impaired biliary uptake and transport by the liver cell, conjugation, excretion, or transport by the biliary system. Alcohol, drug toxicity, and viral hepatitis commonly cause decreased hepatobiliary excretion as well as obstruction. Cholelithiasis and malignancy often lead to obstructive cholestasis. Examples of cholestasis include viral or alcoholic hepatitis, drug-induced hepatitis, primary biliary cirrhosis, congestive heart failure, sepsis, pregnancy, neoplasm, or gallstones (2).

II. **History**

  A. Does the patient have exposure risk to alcohol, drugs, toxins, or medications? A history of nonprescription and prescription drugs and potential chemical toxins at home or work must be elicited.

  B. Recent trauma can result in hemolysis. Pruritus, dark urine, and clay-colored stools suggest cholestasis. If the patient presents with right upper quadrant pain and nausea following a fatty meal, think cholelithiasis. A fever with right upper quadrant pain suggests cholangitis or, with a history of exposure, hepatitis. Jaundice, vague epigastric discomfort, and weight loss suggest pancreatic cancer. A family history of liver disease points to a hereditary cause (e.g., Gilbert's or Wilson's syndromes).

C. Is the jaundice acute or chronic? Acute onset of jaundice suggests a viral hepatitis, acute liver failure, or an acute biliary tract obstruction. Gradual onset of jaundice points to chronic liver failure, alcohol toxicity, or malignancy. A lifelong history of jaundice suggests an inherited metabolic or hemolytic cause.

III. **Physical examination.** The physical examination should focus on the following: Eyes should be examined for icterus or Kayser-Fleischer rings, which are copper-colored rings suggestive of Wilson's disease. Heart and lung examination revealing S_3 gallop or rales is suggestive of congestive heart failure, which leads to passive liver congestion. Ascites, hepatosplenomegaly, venous hum, and tenderness on abdominal examination points to portal hypertension and indicates liver cirrhosis (Chapters 9.2 and 9.9). Suspect pancreatic carcinoma when a nontender, palpable mass is found on upper abdominal examination. Signs of cirrhosis include excoriations, spider nevi, caput medusa, Dupytren's contracture, gynecomastia, and palmar erythema. Delirium, drowsiness, asterixis, and tremor occur with liver failure.

IV. **Testing**
   A. **Laboratory tests.** Laboratory assays measure bilirubin as indirect (unconjugated) and direct (conjugated) fractions. An elevated indirect bilirubin level is consistent with overproduction of bilirubin or decreased uptake, transport, or conjugation by the hepatocyte. Elevation of direct bilirubin points to decreased excretion or transport by the biliary system (3). Transaminase levels (aspartate aminotransferase and alanine aminotransferase) increase from hepatocellular necrosis or inflammation from the release of aspartate aminotransferase from lysed hepatocytes. Hepatocyte damage and cholestasis increase alkaline phosphatase levels. γ-Glutamyl transpeptidase levels increase in cholestasis and alcohol abuse. Pancreatitis, pancreatic carcinoma, or common bile duct stones elevate amylase levels. With hepatocellular damage, coagulation studies can be prolonged. Antimitochondrial antibodies are present in primary biliary cirrhosis. Hepatitis B serologic tests are summarized in Table 9.8. Hepatitis A IgM antibody detects acute stage hepatitis A and IgG detects chronic stage hepatitis A. Anti-hepatitis C virus indicates hepatitis C infection. Hepatitis D only occurs with hepatitis B infection and is detected by anti-hepatitis D (4).
   B. **Diagnostic imaging** has limited uses. Plain films of the abdomen rarely provide useful information. Cholelithiasis or pancreatic mass are best detected by ultrasound. Magnetic resonance imaging or computed tomography scans are used to examine the liver, pancreas, biliary tree, and suspected obstruction not identified by ultrasound. Hepatoiminodiacetic acid scanning is useful in a patient with suspected acute cholecystitis. Percutaneous transhepatic cholangiography and endoscopic retrograde cholangiopancreatography are used if obstructive jaundice is suspected to show the cause, location, and extent of involvement (5).
   C. **Other tests.** Percutaneous liver biopsy is not indicated in the routine workup of jaundice but may prove useful in diagnosing the cause of jaundice when the above-mentioned tests are inconclusive. Iron levels are increased in hemochromatosis. Copper levels are increased in Wilson's disease.

Table 9.8 Hepatitis B serologic tests

	Acute infection	Chronic infection	Convalescent	Immunized
HBsAg	+	−	−	−
HBsAb	−	−	+	+
HBcAb	+	+	+	−
HBeAg	+	+	−	−

V. Diagnostic assessment. The patient's history and associated symptoms guide the initial differential diagnosis of jaundice. Physical examination further narrows the causative choices and analysis of hepatic enzyme levels and viral serologies should confirm the initial diagnosis. Imaging studies play a limited role, except in suspected cases of malignancy or biliary obstruction.

Most patients have acute viral hepatitis as the cause of jaundice. Consultation is indicated when testing is inconclusive, when a surgical cause is suspected, or as needed for treatment.

References

1. Scharschmidt BF, Goldberg HI, Schmid R. Approach to the patient with cholestatic jaundice. *N Engl J Med* 1983;308:1515.
2. Lucas WB, Chuttani R. Pathophysiology and current concepts in the diagnosis of obstructive jaundice. *Gastroenterologist* 1995;3:105–118.
3. Fevery J, Blanckaert N. What can we learn from analysis of serum bilirubin? *J Hepatol* 1986;2:113–121.
4. Bakerman S. *ABC's of interpretive laboratory data*, 3rd ed. Myrtle Beach, SC: Interpretive Data, Inc., 1994:279–286.
5. Barloon TJ, Bergus GR, Weissman AM. Diagnostic imaging to identify the cause of jaundice. *Am Fam Physician* 1996;54:556–562.

9.11 Rectal Bleeding

Ted Epperly

Rectal bleeding is a common problem encountered by primary care providers across the United States. Annually, approximately 3% of the general population will report seeing blood in the toilet bowl and roughly 12% to 20% will note blood on the toilet paper (1–3). The prevalence of rectal bleeding is significantly higher in persons aged 20 to 40 years (18.9%) than in those aged more than 40 years (11.3%) (2). Only 14% to 28% of patients with rectal bleeding consult their doctor for this problem (2,3).

I. **Approach.** The key issue for the primary care provider is to determine which patients need aggressive diagnostic evaluation and which patients can be reassured and followed over time. The diagnostic approach is based on history, physical examination, and risk factor assessment. The differential diagnosis of rectal bleeding is presented in Table 9.9.

II. **History**

A. **Initial history.** The history is an important tool for risk stratification. Important questions to ask: What is the color of blood passed? Is the bowel movement associated with pain? How long has the bleeding occurred? Is there blood on toilet tissue versus mixed with stool, or dripping into the toilet bowl? Have there been prior episodes? Is abdominal pain, constipation, diarrhea, medication use, or weight loss present? What medications do you take? The only historical questions that have evidence-based data to support benign versus serious pathology are the presence of constipation, diarrhea, age less than 50 years, and bleeding longer than 2 months (1,2) (Chapters 9.3 and 9.4). These findings are associated with more benign causes. An exception to this is in the pediatric age group where bleeding in children can represent hereditary and anatomic anomalies (4).

B. **Other questions** that can help discriminate serious from benign causes are a change in bowel habit to persistent loose stools for more than 1 month, absence of perianal symptoms in the presence of rectal bleedings, first time rectal bleeding, and the appearance of dark red blood (3). These are especially likely to be associated with more serious causes.

III. **Physical examination.** Assess the patient's weight, general condition, and vital signs. Orthostatic blood pressure changes with a drop of 10 mm Hg or an increase

Table 9.9 Differential diagnosis of rectal bleeding

Benign anorectal disorders
  Hemorrhoids (internal and external)
  Anal fissures
  Varices
Diverticular disease
Inflammatory bowel disease
Ulcerative colitis
Crohn's disease
Infectious colitis or enteritis
  Viral
  Bacterial
Ischemic colitis
Neoplasia
  Benign adenomatous polyps
  Adenocarcinoma
Coagulopathies
Arteriovenous malformations
  Vascular ectasias, angiomas,
    angiodysplasia
	Upper gastrointestinal hemorrhage
	  Gastritis
	  Gastric ulcer
	  Duodenal ulcer
	  Mallory-Weiss tear
	  Esophageal varices
	  Neoplasms
	  Hereditary hemorrhagic telangiectasia
	    (Rendu-Osler-Weber disease)
	  Epistaxis
	  Aortoenteric fistula
	Small intestinal hemorrhage
	  Arteriovenous malformations
	  Diverticula (Meckel's)
	  Regional enteritis
	  Neoplasia
	  Aortoenteric fistula

in heart rate of 10 beats/minute indicates a blood loss of at least 1,000 ml (20% of circulating blood volume) (5). It is important to perform an external anal inspection, (checking for external hemorrhoids, fissures), digital rectal examination (checking for a rectal mass, polyp or anal pain), abdominal examination (checking for tenderness or mass), and nasopharyngeal examination (checking for a bleeding source).

IV. Testing

    A. Anoscopy. The anoscope allows inspection for fissures, fistulas, bleeding and nonbleeding hemorrhoids, and rectal friability.

    B. Rigid proctosigmoidoscopy has given way to flexible sigmoidoscopy; it visualizes well the distal 25 cm of the proctosigmoid area for neoplasia, friability, polyps, ulcers, or hemorrhoids. Rigid sigmoidoscopy has a sensitivity of 69% and specificity of 95% in determining the presence or absence of disease (1).

    C. Flexible sigmoidoscopy is much better tolerated by the patient than rigid proctosigmoidoscopy. It visualizes the distal 60 to 70 cm of the colon and detects similar findings as rigid proctosigmoidoscopy with similar sensitivity and specificity.

    D. Air contrast barium enema demonstrates polyps, masses, mucosal irregularities, diverticulae and inflammatory bowel disease with a sensitivity of 52% and a specificity of 98% (1). When used in combination with sigmoidoscopy, it has a sensitivity of 96% and specificity of 76% with a positive predictive value of 55% (1).

    E. Stool guaiac testing. As a test for occult bleeding in determining serious pathology, the guaiac card has a sensitivity of 44% to 75% and a specificity of 85%. As a screening tool, it has received mixed blessings, being promoted by the American Cancer Society and National Cancer Institute, but with insufficient evidence to recommend for or against by the US Preventive Services Task Force.

    F. Colonoscopy. The diagnostic procedure of choice to visualize the entire colon. It allows only one bowel preparation and has identification rates of 74% to 82% of lower GI bleeding sources (5). The sensitivity of this examination approaches 98%.

G. Nuclear scintigraphy. ^{99m}Technetium-labeled red blood cells detects occult bleeding sources when the above-mentioned methods fail. Sensitivity ranges from 80% to 98% in the colon with specificity of 41% to 97% (5).

H. Mesenteric angiography uses a transfemoral placement to selectively evaluate the superior mesenteric, inferior mesenteric, and celiac axis. The sensitivity is 40% to 86% with a complication rate of 2% (5). Treatment interventions include arterial infusion of vasopressin and embolization with coil springs or gel foam.

I. Enteroscopy. Small bowel enteroscopy uses a special enteroscope or pediatric colonoscope. This scope is passed orally and has a diagnostic yield of 25% (5).

V. Diagnostic assessment. The answers provided in the patient's history and physical examination are important to risk stratify this common problem. If a workup is believed necessary to deal with diagnostic uncertainty, then the entire colon should be visualized. This approach should consist of a digital rectal examination, anoscopy, rigid or flexible sigmoidoscopy, and the use of air contrast barium enema as deemed necessary. Alternatively, exploration by colonoscopy can be used, based on the provider's discretion. The latter makes most sense as two bowel preparations can be reduced to one with enhanced patient comfort. Further workup, including nuclear scintigraphy, mesenteric angiography, enteroscopy, and referral to a surgeon or a gastroenterologist, depends on the clinical situation and seriousness of the bleed encountered. Serious pathology occurs in approximately 25% of rectal bleeding patients with 6.5% to 10% having cancer, 13% to 25% having polyps, and 4% to 11% having inflammatory bowel disease (1,2). Ten year follow-up of patients with benign anorectal disease or no evident cause of bleeding found no difference in the incidence of cancer compared with similarly aged cohort in the general population (1).

References

1. Helfant M, Marton KI, Zimmer-Gembeck MJ, Sax HC. History of visible rectal bleeding in a primary care population: initial assessment and 10-year follow-up. *JAMA* 1997;277(1):44–48.
2. Talley NJ, Jones M. Self reported rectal bleeding in a United States community: prevalence, risk factors, and health care seeking. *Am J Gastroenterol* 1998;93: 2179–2183.
3. Thompson M, Prytherah D. Rectal bleeding: when is it right to refer. *Practitioner* 1996;240:198–200.
4. Colletti RB, Compton CC. Weekly clinicopathological exercises: case 7-1997. A 14-year-old girl with recurrent painless rectal bleeding. *N Engl J Med* 1997;336(9): 641–648.
5. Vernava AM, Moore BA, Longo WE, Johnson FE. Lower gastrointestinal bleeding. *Dis Colon Rectum* 1997;40:846–858.

9.12 Steatorrhea

Charles L. Bryner, Jr.

Steatorrhea, the third most common cause of chronic diarrhea, manifests as a history of greasy, foul-smelling stools that leave an oily residue in the toilet bowl, increased flatulence, and weight loss.

I. Approach. A simple diagnostic approach is to divide the causes of steatorrhea into two categories: Does the malabsorption result from intraluminal digestion abnormality or from mucosal disease blocking absorption? Although crossover occurs between the categories, this categorization is a clinically expedient starting point.

II. History. A careful history and physical examination provide clues to probable diagnoses and guides the astute clinician to tests most likely to provide a definitive diagnosis. How frequent are stools? How long have symptoms been present? Any recent travel or pancreatitis (ask about level of alcohol intake)? Weight loss (Chapter 2.13)? Are there food intolerances or family history of similar problems?

A. Liver disease. Does the patient have liver disease? Acute or chronic liver disease can cause steatorrhea. Impaired synthesis or excretion of conjugated bile salts results in a bile salt deficiency and maldigestion of fats. Hepatitis, primary biliary cirrhosis, alcohol-induced liver diseases, or extrahepatic biliary obstruction (including cancer of the head of the pancreas) may be culprits in steatorrhea (Chapter 9.8). Liver function testing and appropriate use of ultrasonography or computed tomography (CT) may delineate the problem. Prolonged, severe cardiac failure or hemochromatosis can cause cirrhosis, which can produce steatorrhea.

B. Medications. Has the patient been taking any medications? Laxative abuse occurs more frequently in women than in men. Laxative abuse hastens gastrointestinal (GI) transit and can preclude adequate absorption of fats. Other drugs that can cause steatorrhea include bile acid sequestering resins (cholestyramine and colestipol), colchicine, paraaminosalicylic acid, paromomycin sulfate (Humatin), and antibiotics (e.g., tetracycline and neomycin).

C. GI problems. Is there a history of GI surgery or disorder affecting gastrointestinal motility? The short bowel syndrome following gastrectomy is a well-known cause of steatorrhea (5). Pancreatic enzymes can be inactivated by exposure to gastric acids or by bacterial overgrowth secondary to stasis of intestinal contents in a blind loop. Segmental stasis of intestinal contents can occur in diabetes or scleroderma. Stasis permits bacterial overgrowth of the affected segment. The bacteria subsequently deconjugate and metabolize the bile acids in the small bowel rather than the colon.

D. Foods. Ingestion of certain foods has been shown to cause steatorrhea. Ingestion of a large amount of peanuts or using liquid paraffin to treat constipation can result in significant steatorrhea.

III. Physical examination. Physical findings associated with steatorrhea are limited. Thoroughly examine the abdomen to exclude palpable masses and search for signs of alcoholic liver disease. Testing of the stool for occult blood can be helpful.

IV. Testing. The Sudan III spot test for stool fat or quantitative determination of fecal fat in the total stool collected over 72 hours confirms steatorrhea (1,2). More than 7 g/day of fat excreted while the patient consumes a diet containing no more than 100 g/day of fat defines steatorrhea.

How severe is the steatorrhea? More than 35 g/day of fat excreted is more likely maldigestion of fats from pancreatic disease than malabsorption disorders of the intestinal mucosa.

How can the clinician differentiate mucosal disease from intraluminal digestive problems? The D-xylose test measures the absorptive capacity of the proximal small bowel mucosa. D-xylose does not require pancreatic exocrine function to be absorbed. Disorders of the intestinal mucosa that impede absorption lead to low levels of sugar in both serum and urine samples. Inadequate renal function, dehydration, or hypothyroidism can also depress urine levels, which warrants determinations of serum thyroid-stimulating hormone, blood urea nitrogen, and serum creatinine. Bacterial overgrowth of the small intestine can also produce an abnormal D-xylose test.

An abnormal D-xylose test should prompt referral for small intestine biopsy to search for evidence of mucosal diseases, including celiac sprue (3), Whipple's disease, giardiasis, tropical sprue, or intestinal lymphoma. A biopsy is more likely to detect diseases with diffuse rather than patchy involvement of the mucosa. Some of these entities can also be diagnosed by their characteristic appearance on an upper GI series.

Serum antibody testing can now identify celiac sprue (4). Sweat chloride testing is indicated in young children because cystic fibrosis is the leading cause of steatorrhea in this age group.

What if the D-xylose test is normal? A normal test indicates proper mucosal function and so the problem is the digestion of fats within the intestinal lumen. The most frequent cause is pancreatic insufficiency (Table 9.10). Confirmation

Table 9.10 Causes of pancreatic exocrine insufficiency

Alcohol-induced liver diseases	Cystic fibrosis
Chronic pancreatitis	Zollinger–Ellison syndrome
Hypertriglyceridemia	Gastrectomy
Pancreatic cancer	Vagotomy
Resection of the pancreas	Hemochromatosis
Pancreatic duct blockage	Shwachman–Diamond syndrome
Traumatic pancreatitis	Trypsinogen deficiency
Hereditary pancreatitis	α_1-antitrypsin deficiency
Enterokinase deficiency	Somatostatinoma

once relied on intubation of the intestine to directly measure pancreatic secretions. The newer noninvasive NBT-PABA (bentiromide) test requires pancreatic enzymes to cleave a peptide, allowing its absorption and subsequent measurement when excreted in urine. Occasionally, a secretin test will be required to measure pancreatic function. A therapeutic trial of pancreatic enzymes with improvement in symptoms is considered presumptive proof of the diagnosis. Abdominal ultrasonography, CT, or endoscopic retrograde cholangiopancreatography can also be useful in the evaluation of suspected pancreatic disease.

Disorders of the terminal ileum (Crohn's disease, granulomatous ileitis, prior ileal resection) result in poor absorption of bile salts which then pass into the colon where bacteria deconjugate them. Poor absorption depletes the supply of bile salts, resulting in maldigestion of fats (5). The bile salt breath test, a nuclear medicine study, measures bile acid absorption. Because the terminal ileum is also the site of vitamin B_{12} absorption, the Schilling test can also be used to search for disorders of absorption.

How to test for bacterial overgrowth in the intestine? The upper small intestine is normally bacteriologically sterile, except for contaminants from the mouth and upper respiratory tract. This is maintained by peristalsis. Aspiration of fluid through an endoscope or a small-intestine tube placed under fluoroscopic guidance that yields a bacterial colony count greater than 100,000/ml is diagnostic. Noninvasive testing is available by the C-xylose breath test, the bile acid breath test, or the breath hydrogen test. A therapeutic trial of oral tetracycline with subsequent resolution of steatorrhea is presumptive confirmation of bacterial overgrowth, which may avoid more costly testing.

V. **Diagnostic assessment.** The differential diagnosis for steatorrhea is extensive. The degree of steatorrhea can lend clues to the source. Mild steatorrhea can occur with any disorder that causes rapid transit of intestinal contents as the shortened exposure of the fats prevents proper absorption. The proper workup of this symptom will frequently require specialized testing and procedures necessitating consultation with a gastroenterologist when the initial history and more readily available tests fail to reveal its source.

References

1. Wilson FA, Dietschy JM. Differential diagnostic approach to clinical problems of malabsorption. *Gastroenterology* 1971;61:911–931.
2. Olsen WA. A practical approach to diagnosis of disorders of intestinal absorption. *N Engl J Med* 1971;285:1358–1361.
3. Pruessner HT. Detecting celiac disease in your patients. *Am Fam Physician* 1998;57: 1023–1034.
4. Murray JA. Serodiagnosis of celiac disease. *Clin Lab Med* 1997;17:445–464.
5. Toffolon EP, Goldfinger SE. Malabsorption following gastrectomy and ileal resection. *Surg Clin North Am* 1974;54:647–653.

10. RENAL AND UROLOGIC PROBLEMS

R. WHITNEY CURRY, JR.

10.1 Dysuria

David M. Quillen

I. **Approach.** Dysuria is defined as "painful urination." Acute dysuria is a frequent problem seen in ambulatory practices, accounting for more than three million office visits a year. The most common diagnosis given for patients with dysuria is a urinary tract infection (UTI). Estimated cost for traditional management of acute UTIs approaches $1 billion per year in the United States. Although a UTI is the most common cause for dysuria symptoms, many other causes need to be accurately diagnosed. The differential diagnosis for patients with dysuria can be separated into broad categories. With a few notable exceptions, the differential diagnoses for men and women are similar, although the incidences are much different and change with age (1–2).

  A. **Causes of dysuria—Female**
    1. Infectious
      a. Cystitis, lower UTI, with or without pyelonephritis
      b. Urethritis caused by a sexually transmitted disease (STD): chlamydia, *Neisseria gonorrhoeae*, herpes simplex virus (HSV)
      c. Vulvovaginitis: bacterial vaginosis, trichomoniasis, yeast, genital HSV
    2. Noninfectious
      a. Trauma, irritant, allergy, sexual abuse

  B. **Causes of dysuria—Male (3)**
    1. Infectious
      a. Urethritis caused by chlamydia, *N. gonorrhoeae*, yeast (uncircumcised, balanitis), HSV (Chapter 10.9)
      b. Cystitis (if culture positive, possible anatomic abnormality, further workup indicated)
      c. Prostatitis, acute more common than chronic (4)
    2. Noninfectious
      a. Penile lesions, trauma, sexual abuse

II. **History.** A good general history is critical and can help direct further questions.

  A. **Distinguishing between symptoms of "internal" dysuria and "external" dysuria** is often helpful. Internal dysuria is where the discomfort seems to be centered inside the body and begins before or with the initiation of voiding. External dysuria is when the discomfort appears after voiding has initiated. Symptoms of internal dysuria suggest inflammation of the bladder or urethra, whereas those of external dysuria suggest vaginitis, vulvar inflammation, or external penile lesions.

  B. **Careful questioning about other associated symptoms and risk factors** is the key to sorting out the diagnosis. The history of a new sex partner may support an STD cause. Diaphragm usage may support a bladder infection as well as associated symptoms of frequency, urgency, voiding small volumes, hematuria, and abrupt onset. Gradual onset is more suggestive of urethritis and external causes. Other symptoms of suprapubic pain, costovertebral angle tenderness, fever, flank pain, and so on should be asked about and can direct the diagnostic workup.

III. **Physical examination.** The physical examination is essential in narrowing the diagnosis. It helps to rule out pyelonephritis and other systemic infections in patients with dysuria, allowing the physician to search for the less severe causes. Fever, flank tenderness, and suprapubic tenderness are useful findings. A careful genital examination (speculum in women, foreskin retraction and prostate examination in uncircumcised men) can point to specific localized causes. The genital examination also allows collection of samples for testing. Attention to localized lesions (e.g., HSV lesions), discharge (yeast, bacterial vaginosis, gonorrhea, and trichomoniasis) and trauma also help make the diagnosis.

IV. **Testing.** The history and physical examination usually suggests which tests are most appropriate. A urinalysis is the most common study performed. It is important also to gather samples for gonorrhea, chlamydia, and HSV, using wet preparations and potassium hydroxide testing when appropriate. Rapid tests on urine samples for the detection of bacteria and leukocytes can be done while patients wait. Direct microscopic examination of the urine can isolate bacteria and leukocytes. Rapid dipstick biochemical tests can isolate leukoesterase and nitrate, which are consistent with leukocytes and urea-fixing bacteria. Urine cultures require overnight to 48 hours of incubation to detect specific bacterial pathogens. Pyuria (defined as white blood cell count >10/mm^3 of urine) is seen in more than 95% of patients with acute UTI but is uncommon in the absence of infection. Pyuria without bacteriuria suggests a chlamydia infection. Urine dipstick testing is generally less sensitive for pyuria than microscopic examination, but it is more convenient (5).

V. **Diagnostic assessment.** Given the many causes of dysuria, an accurate diagnosis can be difficult without a thorough approach to each patient. Because most causes have other associated symptoms and findings, a diagnosis can usually be made with a carefully taken history, a focused physical examination, and appropriate laboratory tests. Separating an uncomplicated UTI or STD from the more serious pyelonephritis and other possible diagnoses is the challenge in these patients.

References

1. Carlson KJ, Mulley AG. Management of acute dysuria. *Ann Intern Med* 1985;102: 244–249.
2. Johnson JR, Stamm WE. Diagnosis and treatment of acute urinary tract infections. *Infect Dis Clin North Am* 1987;4(1):773–791.
3. Ainsworth JG, Weaver T, Murphy S, Renton A. General practitioners' immediate management of men presenting with urethral symptoms. *Genitourin Med* 1996;72(6):427–430.
4. Roberts RO, Lieber MM, Rhodes R, Girman CJ, Bostwick DG, Jacobsen SJ. Prevalence of a physician-assigned diagnosis of prostatitis: the Olmsted County Study of Urinary Symptoms and Health Status Among Men. *Urology* 1998;51(4):578–584.
5. Kurowiski K. The woman with dysuria. *Am Fam Physician* 1998;57(9):2155–2164, 2169–2170.

10.2 Hematuria

Siegfried Schmidt and Ku-Lang Chang

Hematuria, defined as "blood in the urine," is encountered frequently in family practice. It can occur as gross (macroscopic) hematuria with obvious reddish discoloration or can be seen microscopically, detected only with dipstick or microscopic examination. Routine urinalysis in 1,000 men aged between 18 and 33 years reported a 40% incidence (1). The extent of the workup can be determined by considering factors such as the likelihood of association with a severe underlying illness, complications of procedures, and expenses affecting the patient.

I. **Approach**

A. **General approach.** The overall objective dealing with hematuria is to discover potentially serious diseases (including glomerulonephritis and malignancies). In general, the degree of hematuria is of little diagnostic or prognostic value. As little as 1 ml of blood can cause a visible color change. In addition, a variety of drugs, foods, and food coloring can discolor the urine. The use of a benzidine dipstick allows differentiation of these discolorations from those of hematuria and myoglobinuria. The timing of hematuria during micturition can be helpful.

Other associated symptoms will help to narrow the diagnosis and direct the workup. A detailed history is essential and it will help pinpoint other causes of hematuria (e.g., specific drugs, parasites, and congenital or hereditary factors). It is helpful to know that hematuria in the adult is more often urologic than nephritic in origin. Mariani and Mariani determined the cause for asymptomatic, isolated hematuria in 1,000 adult cases and found that only 1.5% were glomerular in origin; 75% were caused by urethritis, prostate disease, bladder malignancies, and cystitis (2). Strategies for further diagnostic tests depend on the history and physical examination findings, which should give some idea as to whether the cause is nephritic, renal parenchymal, urologic, extrarenal in origin.

B. **Red flags.** Painless gross hematuria in an elderly man, in the absence of infection, is caused by a malignancy until proved otherwise. Hematuria associated with "sterile" pyuria is genitourinary tuberculosis or interstitial nephritis until proved otherwise. The presence of hematuria in patients on anticoagulation treatment warrants a complete evaluation. To avoid missing a malignancy, repeat evaluations are indicated for those patients in whom a malignancy is suspected (mainly older adults) and for those with a negative evaluation. The time interval is subject to debate and a reasonable time frame appears to be 3 to 6 months for less invasive tests and 1 year for more invasive tests (3).

II. **History.** A thorough history is of utmost importance!

  A. **General aspects**

   1. Type of hematuria (macro/gross or microscopic).
   2. Relationship to urination or timing of hematuria. The three-container method will help to separate the micturition into three portions with an initial, middle, and final portion.

      Predominantly, initial hematuria results from anterior urethral disease; final hematuria results from disease of the bladder neck or posterior urethra; and hematuria throughout the stream suggests a disease site higher in the bladder, ureter, or kidney.
   3. Urine color. Color can be affected by the following: Phenazopyridine (orange); nitrofurantoin (brown); rifampin (yellow-orange); L-dopa, methyldopa, and metronidazole (reddish-brown); phenolphthalein in laxatives, red beet and rhubarb consumption, food coloring, and vegetable dyes (red).
   4. Clots, especially wormlike clots, suggest a location above the bladder neck.
   5. Associated symptoms (e.g., recent sore throat, fever, chills, and flulike symptoms) may be the first sign of IgA nephropathy or postinfectious glomerulonephritis. Urinary frequency, dysuria, fever, chills, and urgency point to an infectious process. Diminished urine flow and abdominal pain or flank pain radiating into the groin can indicate the presence of urinary tract obstruction (Chapter 10.5). Vaginal discharge or bowel movement changes may hint at a nonurinary tract cause such as a foreign body (especially in children). A rash, joint pain, photosensitivity, flulike symptoms, and Raynaud's phenomenon point to a collagen vascular disease.

  B. **Past medical history** should lead to a suspicion of parasites (e.g., *Schistosoma heamatobium*) if the patient has traveled to endemic areas; of bladder tumor if there was exposure to chemical carcinogens (e.g., aniline dyes), or tobacco smoke. Other causes of hematuria detected in the history include drug ingestion and anticoagulation, and medical problems such as prostatic hypertrophy, diabetes mellitus (nephrosclerosis), analgesic medication abuse (renal papillary necrosis), nephrolithiasis, trauma (including vigorous masturbation), chemotherapy exposure with cyclophosphamide (chemical cystitis), antibiotic use (interstitial nephritis), previous urinary tract malignancies suggesting recurrence, and sickle cell disease (papillary necrosis).

C. **Family history.** Delineate any family history of polycystic kidney disease, sickle cell trait and disease, nephrolithiasis, various glomerular diseases, tuberculosis, and benign familial hematuria. The combination of renal failure, deafness, and hematuria suggests Alport's hereditary nephritis.

III. **Physical examination** should focus on signs of systemic disease (fever, rash, lymphadenopathy, joint swelling, and abdominal or pelvic mass), and underlying medical or renal disease (hypertension, edema). Multiple telangiectasias and mucous membrane lesions indicate hereditary hemorrhagic telangiectasia (Rendu-Osler-Weber disease). An abdominal mass in children requires exclusion of Wilms tumor.

IV. **Testing**

A. **Initial evaluation.** Hematuria is usually detected by dipstick or microscopic examination. The dipstick test relies on detecting hemoglobin and should always be confirmed by microscopic examination of the urine sediment. Some controversy exists about the abnormal number of red blood cells in urine. Most clinicians consider more than three to five red blood cells per high power field (40 × lens) as definitely abnormal. When dipstick testing is positive for blood but urine microscopy reveals no red blood cells, hemoglobinuria or myoglobinuria should be considered. The next step is a urine culture. Baseline blood tests include a renal panel, complete blood count with differential, sedimentation rate, prothrombin time, and partial thromboplastin time.

B. **Further evaluation** is highly dependent on the suspected cause. Further blood tests can include serum complement titer (significant if low), antistreptolysin-O titer (high), antinuclear antibody and extended panels with anti-deoxyribonuclease B titer (high), and hemoglobin electrophoresis. A tuberculin skin test or chest x-ray study can be done to detect tuberculosis. Further tests can include imaging studies and cytology. Intravenous pyelogram and abdominal and pelvic ultrasound or computed tomography scanning may detect malignancies of the various anatomic areas as well as benign conditions such as urolithiasis, obstructive uropathy, renal cysts, parenchymal abnormalities, and nonurinary tract lesions. To complete the workup, send the urine for cytology study and proceed with cystoscopy looking for abnormalities of the urethra and bladder. Biopsies of various areas, including kidney and bladder, and invasive vascular studies may be needed. Unless a diagnosis is made, patients will need referral to subspecialists.

V. **Diagnostic assessment.** The key to the diagnosis of hematuria is the clinical history and physical examination. Laboratory and imaging studies only confirm or rule out initial suspicions. The goal is to diagnose a variety of serious illnesses, including malignancies and renal parenchymal diseases. In general, keep in mind that transient hematuria, especially in a young person, is quite common and rarely indicative of significant pathology (4). When present in patients aged more than 50 years, however, transient hematuria always warrants a comprehensive evaluation to rule out malignancy. Similarly, a diagnostic workup should be performed when persistent hematuria is found in patients of any age.

References

1. Froom P, Ribak J, Benbassat J. The significance of microhematuria in young adults. *BMJ* 1984;288:20–28.
2. Mariani AJ, Mariani MC. The significance of adult hematuria: 1000 hematuria evaluations including a risk-benefit and cost-effectiveness analysis. *J Urol* 1989; 141:350–355.
3. Messing EM, Young TB, Hunt VB, et al. Hematuria home screening: repeat testing results. *J Urol* 1995;154(1):57–61.
4. Murakami S, Igarashi T, Hara S, et al. Strategies for asymptomatic microscopic hematuria: a prospective study of 1034 patients. *J Urol* 1990;144:99–106.

10.3 Impotence

Louis Kuritzky

I. **Approach.** Impotence, defined as the consistent inability to get or maintain an erection sufficient for intercourse, is a patient-defined diagnosis. Because up to one-third of men aged more than 65 years have erectile dysfunction (ED), sheer volume merits accurate clinical definition. The role of the clinician is to confirm impotence, rule out correctable secondary causes, and expeditiously restore sexual function. Although current consensus suggests the term impotence should be replaced with ED because of the alleged pejorative connotations of the former, clinicians should feel comfortable using either term. In fact, technical terms that might cause confusion or be discordant with the patient's educational or cultural status should be particularly avoided.

Having self-diagnosed impotence, men usually are seeking restoration of sexual function, not further confirmation of the diagnosis. Most healthy men will occasionally experience an isolated episode of inability to perform sexually as a result of fatigue, depression, boredom, anxiety, sleep deprivation, or relationship conflict, but do not fit the consistent portion of the definition. To encourage hopefulness, explain at the outset that essentially 100% of men may have sexual function restored using currently available treatments. Impotence is broadly divided into psychogenic and organic categories, although often a substantial degree of overlap is seen (1).

A. **Psychogenic impotence** can reflect depression, relationship conflict, performance anxiety, or partner-directed hostility. The history is definitive in most cases. Sudden, complete loss of function, situation or partner variability, and maintenance of morning or masturbatory erections are typical. Good rigid morning erections indicate an intact erectile circuitry sufficient for sexual responsivity, hence circumstantial erectile capacity is psychogenic. Occasionally, patients with dysfunctions other than impotence will seek advice, for instance believing that premature ejaculation is impotence. In such cases, corrective education combined with appropriate attention to the alternate diagnosis is the logical next step.

B. **Organic sexual dysfunction** is characterized by incremental loss of erectile function. In middle age, men with organic ED note reduced erectile turgidity, increasing requirement for tactile stimulation to produce an erection, and a lengthening refractory period (i.e., the amount of time after ejaculation required before the male is receptive to restimulation and erection). Such stepwise loss of sexual function corroborates organicity.

Most organic impotence is on a vascular basis. Because integrity of the endothelium is necessary to provide adequate dilation of the sinusoids of the corpora cavernosa via the arteries supplying the penis, predictably, disorders causing endothelial dysfunction are associated with ED. For instance, diabetes causes a marked shift "to the left" in the incidence of impotence, so that by age 30, almost one of seven men who are diabetic manifest erectile insufficiency (Chapter 14.1). Unfortunately, improved glycemic control rarely reverses the endothelial or neurologic pathologies sufficient to fully restore erectile function. Smoking, hypertension, atherosclerosis, hyperlipidemia, and peripheral vascular disease all impair endothelial function and, hence, induce ED. Unless a correctable cause of impotence is suspected, it is usually unnecessary to determine the exact underlying cause. On the other hand, all the commonly used treatment tools (i.e., vacuum constriction pumps, intracavernosal injection, intraurethral prostaglandin, sildenafil) can be used, regardless of the underlying cause.

II. **History**

A. **Basic history.** Although written questionnaires may elicit sexual dysfunction, most patients prefer to communicate such issues in the privacy of verbal communication with their primary care provider. For the initial inquiry, simply ask: "Are you sexually active?" For sexual dysfunction evaluation, gender orientation is not relevant to diagnosis or therapy, so that whether the patient is homosexual, heterosexual, or bisexual has no distinct bearing on the diagnostic or therapeutic direction. For persons who are not sexually active, next determine whether this is a matter of choice or an obstacle that prevents sexual activity (e.g., lack of partner, ED, physical disorder).

For persons who are sexually active, a series of follow-up questions will uncover most relevant psychosexual pathology. Begin with: "How would you rate your sex life on a scale of 1 to 10?" If the response is 10, sexual dysfunction is decidedly unlikely. However, most individuals respond, "Oh, about a 7." Follow with, "What would have to be different to change your sex life from a 7 to a 10?" This forced-choice inquiry often produces responses which directly indicate problematic underlying issues: "Well, if I could just get a good erection." "If my erection could last more than 30 seconds." "If my partner didn't always pick a fight with me and then expect to have sex."

For impotent men, their response is usually direct and simple, indicating an inability to get or maintain an erection. Follow-up questions should determine the duration and nature of onset. Absence of morning erections should be sought, as this typifies organic impotence. Men who are much more likely to have psychogenic ED are those who report sudden, complete loss of sexual function, or "circumstantial" impotence, for example, (a) good function with one partner, but not another; (b) good erections with masturbation but not with interactive sex; (c) good morning erections, but not at times of interactive sex; or (d) overt anxiety or relationship conflict. Because organic ED generally leads to psychological consequences, many patients suffer a combination of psychogenic and organic impotence.

- B. **Inquiry about libido** is a crucial diagnostic point for testosterone deficiency. Testosterone is necessary for libido, but not erections. Men who present with good libido have only a remote possibility of having testosterone deficiency.
- C. **A medication history** should be taken for all men complaining of impotence, recalling that most medication-induced impotence is evident by the temporal relationship between onset of impotence and medication initiation. On the other hand, agents such as thiazides can produce impotence after months of use. Similarly, some antidepressants can produce sexual dysfunction either early or after weeks of therapy. The relationship of medications to impotence can often be clarified by a drug holiday.

III. **Physical examination.** Although physical examination is usually not enlightening, general agreement is seen that the genitals should be examined for evidence of overt testicular atrophy, and the penis for Peyronie's disease. In the latter, inflammatory plaques in the corpora cavernosa produce an area of limited expansile capacity, with subsequent penile deviation on erection which can prevent intromission. A rectal examination to document rectal sensation as well as tone can be complemented by the bulbocavernosus reflex. This reflex is elicited by briskly squeezing the glans penis in one hand while a single digit from the other is in the rectum. A normal examination, indicating an intact reflex arc, is manifest as a rectal contraction in response to the glans squeeze. Prostate examination is pertinent at this point, in the event testosterone therapy is required.

IV. **Testing.** Reasonable screening tests for impotence include a complete blood cell count, testosterone level, and a urinalysis. If testosterone is low, luteinizing hormone and follicle stimulating hormone levels should be measured, as an increase in either of these indicates gonadal failure, for which testosterone replacement is indicated; a decrease, however, indicates hypothalamic or pituitary insufficiency, necessitating central nervous system imaging to rule out a mass lesion. Similarly, low testosterone merits a serum prolactin level, as elevations of prolactin result in testosterone suppression. Other diagnostic testing, such as penile Doppler flow or nocturnal penile tumescence testing, add little to the options for therapy, but much to the expense.

V. **Diagnostic assessment.** In primary care, 98% of patients will have no testosterone deficiency, prolactin excess, or physical abnormalities (1). Such patients should be reassured that although they have no readily correctable cause for their impotence, effective therapy can be immediately begun. Patients who fail to respond to the standard tools for potency restoration (oral agents, vacuum constriction devices, and so on), or who desire more definitive delineation of their underlying pathology (as might be determined by Doppler studies) should be referred to specialty diagnostic centers.

Reference

1. Kuritzky L, Ahmed O, Kosch S. Management of impotence in primary care. *Compr Ther* 1998;24(3):137–146.

10.4 Nocturia

Anna M. Wright and Vincent H. Ober

I. **Approach.** Nocturia, defined as awakening from sleep to urinate, is a frequent symptom in patients of all ages and it is associated with many disease processes. Nocturia is usually caused by increased urine output, sleep-related difficulties, or urinary tract dysfunction (1). A careful history with a focused physical examination and laboratory tests are the most important diagnostic tools.

II. **History.** Possible causes of nocturia include:
   A. **Increased urine output.** The history should include questions concerning the following causes of increased urine output:
      1. Excess intake of fluids
      2. Drugs (i.e., caffeine, alcohol, diuretics, nonsteroidal antiinflammatory drugs, calcium channel blockers, lithium)
      3. Diabetes mellitus (Chapter 14.1)
      4. Diabetes insipidus (central or nephrogenic)
      5. Hypercalcemia (Chapter 17.4)
      6. Peripheral edema (from any cause) (Chapter 2.3)
      7. Congestive heart failure (Chapter 7.5)
      8. Renal disease
      9. Aging (1)
   B. **Sleep-related nocturia.** Disrupted sleep will cause a patient to arise and empty a partially filled bladder. Causes of disrupted sleep include:
      1. Use of a short-acting sedative hypnotic
      2. Pain (acute or chronic)
      3. Dyspnea (from pulmonary or cardiac disease) (Chapter 8.7)
      4. Anxiety or depression
      5. Drugs that interfere with the sleep cycle (2)
      6. Parkinson's disease
   C. **Dementia**
   D. **Sleep apnea (3)**
   E. **Urinary tract dysfunction.** Causes of lower urinary dysfunction include:
      1. Lower urinary tract infection
      2. Small bladder capacity
      3. Detrusor hyperactivity
      4. Prostatic hypertrophy
      5. Urinary retention for any reason
      6. Decreased bladder compliance (interstitial cystitis, radiation, tuberculosis) (2)
      7. Sensory stimulation in a paraplegic
      8. Neurogenic bladder (spastic or atonic) from multiple sclerosis, cerebrovascular accidents, herniated disks, or spinal cord injury
      9. Obstetric, gynecologic, or urologic disease or injury
      10. Chronic obstructive pulmonary disease (COPD) (4)
      11. Fecal impaction

III. **Physical examination.** The extent of the physical examination will be guided by the history. Essential for all patients is a genitourinary examination to identify lower urinary tract abnormalities such as bladder distention, cystocele, or rectocele. Examination of the heart, lungs, and extremities will identify pulmonary, cardiac disease, and peripheral edema. A rectal examination (with sphincter contraction during the examination) will identify sphincter laxity, fecal impaction, tumors, and prostate abnormalities. Absence of the anal wink (S4-5) or bulbocavernosus reflex (S2-3) can indicate spinal cord pathology. (In older patients, the absence of these reflexes is not always pathologic.) An expanded neurologic examination will be necessary in patients with other neurologic symptoms.

IV. **Testing.** A routine urinalysis by dipstick testing will identify infection and some types of renal disease. A low specific gravity can indicate increased fluid intake or renal disease with the inability to concentrate urine. Microscopic evaluation and urine culture can be helpful in selected cases. Serum blood urea nitrogen and creatinine can be elevated in renal disease. Urine electrolytes can help to diagnose diabetes insipidus. Measurement of postvoid residual urine will evaluate for urinary retention. A voiding diary with measurement of urine volume can be helpful. If the nighttime voided urine volume is high, the cause is excessive urine production. If the volume is less than bladder capacity (highest daytime voided volume), the nocturia is caused by a sleep-related problem or lower urinary tract pathology. Cystoscopy, renal ultrasound, intravenous pyelogram, and urodynamic studies are not usually needed in the evaluation of nocturia.

V. **Diagnostic assessment.** Patients with excessive fluid intake or use of alcohol or caffeine near bedtime or patients on medications (e.g., diuretics, theophylline, or calcium channel blockers) may complain of nocturia. Aging is associated with a loss of the nocturnal increase in vasopressin and increased nocturnal urine production (2). Nocturia, frequency, urgency, and dysuria coupled with a positive urinalysis indicate a urinary tract infection. Findings of rales on lung examination, an S_3 gallop, and lower extremity edema suggests congestive heart failure. COPD can cause respiratory acidosis and increased excretion of hydrogen ion with the production of an acid urine and bladder irritation (4). In a male patient, a diminished urinary stream and an enlarged prostate suggest prostatic hypertrophy and obstructive uropathy. Patients with insomnia from any number of causes (depression, pain, dyspnea, and so on) may experience nocturia. Be alert for the patient with nocturia secondary to neurologic conditions, which can cause inadequate secretion of vasopressin (diabetes insipidus).

References

1. Resnick NM. Urinary incontinence. In: Cassel CK, Cohen HJ, Larson EB, et al., eds. *Geriatric medicine*, 3rd ed. New York: Springer-Verlag, 1997:562–566.
2. Donahue JL, Lowenthal DT. Nocturnal polyuria in the elderly person. *Am J Med Sci* 1977;314(4):232–237.
3. Pressman MR, Figueroa WG, Kendrick-Mohamed J, Greenspon LW, Peterson DD. Nocturia. A rarely recognized symptom of sleep apnea and other occult sleep disorders. *Arch Intern Med* 1996;156(5):545–550.
4. McAninch JW. Symptoms of disorders of the genitourinary tract. In: Tanagho EA, McAninch JW, eds. *Smith's general urology*, 14th ed. Norwalk, CT: Appleton & Lange, 1995:36–38.

10.5 Oliguria and Anuria

Marcia W. Funderburk

Oliguria and anuria are important clinical signs that should be recognized quickly so that the cause can be identified and treatment initiated promptly to preserve renal function and prevent life-threatening complications.

I. **Approach.** The amount of urine output must first be established (most reliably measured using an indwelling catheter). Oliguria is defined as urine volume less than 500 ml/24 h or less than 20 ml/h (in small children, less than 0.8 ml/kg/h). Anuria is strictly defined as the total absence of urine; in the clinical setting, however, a urine output of less than 50 to 100 ml/24 h is often considered anuria (1).

   A. **Oliguria.** It is helpful to think of oliguria as being either (a) prerenal, (b) renal, or (c) postrenal.

   1. Prerenal disorders are characterized by decreased renal perfusion, leading to decreased glomerular filtration rate such that the daily endogenous load of nitrogenous wastes cannot be excreted, thus the term prerenal azotemia.

   2. Renal disorders are characterized by pathology within the kidney parenchyma itself, which can be the end result of prolonged decreased renal perfusion.

   3. Postrenal disorders causing oliguria are characterized by partial obstruction of the urinary tract at an anatomic position distal to the kidney. This can be confusing because these disorders can also cause polyuria.

   B. **Anuria** results from total obstruction of the urinary tract or as an end result of the prerenal and renal causes of oliguria. A sudden cause of anuria, especially in the elderly, is bilateral renal artery occlusion (or unilateral occlusion in a single kidney) typically caused by embolism. Early recognition of this entity is imperative to restore blood flow to the ischemic kidney(s).

II. **History**

   A. **Pertinent present history.** A patient may complain of decreased urine output in some clinical situations. More often, however, the clinical situation and pertinent history should lead to an evaluation of the presence of oliguria or anuria.

   1. Are there symptoms of illness or trauma leading to hypotension?

      a. Hypovolemia (e.g., hemorrhage, diuretic overuse, gastrointestinal fluid loss, skin fluid loss owing to burns or heat exposure, third spacing, secondary to burns, peritonitis, pancreatitis, or trauma)?

      b. Decreased cardiac output (e.g., congestive heart failure, myocardial infarction, pericardial tamponade, or acute pulmonary embolus)?

      c. Peripheral vasodilatation (e.g., septic shock, anaphylactic shock)?

   2. Are there symptoms of vascular disease? Consider bilateral renal vascular obstruction due to severe renal artery stenosis, thrombosis, or embolism.

   3. Is there any history consistent with renal parenchymal injury [e.g., recent radiocontrast agent, nephrotoxin exposure such as ethylene glycol, nonsteroidal antiinflammatory drug overdose, acute nephritis, acute vasculitis, pyelonephritis (in the elderly), papillary necrosis (in diabetic patients), or prolonged hypotension with hypoperfusion of the kidney]?

   4. Is there any history consistent with urinary tract obstruction?

      a. Bladder neck obstruction (e.g., benign prostatic hypertrophy, prostate cancer, bladder cancer, or functional obstruction due to drug side effects)?

      b. Obstruction of the urethra or bilateral ureters—internally (2° blood clots, stones, sulfonamide or uric acid crystals, pyogenic debris, necrotizing papillitis or edema), or externally (2° tumor, periureteral fibrosis, accidental ureteral ligation during pelvic surgery, ascites, pregnancy, pelvic abscess, or hematoma)?

   5. Medication use must be considered—diuretics, antihypertensives, anticholinergics, aminogycosides, amphotericin B, or chemotherapeutic drugs.

   B. **Other pertinent past history.** Is there a history of cancer, recent surgery, kidney stones, neurologic disorder, vascular disease, chronic liver disease (hepatorenal syndrome), or kidney transplant?

III. **Physical examination**

   A. **Focused physical examination (PE).** This should include vital signs (notably blood pressure, pulse, and temperature). Orthostatic blood pressure and pulse may be necessary. Signs of hypovolemia, hypotension, and dehydration should be noted—skin turgor and color, mucous membranes, capillary refill, warmth of extremities.

B. Additional PE. Depending on the history (e.g., skin rash, cardiac examination, bruits over kidneys) palpate for a distended bladder; if a cancer or outlet obstruction is suspected, perform a rectal or pelvic examination.

IV. Testing

A. An indwelling urinary catheter serves as a diagnostic tool (if obstruction has occurred at the bladder neck or urethra) and for accurate urine volume measurement. Urine output and blood pressure monitoring can often lead to expedient correction of prerenal causes, thus avoiding further complications.

B. Urinalysis is often normal in prerenal causes of oliguria or anuria, except being highly concentrated with possible qualitative proteinuria because of the high concentration. Microscopic analysis is usually unremarkable (or reveals few hyaline or granular casts) in prerenal causes; whereas proteinuria, casts, and hematuria can point to renal causes.

C. Urine osmolality is typically high in prerenal causes (>500 mOsm/kg H_2O) versus impaired in renal causes (<350 mOsm/kg H_2O) (2).

D. Urine sodium is typically less than 20 mEq/L in prerenal causes (unless diuretics have been used) versus more than 40 mEq/L in renal causes (2).

E. Blood urea nitrogen and creatinine levels are elevated. The ratio must be interpreted considering the entire clinical situation. Urine:plasma creatinine ratio (U:P Cr) is calculated to help differentiate between prerenal (U:P Cr >40) and renal (U:P Cr <20) causes (2).

F. Diagnostic imaging, which may be necessary in some cases, is guided by the history and PE findings [e.g., ultrasound (US), computed tomography (CT), retrograde pyelogram, renal biopsy].

V. Diagnostic assessment. The key to a diagnosis of oliguria or anuria is to actively anticipate when it is likely to manifest and accurately measure using an indwelling catheter. Once recognized and a cause is suggested, (a) prerenal causes can be assessed further by measuring hemodynamic status and administering fluids; (b) renal causes can be assessed further with urinalysis (qualitative and quantitative), renal US, or renal biopsy; and (c) postrenal causes can be assessed further using US, CT, or retrograde pyelography.

References
1. Eliahou HE. Oliguria and anuria. In: Massry SG, Glassock RJ, eds. *Massry and Glassock's textbook of nephrology*, 3rd ed. Baltimore: Williams & Wilkins, 1995:543–546.
2. Lake EW, Humes HD. Acute renal failure including cortical necrosis. In: Massry SG, Glassock RJ, eds. *Massry and Glassock's textbook of nephrology*, 3rd ed. Baltimore: Williams & Wilkins, 1995:984–987.

10.6 Priapism

David B. Feller

Priapism is defined as a persistent, often painful penile erection not associated with sexual stimulation. Although relatively uncommon, priapism represents a urologic emergency. Without prompt recognition and treatment, priapism can result in urinary retention, cavernosa fibrosis, impotence, or even gangrene.

I. Approach. Two types of priapism (low-flow or veno-occlusive and high-flow or arterial) have been described, based on the underlying precipitating event (1). Arterial priapism usually occurs after injury to the cavernous artery from perineal or direct penile trauma. This injury then leads to uncontrolled high arterial inflow within the corpora cavernosa. Veno-occlusive priapism is characterized by inadequate outflow and is by far the most common. Distinction between the two is imperative because ultimate treatment varies significantly.

II. History

A. Specific information. Is there a history of penile or perineal trauma? How much pain does the patient experience? Does the patient take any medications that may predispose to priapism (2)? Is there any history of malignancy? Is there any history of sickle cell disease? How long has the priapism been present?

1. A history of penile or perineal trauma almost always precedes arterial priapism and is the most important historical information distinguishing between the two types of priapism.
2. Moderate to severe persistent pain, which is characteristic of veno-occlusive priapism, results from tissue ischemia. Pain is more frequently mild or transient with arterial priapism.
3. Studies have suggested that up to 41% of patients who present with priapism (veno-occlusive) have taken some type of psychotropic medication, usually neuroleptics or trazodone (2). Prazosin use has also been associated with priapism.
4. Priapism has been reported commonly (4% to 40%) after intracavernous injection with prostaglandin for the treatment of erectile dysfunction (ED) (Chapter 10.3). Subsequently, therapeutically induced prolonged erection has become the primary cause of priapism (3).
5. Any history of malignancy, especially genitourinary or pelvic carcinoma in patients who present with priapism, should result in a workup for penile metastasis. In a recent review, 20% to 53% of patients with penile metastases presented initially with priapism (4).
6. The most common cause of priapism in children is sickle cell disease.

B. Red flag. Priapism lasting longer than 4 hours, regardless of cause, is a true urologic emergency and immediate evaluation and treatment are necessary (3).

III. Physical examination
should include a thorough genitourinary examination to look for trauma or malignancy. The corpora cavernosa, but not the corpora spongiosum, is involved with priapism and, therefore, the glans will remain flaccid while the shaft is erect and tender. Also palpate for inguinal lymphadenopathy [genitourinary (GU) malignancy], and examine the abdomen (abdominal or GU malignancy and trauma).

IV. Testing

A. Clinical laboratory tests. In most instances, the history and physical examination will determine the cause of priapism. A complete blood count and sickle cell screen may be useful, looking for malignancy and sickle cell disease, respectively. Coagulation studies are also recommended (in case aspiration is contemplated for treatment) (5).

B. Diagnostic imaging, in most instances, is not needed. With suspicion of pelvic malignancy, computed tomography is generally the next step. If trauma preceded priapism, arteriography may be indicated.

V. Diagnostic assessment.
The key to determining the cause of priapism is the clinical history. Examination will reveal an erect, usually tender penis with flaccid glans. Distinguish early between arterial and veno-occlusive priapism; the former is often associated with trauma and less painful or painless erections. In evaluating priapism, aim at determining how long it has been present because permanent damage can occur within as little as 4 hours, and what is causing it. The most common causes are result from effects of psychotropic medications or medications for ED. Less common causes include trauma, sickle cell disease, and pelvic malignancy. Priapism is considered a urologic emergency and should be managed aggressively. Treatment within 4 to 6 hours of onset has been shown to decrease morbidity, need for invasive procedures, and impotence (2).

References

1. Brock G, Breza J, Lue TF, et al. High flow priapism: a spectrum of disease. *J Urol* 1993;150:968–971.
2. Thompson JW Jr, Ware MR, Blashfield RK. Psychotropic medication and priapism: a comprehensive review. *J Clin Psychiatry* 1990;51:430–433.

3. Broderick GA. Intracavernous pharmacotherapy—treatment for the aging erectile response. *Urol Clin North Am* 1996;23:111–126.
4. Chan PT, Begin LR, Arnold D, et al. Priapism secondary to penile metastasis: a report of two cases and a review of the literature. *J Surg Oncol* 1998;68:51–59.
5. Samm BJ, Dmochowski RR. Urologic emergencies. *Postgrad Med* 1996;100:187–200.

10.7 Scrotal Mass

Robert L. Hatch

Scrotal masses are common, occurring in all age groups, from infants to elderly men. In fact, up to 20% of adult males have varicocele (1). Many scrotal masses are benign and require no treatment, whereas others require immediate recognition and emergency treatment.

I. **Approach**. When evaluating scrotal masses, the primary objective is to rapidly identify and refer patients who require immediate intervention. Testicular torsion is a true emergency, as the best results occur if patients are in the operating room within 6 hours of onset of symptoms (1). Strangulated inguinal hernias also present urgent situations, whereas testicular cancers and incarcerated hernias require prompt but less urgent treatment. The diagnosis is often apparent, based on the history and physical examination alone. Ultrasound, laboratory studies, and other imaging procedures can be used to confirm or exclude certain diagnoses (Chapter 10.8).

II. **History**

   A. **Pain.** Is the mass painful? How painful? Testicular torsion usually presents with severe pain. Torsion of a testicular or epididymal appendage, strangulated hernias, orchitis, or epididymitis can also be very painful. Varicocele, hydrocele, spermatocele, and testicular tumors are typically painless, but may at times present with a dull ache or heaviness of the scrotum.

   B. **Inciting event.** Did the mass first appear after vigorous activity or testicular trauma? Torsion is often precipitated by one of these factors, whereas a new swelling following minor trauma can suggest bleeding associated with a tumor.

   C. **Patient age**. Based on a review of 238 testicular masses in children, torsion of an appendage is the most common cause of acute masses in children aged up to 13 years. Above this age epididymitis and testicular torsion become more common (2). The incidence of testicular torsion peaks in the age group 13 to 15 years (2), but it can also occur in both middle-aged males and neonates. Indeed, torsion accounts for 83% of acute scrotal masses in children aged less than 1 year (2). The average age for patients with testicular cancer is 32 years (1). Hydrocele, epididymitis, varicocele, and hernias are more common in adults; as with most scrotal masses, however, they occur over a wide range of ages.

   D. **Duration.** How long has the mass been present? Torsion typically presents with sudden onset of symptoms, leading patients to seek care soon after appearance of the mass. Other acute conditions can also have an abrupt onset. Many benign scrotal masses have been noted for some time by the patient. Abrupt appearance of a varicocele in an older man can signal venous obstruction. In such cases, consider renal tumor with spermatic vein occlusion if the varicocele is on the left and vena cava obstruction if it is on the right.

   E. **Symptoms of infection.** Is there a history of fever, penile discharge, mumps, or any other infection recently? Epididymitis often presents with discharge and mild fever. A high fever often accompanies orchitis. Mumps orchitis typically occurs 3 to 4 days after the parotitis. Many other infections, including tuberculosis and syphilis, can produce epididymitis or orchitis.

F. **Previous history.** Have the symptoms previously appeared? Patients with torsion may have had similar, milder symptoms in the past (torsion that spontaneously resolved). Patients with chronic epididymitis generally describe an initial severe bout that has been followed by milder recurrences.

G. **Other associated symptoms.** Are there any other symptoms? Nausea often accompanies torsion and orchitis.

III. **Physical examination**

A. **Palpation of scrotum and contents:**

1. **Determine the orientation of the testicle.** A torsed testicle is usually retracted upward and rotated to an abnormal position. This may be indicated by an epididymis that appears to lie in an abnormal location (normally, the head of the epididymis lies at the superior pole of the testicle and its body extends posterolateral along the testicle). Comparison with the other testicle may help with this determination. Normal position does not rule out torsion, however, as the testicle may have rotated a full 360°, or swelling can make accurate assessment of the position difficult.

2. **Assess for swelling and tenderness.** Torsion, orchitis, and epididymitis all develop swelling and tenderness soon after onset. The swelling often obscures normal anatomy.

3. **Determine location of mass.** Appendices of the epididymis and testicle can extend from the superior pole of either structure. Spermatocele is most commonly found superior and posterior to the testicle. Varicocele occurs in a similar location, most commonly on the left side. In epididymitis, the epididymis is usually diffusely swollen, which makes it difficult to distinguish epididymis from testicle.

4. **Assess the consistency of the mass.** A varicocele typically has the consistency of a bag of worms. Hydrocele and spermatocele usually have a cystic consistency. Hydrocele can become tenser as the day progresses (because of the dependent position).

B. **Assess the cremasteric reflex.** When the inner thigh is lightly stroked, the testicle on that side should rise noticeably. Absence of this reflex suggests torsion of the testicle (3).

C. **Elevate the testicle.** This usually relieves the pain of epididymitis but not of torsion (3).

D. **Transilluminate the mass.** Hydrocele and spermatocele will transilluminate.

E. **Examine the patient in both the supine and standing positions.** Hernias and varicocele usually become more prominent on standing. Have the patient perform the Valsalva maneuver while standing, which may further accentuate these findings.

F. **General examination.** Tumors can be associated with metastases or gynecomastia (Chapter 14.2).

IV. **Testing.** Either radioisotope scans or color Doppler ultrasound can be used to confirm or rule out testicular torsion. Specificities of 95% and 97% are reported (2). False-negative results do occur, however, producing lower sensitivities (86% and 80%, respectively) (2). In this series, most false-negative results occurred either in cases of prolonged torsion in which the testicles were no longer salvageable or in cases of intermittent torsion. Ultrasound can be helpful in differentiating some masses (e.g., hydrocele from solid mass, testicular from extratesticular). However, ultrasound showed a disappointing ability to differentiate malignant from benign masses in children (4). Aspiration of a spermatocele usually reveals dead sperm (1). Pyuria is almost always present in epididymitis, but it has also been found in up to 27% of patients with torsion (>five white blood cells per high power field) (5). Similarly, leukocytosis suggests an infectious cause but it has also been found in 33% of patients with torsion (5).

V. **Diagnostic assessment.** Each type of scrotal mass has a typical presentation, and most can be readily diagnosed based on history and physical examination. However, considerable overlap is seen in the presentation and laboratory or imaging studies of these conditions, which makes establishing a diagnosis challenging in some cases. If the diagnosis of testicular torsion cannot be rapidly and confidently excluded, emergent referral is strongly recommended. If testicular torsion is not suspected but a diagnosis is not clear after the history, physical examination, and appropriate studies, less urgent consultation is recommended.

References
1. Junnila J, Lassen P. Testicular masses. *Am Fam Physician* 1998;57:685–692.
2. Lewis AG, Bukowski TP, Jarvis PD. Evaluation of acute scrotum in the emergency department. *J Pediatr Surg* 1995;30:277–282.
3. Son KA, Koff SA. Evaluation and management of the acute scrotum. *Prim Care* 1985;6:637–646.
4. Aragona F, Pescatori E, Talenti E. Painless scrotal masses in the pediatric population: prevalence and age distribution of different pathological conditions—a 10-year retrospective multicenter study. *J Urol* 1996;155:1424–1426.
5. Kattan S. Spermatic cord torsion in adults. *Scand J Urol Nephrol* 1994;28:277–279.

10.8 Scrotal Pain

George R. Wilson

I. **Approach.** Most patients seen with scrotal pain are adults and have either epididymitis (1) or varicocele. However, the patient presenting with testicular torsion represents a surgical emergency requiring rapid diagnosis and intervention if the testicle is to be saved. The most important step in evaluating the patient with scrotal pain is to carefully document the time since onset of pain (2). Early determination of symptom onset not only helps make the diagnosis, it has a significant impact on how rapidly various tests need be accomplished in the process. The greatest opportunity to salvage a testicle with torsion occurs in the first 6 hours (3). After 6 hours, it drops off rapidly and approaches zero by 48 hours (3).

II. **History**
   A. **Trauma** rarely causes significant damage to the testicle. Traumatic damage is extremely rare in prepubertal patients (4). Unless the testicle is ruptured or a secondary torsion occurs, pain from trauma usually resolves in less than 1 hour (4). Severe pain or evidence of testicular rupture associated with minor trauma is suggestive of occult tumor (1,4).
   B. **Symptoms and disease course**
      1. **Testicular torsion** is the most common cause of scrotal pain in first year of life (3). It is frequently misdiagnosed as colic, or an intraabdominal disorder. The highest incidence occurs between the ages of 12 to 18 years (5). Testicular torsion causes acute pain with testicular swelling and scrotal erythema, and nausea and vomiting are common.
      2. **Torsion of testicular appendage.** Torsion is common between the ages of 10 to 15 years; however, it is rare in neonates and adults (5). Pain can last several days with malaise and may not localize to the scrotum initially, but presents as lower abdominal pain.
      3. **Epididymitis** is the most common cause of acute scrotal pain in adults (1). It is rare in prepubertal children (5). In infants or young children, suspect urogenital anomaly or dysfunction (3). The onset can be abrupt or insidious. Fever, voiding symptoms, or both are common (4). Scrotal edema and erythema can occur, but less commonly than that seen with torsion (5).
      4. **Orchitis** is usually caused by extension of epididymitis inflammation to the testis (4). Mumps orchitis, which is seen only after puberty in 20% of mumps cases, is usually unilateral (70%). It is declining in the United States because of immunization (5).

C. **Sexual activity** is an important factor in all age groups. In prepubertal children, rule out abuse or self-experimentation. In adolescents and adults, infection and trauma can occur from sexual practices. A good history is especially important.

D. **Recurrent pain.** A history of previous ipsilateral pain is associated with a 44% incidence of testicular torsion (1). Consider multiple causes. Is previous pain similar or different from the current episode?

E. **Infection.** Look for a history of urinary tract infection (UTI), dribbling, urgency, dysuria, and incomplete emptying (Chapter 10.1). Consider reflux, obstruction, chronic prostatitis, and unusual sexual practices.

F. **Concurrent illness.** Possibilities include Henoch–Schönlein purpura, mononucleosis, Buerger's disease, coxsackie B virus, and polyarteritis nodosa (1,4). Also consider incarcerated hernia or thrombosed varicocele (1).

III. **Physical examination**

A. **Observation.** Especially in the very young, it is important to quietly observe the patient before initiating an examination (4). Is he quiet or active? Playing or fussing? Is there guarding?

B. **Referred pain.** The neonate or young child with abdominal pain *always* deserves an examination of the scrotum (2,4).

C. **Scrotum.** Edema and redness are found in torsion and epididymitis. They occur early in testicular torsion. If pain is present longer than 24 hours and no scrotal changes are noted, torsion is unlikely (4). Discoloration suggests trauma but it can also be seen with delayed diagnosis of torsion and epididymitis. Check for the cremasteric reflex, which rules out testicular torsion if present on the painful side (2,4). Its presence must be demonstrated on the nonpainful side to be reliable indicator. Unilateral swelling without skin changes suggests hernia or hydrocele (4). In torsion, pain increases when the scrotum is elevated; it decreases with epididymitis (Prehn's sign) (5) (Chapter 10.7).

D. **Penis.** Look for discharge, redness, and trauma. Partial hypospadius suggests possible other genitourinary anomalies. A higher incidence of UTI is seen in the uncircumcised neonate.

E. **Testes.** Are they present or absent? Examine the inguinal canal. Evaluate for high versus low, transverse versus vertical lie. High, transverse testicle suggests torsion (4). Evaluate size, shape, and tenderness. The testicle with torsion will become swollen early in the process, however, the appendage with torsion does not cause a difference is testicular size (2). Feel and look for a palpable mass on the margin of the testis. Transilluminate for the "blue dot sign" to diagnosis torsion in the appendage (4,5). Does tenderness involve the entire testicle or is it asymmetric (4)?

F. **Other.** Rule out other causes, examine skin for petechiae, and look for adenopathy. Examine the abdomen and flank for a source of referred pain or signs of trauma. Fever is not usually present with a testicular torsion (unless delayed), but can be found in epididymitis (4).

IV. **Testing**

A. **Clinical laboratory tests**

1. **Urinalysis** is not usually helpful. It is negative in most cases. If positive, the diagnosis is more likely epididymitis than torsion in the testicle or appendage (3,4).

2. **White blood cells (WBC).** The finding of a leukocytosis is nonspecific. The WBC count is more commonly elevated in epididymitis. It can be elevated in appendiceal torsion and testicular torsion, especially after 24 hours (4).

3. **Serology and erythrocyte sedimentation rate** are not helpful in the assessment of acute pain.

B. **Imaging**

1. **Doppler ultrasound**

a. **Gray-scale ultrasound.** Real time, gray-scale ultrasound findings are nonspecific and not reliable for either epididymitis or testicular torsion. The testicle may appear normal early in torsion. Once changes are seen, irreversible damage may be present (5).

    b. Color Doppler imaging is much more reliable for the diagnosis of both torsion and epididymitis. In torsion there is a total absence of blood flow on the affected side as compared with the contralateral side; in epididymitis there is a marked increase in arterial blood flow as compared with the contralateral side (5).

  2. Nuclear scanning is of questionable value in the acute setting. It is declining in use as color Doppler becomes a primary diagnostic modality (5). It may effectively demonstrate ischemia but too late to save the testicle. It is useful in cases of trauma, asymptomatic mass, and when elective surgical exploration is contraindicated and Doppler studies are equivocal (2).

  3. Magnetic resonance imaging provides a good view of the anatomy but is not useful in the acute setting (5).

V. Diagnostic assessment. The two most important pieces of clinical history that determine the course and outcome in scrotal pain are the age of the patient and the time elapsed since pain onset. Severe unilateral pain of less than 6 hours duration, worsened by elevation of the testicle in an adolescent, is testicular torsion until proved otherwise at surgery. In the neonate, it is important that the scrotum be examined any time abdominal symptoms are present. Epididymitis in the infant or child is rare. When present, rule out congenital and functional anomalies. In adults, the primary cause of scrotal pain is epididymitis and the course is chronic. Unless the testicle is ruptured, trauma rarely causes scrotal pain that lasts longer than 1 hour. Testicular rupture from mild trauma must be evaluated for tumor. The best tool for evaluation of acute, unilateral pain is color Doppler ultrasonography. Laboratory tests are nonspecific and are helpful only as confirmatory in some causes. Most importantly, if there is any doubt to the diagnosis, then it is always appropriate to refer to a surgeon for exploration.

References

1. Morgan RJ, Parry JRW. Scrotal pain. *Postgrad Med* 1987;63(741):521–523.
2. Galejs LE. Diagnosis and treatment of the acute scrotum. *Am Fam Physician* 1999;59(4):817–824.
3. Lewis AG, Bukowski TP, Jarvis PD, Wacksman J, Sheldon CA. Evaluation of acute scrotum in the emergency department. *J Pediatr Surg* 1995;30(2):277–282.
4. Kass EJ, Lundak B. The acute scrotum. *Pediatr Clin North Am* 1997;44(5):1251–1266.
5. Sandock DS, Herbener TE, Resnick MI. Disorders of the scrotum and its contents. In: Resnick MI, Older RA, eds. *Diagnosis of genitourinary disease*, 2nd ed. New York: Thieme-Stratton Inc.; 1997:465–483.

10.9 Urethral Discharge

George P.N. Samraj

Discharge from the urethra is a common symptom. The characteristics and the cause of urethral discharge (UD) vary widely. Discharge can be profuse or scanty; clear, yellowish, or white; mucopurulent or serous; bloody, watery, or frank pus. UD can be from an acute or chronic condition and patients may or may not have symptoms.

  I. Approach. The causes of UD are summarized as follows:
    A. Sexually transmitted diseases
      1. Gonococcal (GC)
      2. Nongonococcal (NGC):
        a. *Chlamydia trachomatis*
        b. *Ureaplasma urealyticum*
        c. *Mycoplasma genitalium*

   d. Other organisms linked to UD:
   - **(1)** Bacteria: *Gardnerella vaginalis, Escherichia coli*, tuberculosis, *Corynebacterium* species, bacterioides, mycoplasmas
   - **(2)** Viruses: herpes simplex virus, adenoviruses, cytomegalovirus, human papilloma virus, and others
   - **(3)** Protozoal: *Trichomonas vaginalis*; approximately 5 million cases occur annually in the United States
   - **(4)** Fungal: *Candida* species

B. Nonsexually transmitted diseases
   1. Infections: cystitis, prostatitis
   2. Anatomic abnormalities: urethral stricture, phimosis
   3. Congenital abnormalities of the urogenital system
   4. Iatrogenic: catheterization, instrumentation, and other procedures
   5. Chemical irritation from use of douches, lubricants, and other chemicals
   6. Tumors and malignant lesions and new growths
   7. Foreign bodies: common in children, teenagers
   8. Substance abuse: chronic use of amphetamines or other stimulants produces a serous discharge. Caffeine and alcohol are also implicated in UD
   9. Miscellaneous factors linked to UD: sexual practices, masturbation, oral sex
   10. Unknown: no organisms may be found in up to one-third of patients

II. History. A detailed medical history is essential for the evaluation of UD. The essential symptoms addressed at the time of interview are (a) dysuria, (b) urethral discharge, (c) itching at the urethra, (d) hematuria, (e) rectal symptoms, (f) contact with infectious agents, and (g) sexual history. The characteristics of UD are noted in relation to color, quantity, odor, consistency, frequency, and relationship to urination. Profuse, yellowish UD occurring 3 to 7 days after sexual exposure is characteristic of GC. GC infection is more common in men than in women. In 1997, 324,901 cases of gonorrhea were reported to the Centers for Disease Control, with a case rate of 122/100,000 (1). Clear to white, scanty, or mucopurulent UD (23% to 55%) that develops gradually at least a week after exposure, with waxing and waning in intensity, suggests chlamydial infection. This is the most common sexually transmitted disease (STD) in the United States, with 3 million new cases occurring annually (2). As many as 85% of women with chlamydial infections and 40% of infected men are asymptomatic (3). Sexual history should include sexual behaviors, condom usage, number of sexual partners, recent sexual contacts, and the orifices used for sexual contacts. Consistent usage of condoms prevents sexually transmitted urethritis. Oral sex increases UD from oral flora infections.

III. Physical examination
   A. Focused physical examination (PE) should include vital signs, and urologic and rectal examination. In men, this should include examination of the penis, perimeatal region (for evidence of erythema), urethral meatus, scrotum, testicles, epididymis, prostate, and perianal and inguinal region. Stains present on the patient's underwear may indicate the characteristics of the discharge, which is particularly useful in a patient who has urinated shortly before examination. Recent micturition can eliminate much inflammatory discharge. Sometimes it is necessary to examine the patient in the morning before voiding to enhance the diagnosis. Perform a complete gynecologic and urologic examination in women.
   B. Abdomen. Completely examine the abdomen to rule out intraabdominal pathology, including masses and inflammation, obstruction, or distention of organs.
   C. Additional physical examination should include the skin and other systems, as needed. If a patient is suspected of gonococcal infection, it may be essential to check the patient's joints, skin, throat, eye and other organs.

IV. Testing
   A. UD sample collection. Proper collection and handling of UD sample is essential for the diagnosis. When the discharge is not spontaneous, the urethra should be gently stripped. This is best accomplished by grasping the

penis firmly between the thumb and forefinger with the thumb pressing on the ventral surface. Then move the hand distally, compressing the urethra. This maneuver may express a small amount of discharge. The urethral meatus can be gently spread and if no urethral discharge is expressed, a calcium-alginate urethral (or nasopharyngeal) swab should be inserted at least 2 cm into the urethra and the discharge collected. The use of cotton-tipped swabs is contraindicated because their large size makes the insertion extremely uncomfortable and the cotton fibers can inhibit the growth of certain fastidious organisms (4).

- B. **Clinical laboratory investigations**
  1. **UD Gram's stain.** The test involves staining the UD with Gram's stain and examining it under a microscope. The presence of polymorphs with intracellular diplococci is diagnostic of GC. Polymorphs without the intracellular diplococci are suggestive of NGC disease. Few or no polymorphs are suggestive of other causes. The Gram's stain is quite accurate for men but it is not very sensitive for women (50%).
  2. **UD culture** is essential to identify specific organisms. Other useful tests are:
     a. Detection of bacterial DNA by polymerase chain reaction (PCR)
     b. DNA probes
     c. Direct monoclonal testing and enzyme-linked assays. These tests have a high sensitivity and specificity. Cultures of throat, rectum, and sometimes conjunctivae may be required to establish the diagnosis.
  3. **UD wet preparation** is done to establish the diagnosis of trichomoniasis, candidiasis, and some viral and bacterial infections.
  4. **Urine analysis and urine cultures** are essential for the diagnosis of urinary infections. Collect the urine specimen [as described by Stamey (5)] with four sterile containers (before and after prostatic massage), which is useful to identify the site of infection in men.
  5. **Urinary leukocyte esterase** is a useful screening test for chlamydial and GC infections in asymptomatic men. The usefulness of other **neutrophil enzyme (elastace, myeloperoxidase) studies** of urine have been reported.
  6. **Blood studies,** including a complete blood count, serum chemistry profile, serologic test for syphilis, blood test for human immunodeficiency virus infection, and immunologic studies, may be required in an appropriate clinical setting.
- C. **Diagnostic imaging.** Urethrogram, urologic diagnostic studies, and pelvic, vaginal, and rectal ultrasound studies are indicated in some clinical conditions.
- D. **Diagnostic procedures.** Children and elderly patients may need to be examined under anesthesia to evaluate UD. Anoscopy is done for patients who have had anal intercourse or for those with anal and rectal symptoms. Cystourethroscopy and laparoscopy are also useful in certain conditions.
- V. **Diagnostic assessment**
  - A. **Special concerns.** *Neisseria gonorrhoeae* and *C. trachomatis* infections are reportable to State Health Departments and a specific diagnosis is essential. UD secondary to STD involves many psychosocial and medicolegal implications to the patient, his or her partner, their families, and society. Sexual partners can be traced, tested, and treated. In children with UD, sexual abuse may be suspected. Pregnant women with gonococcal infection or chlamydia can infect the infant at birth (ophthalmia neonatorum).
  - B. **Complications following UD and urethritis.** Some of the complications following UD are postgonococcal urethritis, pelvic inflammatory disease (in women) and infertility, perihepatitis, chronic pelvic pain (Chapter 11.3), adhesions of the intraabdominal organs, obstructions in the gastrointestinal and genitourinary tracts, chronic urethritis, periurethral abscess, fistula, prostatitis, epididymitis, orchitis, urethral syndrome, psychosexual problems, and Reiter's syndrome.

References
1. Centers for Disease Control and Prevention. National Center for HIV, STD, and TB Prevention. *Sexually Transmitted Disease Surveillance.* Atlanta: CDC, 1997.
2. American Social Health Association. *Sexually transmitted diseases in America: how many cases and at what cost?* Menlo Park, CA: Kaiser Family Foundation, 1998.
3. Institute of Medicine. Committee on Prevention and Control of STD. Eng TR, Butler WT, eds. *The hidden epidemic: confronting STD.* Washington, DC: National Academy Press, 1997.
4. Williams R, Kreder KJ Jr. Examination of UD and vaginal exudates. In: Tanagho EA, McAninch JW, eds. *Smith's general urology,* 14th ed. Norwalk, CT: Appleton & Lange, 1995.
5. Stamey TA. Diagnosis, localization, and classification of urinary infections. In: Stamey TA, ed. *Pathogenesis and treatment of urinary tract infections.* Baltimore: Williams & Wilkins, 1980:262.

10.10 Urinary Incontinence

Richard Rathe

Urinary incontinence (UI) in adults is one of the most prevalent and underdiagnosed afflictions in the United States (>25 million effected individuals, >50% of nursing home residents). The economic impact is estimated to be more than $16 billion (1). It is a major cause of social withdrawal and loss of independent living. Patients are often too embarrassed to discuss this problem, even with their physician. Some even view it as a natural part of aging, but this is not the case. Urinary incontinence is a symptom, not a disease. Understanding the types of disorders that cause incontinence is the key to correct diagnosis and effective treatment (2–5).

I. **Approach**
   A. **Definition.** Urinary incontinence is the involuntary loss of urine at times and in amounts that interfere with hygiene and activities of daily living.
   B. **Classification. The classification of urinary incontinence is presented in Table 10.1.**
   C. **Urinary incontinence can be acute or chronic.** Acute causes include infection, medications, delirium, and exacerbation of systemic diseases (e.g., diabetes mellitus, diabetes insipidus, congestive heart failure, or stroke). Chronic conditions that are associated with UI fall into two categories: (a) local (pelvic floor weakness following childbirth, bladder tumor or deformity, tumors, obstruction by an enlarged prostate or cystocele, postsurgical) and (b) systemic [menopause, neuropathy (diabetes, alcoholism), dementia, depression, stroke, tumor, Parkinson's disease].
   D. **The DRIP mnemonic** is often cited as a way to remember the reversible (and curable) causes of UI:
      1. **D:** Delirium and drugs
      2. **R:** Restricted mobility and retention
      3. **I:** Infection, inflammation, and (fecal) impaction
      4. **P:** Polyuria from uncontrolled diabetes and other conditions
II. **History**
   A. **Voiding history.** It is important to fully characterize the patient's problem by taking a detailed history, including the duration of the symptoms, timing of voluntary or involuntary voiding, amounts voided involuntarily, and the relationship to voluntary voiding. Focus on the following areas:
      1. Need for pads or diapers (measure of severity)
      2. Loss of urine with coughing or laughing (suggests stress type)
      3. Inability to hold urine after having the urge to urinate (suggests urge type)

Table 10.1 Types of incontinence

Type	Definition	Mechanism	Disorders
Urge	Inability to delay voiding once the urge occurs	Detrusor hyperactivity	Idiopathic (common in the elderly) Genitourinary conditions (cystitis, stones)
Stress	Loss of urine with increased abdominal pressure	Sphincter failure	Weak or injured pelvic muscles Sphincter weakness
Overflow	Partial retention of urine behind an obstruction	Outlet obstruction Loss of innervation	Obstruction (prostate, cystocele) Neuropathic (diabetes, nerve injury)
Functional	Inability to get to the toilet in time	Physical or cognitive impairment	Dementia or delirium Physical limitations (lack of mobility) Psychological or behavioral causes
Mixed	Any combination of the above		

4. Pain or discomfort (suggests infection or inflammation) (Chapter 10.1)
5. Inability to fully empty bladder (suggests obstruction)
6. Decreased urinary stream (suggests obstruction)
7. What impact does UI have on the patient's life?
8. What does the patient think is going on?

B. **Major medical problems.** Does the patient have any known condition that is associated with UI? These include diabetes, heart failure, menopause, and neurologic problems. Does the patient have other genitourinary symptoms? In female patients, be sure to take a detailed obstetric history.

C. **Medication history.** Since medications are a major cause of incontinence, a thorough medication history is essential. Offending agents include diuretics, older antidepressants, antihypertensives, narcotics, and alcohol.

D. **Special concern.** Central and nephrogenic diabetes insipidus can present with UI because of increased urine output (many liters per day). These patients frequently have a concomitant polydypsia that closely matches their water loss (Chapter 14.5). Consider this diagnosis when the patient gives a history of voiding large volumes of urine.

III. **Physical examination.** The physical examination is often normal in cases of UI. Focus efforts in an attempt to uncover the underlying cause(s):

A. **General.** Is the patient physically capable of getting to the toilet?

B. **Mental status.** Can the patient understand and act on the urge to void?

C. **Neurologic**, including the anal reflex; focal signs suggest a neurologic cause.

D. **Abdominal examination.** Is the bladder distended?

E. **Rectal or prostate.** Does the patient have a fecal impaction or an enlarged prostate?

F. **Pelvic examination.** Look for atrophic vaginitis, uterine prolapse, or a pelvic mass.

IV. **Testing**

A. **Voiding journal.** A voiding journal is a good way to get additional information about the patient's problem. Have the patient record the time and approximate amount of each voiding, and whether they were wet or dry.

B. Urinalysis. Be cautious when interpreting the urine analysis: in the absence of other symptoms, bacteriuria is seldom the primary cause of UI. Treat cystitis or urethritis when the rest of the clinical picture confirms them. Unexplained, persistent microhematuria requires investigation (Chapter 10.2).

C. Postvoiding urine volume. The patient should be catheterized immediately after voiding. In general, the postvoid urine volume should be less than 50 ml. Volumes in the range of 100 to 200 ml may suggest impaired bladder contractility or obstruction. Volumes greater than 200 ml strongly suggest obstruction.

D. Blood urea nitrogen, creatinine, and glucose are simple blood tests that help rule out underlying renal disease and diabetes.

E. Special tests are available via urologic consultation to further delineate the cause of UI. These include cystoscopy, cystometry, and other voiding studies. Up to two-thirds of patients can be successfully treated without urologic referral.

V. Diagnostic assessment. The clinical history is the most important factor leading to the correct diagnosis and successful treatment of urinary incontinence. However, it is an imperfect tool at best. In one review, clinical history had a sensitivity and specificity for stress incontinence of 0.90 and 0.50, respectively. For detrusor instability, the figures were 0.74 and 0.55 (2).

The task becomes even more problematic when considering the reluctance of patients to talk about their symptoms and the tendency for UI to be of a mixed type. Response to therapy (or lack thereof) often drives the practical management of this condition. Lack of response to multiple trials of therapy is a good indication for consulting a urologist. Remember, that your initial assessment will often be incorrect, so keep an open mind and consider all possible diagnoses. Finally, recall that UI frequently involves more than one causal factor. For example, many elderly people have a functional component (can't get to the toilet quickly) in addition to one of the other types.

References

1. Urinary incontinence in adults: acute and chronic management. *AHCPR Clinical Practice Guideline*, No. 2 (1996 Update) Accessed August 1999; http://text.nlm.nih.gov/ftrs/gateway/
2. Jensen JK, Nielsen FR, Ostergard DR. The role of patient history in the diagnosis of urinary incontinence. *Obstet Gynecol* 1994;83(5):904–910.
3. Finding out about incontinence. *AAFP Patient Information Handout* (1998) Accessed August 1999; http://www.aafp.org/patientinfo/incont.html
4. Goode PS, Burgio KL. Pharmacologic treatment of lower urinary tract dysfunction in geriatric patients. *Am J Med Sci* 1997;314(4):262–267.
5. Weiss BD. Diagnostic evaluation of urinary incontinence in geriatric patients. *Am Fam Physician* 1998;57(11):2665–2687. Accessed August 1999; http://www.aafp.org/afp/980600ap/weiss.html

11. PROBLEMS RELATED TO THE FEMALE REPRODUCTIVE SYSTEM

KATHRYN M. ANDOLSEK

11.1 Amenorrhea

L. Allen Dobson, Jr.

Pregnancy is the most common cause of amenorrhea. Evaluation and diagnosis of the other causes of amenorrhea are possible by use of a simple workup scheme (section **V**).

I. **Approach.** Cyclic menstrual bleeding requires an intact hypothalamic-pituitary-ovarian axis, functioning ovaries, a responsive uterine endometrium, and an unobstructed outflow tract. Localizing the specific site of defect is the goal of evaluation.
   A. **Definitions.** Any patient who meets the following definitions of amenorrhea should be evaluated. The differentiation between primary and secondary amenorrhea does not alter the basic evaluation scheme.
      1. No bleeding by age 14 years in the absence of growth or development of secondary sexual characteristics.
      2. No menstrual periods by age 16 years, regardless of the presence of normal growth and development, with the appearance of secondary sexual characteristics.
      3. In a woman who has been menstruating, the absence of periods for a length of time equivalent to a total of at least three of the previous cycles, or 6 months of amenorrhea (1).
   B. **Considerations.** Next to pregnancy, disorders of the hypothalamic-pituitary-ovarian axis are the most common causes of amenorrhea (2). Strict adherence to the aforementioned definitions should not delay evaluation in the presence of obvious characteristics of Turner's syndrome or abnormal genital anatomy.
II. **History**
   A. **Menstrual and reproductive history.** What was the patient's age at menarche? When was the patient's last menstrual period and her previous menstrual pattern? Document pregnancy history with attention to any complications. Is there a history of gynecologic or obstetric procedures?
      1. A history of postpartum infection or curettage (Asherman's syndrome) may suggest destruction of the endometrium and subsequent outflow tract problem.
      2. A history of severe postpartum bleeding requiring transfusion may suggest pituitary failure (Sheehan's syndrome).
   B. **Other history.** Were there any significant medical or psychosocial events preceding amenorrhea? Is there any galactorrhea? Does the patient have any endocrine, metabolic, or eating disorders? Is there a history of recent weight gain or loss? Document the medication history. Is there a history of prolonged and intense exercise? Is there a family history of menstrual problems or endocrine or autoimmune disorders (Section 14)?
      1. Stressful situations or events are often associated with amenorrhea (3).
      2. The incidence of amenorrhea is greatest among competitive endurance athletes and ballet dancers (2).
      3. Premature ovarian failure can be caused by autoimmune disease (4).
      4. Medications associated with amenorrhea include antipsychotics, tricyclic antidepressants, calcium channel blockers, methyldopa, reserpine, digitalis, and chemotherapeutic drugs.
III. **Physical examination.** The purpose of the focused examination is to screen for abnormal anatomy or development and signs of endocrinopathies. A breast examination should document the presence or absence of galactorrhea which, with hair distribution, should provide an evaluation of normal secondary sexual characteristics (Tanner stage). Palpate the thyroid for enlargement or nodules. A careful pelvic examination is essential to detect any structural abnormalities

or lesions. Signs of possible androgenic excess are truncal obesity, hirsutism, acne, male pattern baldness, and clitoral enlargement (Chapter 14.3).

IV. **Testing**

A. **Clinical laboratory tests.** Serum or urine human chorionic gonodotropin, thyroid-stimulating hormone, prolactin, follicle-stimulating hormone, and luteinizing hormone are usually the only tests required to make a diagnosis (section **V**). Additional tests for premature ovarian failure should include free thyroxine (T_4), thyroid antibodies, morning cortisol, calcium, phosphorus and antinuclear antibody, rheumatoid factor, erythrocyte sedimentation rate, and a complete blood count. Further adrenal evaluation of women who exhibit signs of hyperandrogenism with anovulation ("hyperandrogenic chronic anovulation") includes fasting serum testosterone, dehydroepiandrosterone (DHEA)-S, and 17-hydroxyprogesterone (17-HP).

B. **Other laboratory evaluation.** Karotyping is indicated in all women with premature ovarian failure prior to age 30 years or with any physical evidence suggestive of Turner's syndrome (short stature, web neck, shield-shaped chest,

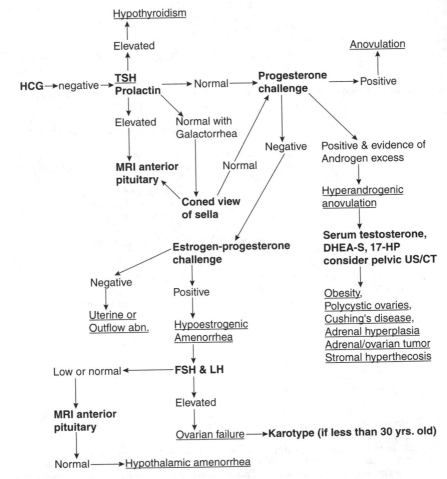

FIG. 11.1 Approach to the evaluation of amenorrhea.

lack of secondary sexual characteristics) (3). Endometrial biopsy should be considered in women with prolonged amenorrhea or with evidence of estrogen or androgen excess to exclude endometrial hyperplasia.

C. Provocative tests

1. Progesterone challenge test. Oral progesterone acetate (10 mg daily for 15 days). A positive test is withdrawal bleeding between days 2 and 7 after finishing medication; alternatively, parenteral progesterone (200 mg) in oil or micronized progesterone 200 mg at bedtime.

2. Estrogen-progesterone challenge test. Oral conjugated estrogen (1.25 mg) or 2 mg estadiol qd for days 1 through 21 with oral progesterone acetate (10 mg) on days 17 through 21. A positive test is withdrawal bleeding between days 2 and 7 after finishing medication.

D. Diagnostic imaging. A coned lateral view of the sella turcica is indicated as a screening examination for galactorrhea if the prolactin level is less than 100 ng/ml. A magnetic resonance imaging scan, which is more sensitive, is indicated for elevated prolactin, abnormal screening x-ray film, or diagnosis of hypothalamic amenorrhea (section **V**).

V. Diagnostic assessment. Use the approach outlined in Figure 11.1 to guide diagnosis (1–3).

References

1. Speroff L, Glass RH, Kase NG. *Clinical gynecologic endocrinology and infertility,* 5th ed. Baltimore: Williams & Wilkins, 1994:401–456.
2. Kiningham RB, Apgar BS, Swenk TL. Evaluation of amenorrhea. *Am Fam Physician* 1996;53:1185–1194.
3. Scott J, DiSaia P, Hammond C, Spellacy W, eds. *Danforth's obstetrics and gynecology,* 7th ed. Philadelphia: JB Lippincott, 1994:665–679.
4. Alper MM, Garner PR. Premature ovarian failure: its relationship to autoimmune disease. *Obstet Gynecol* 1985;66:27–30.

11.2 Breast Mass

Joyce A. Copeland

I. Approach. The goal of the evaluation of a breast mass is to differentiate masses that are cancerous from benign masses in a timely and cost-effective manner.

II. History

A. Current medical history and chief complaint

1. When and how was the mass discovered? Does the patient perform regular breast self-examinations? What, if any, changes have occurred since discovery of the mass?

2. Age and menstrual status. Cancer is more prominent in women aged more than 50 years, although it can be seen in 3% of women who are aged 20 to 29 years. In the postmenopausal age group, 85% of masses prove to be cancer (1). Postmenopausal women have a higher risk for breast cancer (BC). Pregnancy expands the list of possible causes of a mass to include mastitis, galactocele, or a breast abscess.

3. Is the mass painful? If so, is there any cyclic variation in the pain? Has there been any nipple discharge (Chapter 11.6)? Cyclic pain suggests a cystic origin. Persistent pain may represent BC or an inflammatory process.

B. Past medical history

1. What is the reproductive history and current menstrual status? Has the patient ever breastfed an infant? Is she on estrogen replacement therapy (ERT)? A woman who breastfeeds for 2 or more years may decrease her risk for BC. ERT has a controversial role in the cause or advancement of breast cancer.

      2. Breast history. The patient should be questioned about any previous breast mass, breast biopsy, or surgery and the clinical outcome. Has she had a personal history of breast cancer or atypical hyperplasia on a previous biopsy? A prior history of BC or atypical hyperplasia on a biopsy increases the risk for malignancy.

    C. Family history. Is there a family history of breast cancer? If yes, what is the relationship of the family member and at what age was the cancer diagnosed and what was the relative's menstrual status? A mother or sister with premenopausal BC increases risk to the highest level.

III. Physical examination

    A. Inspection. Inspect the breasts for symmetry, contour, skin retraction, rashes, *peau d'orange,* nipple discharge, erythema, or edema.

      1. Symmetry and contour can be disrupted on any breast. Retraction suggests either chronic inflammation or BC caused by skin adherence to the mass.

      2. *Peau d'orange* is a puckering or indentation of the skin over a mass. A rash can be related to Paget's disease with a related ductal carcinoma.

    B. Palpation and compression. Palpate both breasts, including the nipple and areolar region. Palpate the supraclavicular, infraclavicular, and axillary region for adenopathy. Evaluate the consistency, regularity, location, mobility, and tenderness of the mass. Hard, immobile, irregular masses raise the suspicion for BC. Smooth, cystic, or rubbery masses suggest a cyst or fibroadenoma. Fibrocystic changes are often nondiscrete and irregular, but are also mobile and relatively soft. Compressing the nipple may express a discharge (Chapter 11.6).

IV. Testing

    A. Imaging studies. The mammogram is used to characterize the nature of the mass and to provide an assessment of the remainder of the breast tissue and the contralateral breast. It is not a diagnostic procedure. Ultrasound is used to characterize a mass as solid or cystic or to identify masses that may not be identified by mammography. The ultrasound is helpful in evaluating a mass in a patient aged less than 30 years and it can be used as an adjunct in performing aspiration or a biopsy for the indeterminate lesion.

    B. Fine needle aspiration (FNA) (2). The FNA can be used to obtain tissue or fluid in a palpable mass. Fluid aspiration plus resolution of the mass suggests a cystic origin. Grossly bloody fluid demands further evaluation of the mass. A cystic mass in a postmenopausal woman not on ERT requires a more thorough evaluation.

      1. If the mass resolves, reexamine the breast in 4 to 6 weeks. If the fluid reaccumulates, reaspirate.

      2. Residual mass or asymmetry after aspiration requires mammography and biopsy. If no aspirate is obtained, proceed with excisional biopsy.

    C. FNA biopsy (FNAB) (4). The sensitivity of FNAB is 0.65 to 0.98 and the specificity is 0.34 to 1.0. The result of this procedure provides material for a cytologic examination. Correlation with imaging studies must be concordant in conclusion or excisional biopsy is indicated. Imaging guidance is indicated for a nonpalpable mass. Atypia of any degree warrants excisional biopsy.

    D. Triple test for solid mass (3). The triple test includes physical examination, imaging findings, and cytology via FNAB. The technique demonstrates a sensitivity of 97% to 100%, with a specificity of 98% to 100% (3). Concordance for benign findings allows no further testing. Malignant cytopathology requires excisional biopsy. Inconclusive results without concordance requires open excisional biopsy.

    E. Open excisional biopsy. A lesion that is highly suspicious on clinical examination or mammography is best evaluated with open biopsy and excision. Atypical cells on biopsy also require a more definitive tissue diagnosis.

V. Diagnostic assessment.
The evaluation of a breast mass requires knowledge of BC risk factors and the characteristics of benign and malignant lesions. Characterizing the consistency and mobility of the mass combined with information

about the patient's age and menopausal status helps to provide an initial evaluation of the risk for BC. It is important to know what resources and skills are accessible in the community when selecting a diagnostic modality. Sensitivity to the patient's fears, diligent follow-up, and communication are important in the care of the patient and to reduce medicolegal risk. If a patient remains fearful or uncomfortable with the evaluation, referral for a second opinion is a wise move.

References

1. White G, Griffith C, Nenstiel R, Dyess D. Breast cancer: reducing mortality through early detection. *Clinician Rev* 1996;6(9):77–79, 83–84, 100–106.
2. Osuch J, Bonham V, Morris L. Primary care guide to managing a breast mass: step-by-step workup. *Medscape Women's Health* 1998;3:5.
3. The Uniform Approach to Breast Fine-Needle Aspiration Biopsy. [Editorial Opinion]. National Cancer Institute Conference. *Am J Surg* 1997;174(4):371–385.
4. Andolsek KM, Copeland J. Conditions of the breast. In: Taylor RB, ed. *Family medicine: principles and practice*, 5th ed. New York: Springer-Verlag; 1998.

11.3 Chronic Pelvic Pain

Albert A. Meyer

I. **Approach.** A woman has an approximate 5% chance of having chronic pelvic pain in her lifetime (1). It is defined as an episodic or continuous pain that persists for 6 months or longer, sufficiently severe to have a significant impact on her lifestyle and her day-to-day function or relationships. It is less likely to be associated with an identifiable pathophysiologic disorder than is pelvic pain lasting less than 3 months.

II. **History.** As with any pain, the onset, duration, and pattern of the pain must be assessed. The location, intensity, character, and radiation are important historical elements. Aggravating or relieving factors are important, especially as they relate to the urinary, musculoskeletal, or gastrointestinal systems as well as the relationship of pain to sexual activity or menstruation. Systemic symptoms such as fatigue and anorexia are often present. A medication history (e.g., use of birth control pills or over-the-counter medications) should be obtained. The past obstetric, gynecologic, and general surgical histories are extremely important.

It should be noted that women with a history of pelvic inflammatory disease are four times more likely to develop chronic pelvic pain. The list of possibilities for the condition is substantial. A person with intestinal, sexual, urinary, musculoskeletal, and systemic symptoms may be suffering from a psychiatric disorder (e.g., depression) and an acknowledged or remote history of sexual abuse. Often this information is possible to obtain only when the provider creates an atmosphere of mutual respect and trust.

Dyspareunia is often present. Cyclic pain that is related to menstruation usually points to a gynecologic problem. Pain referred to the anterior thigh, pain associated with irregular uterine bleeding, or new onset dysmenorrhea may have a uterine or ovarian cause. Urethral tenderness, dysuria, or bladder pain suggests interstial cystitis or a urethral problem (Chapter 10.1). Pain on defecation, melana, bloody stools, or abdominal pain with alternating diarrhea and constipation can point toward pelvic floor problems, irritable bowel syndrome, or inflammatory bowel diseases.

III. **Physical examination**

    A. **The general condition of the patient** should be noted. Does the patient look chronically ill, which may suggest a pelvic lesion or an inflammatory bowel disorder? Does the patient appear anxious, stressed, or inappropriate?

        1. Can the patient point to the pain with one finger? If so, this can indicate that the pain may have a discrete source.

2. An examination of the lower back, sacral area, and coccyx, including a neuologic examination of the lower extremities, is necessary. Herniated disc, exaggerated lumbar lordosis, and spondylolisthesis can all cause pelvic pain.
3. Examine the abdomen, looking for surgical scars, distension, and palpable tenderness, particularly in the epigastrium, flank, back, or bladder.

B. **A thorough pelvic examination** is the most important part of the evaluation.

IV. **Testing (3).** If no obvious cause is apparent, it is reasonable to obtain a complete blood count, urine analysis, sedimentation rate, and serum chemistry profile. A pelvic ultrasound may be helpful when the pelvic examination is inconclusive. Laparoscopy is best used to diagnose a definite pelvic mass. Laparoscopy has been used extensively in the past but various studies have shown a 66% negative laparoscopy rate for patients with chronic pelvic pain. A multidisciplinary approach using medical, psychologic, environmental, and nutritional disciplines showed decreased pain after 1 year.

V. **Diagnostic assessment.** Chronic pelvic pain has a wide differential diagnosis (1). These complex problems can be assessed using a multisystems approach. Whereas gastrointestinal, gynecologic, musculoskeletal, and psychiatric conditions can cause chronic pelvic pain, a thorough gynecologic history and pelvic examination are the cornerstones of the diagnostic assessment. Few laboratory tests are helpful. A pelvic ultrasound is useful when the pelvic organs cannot be adequately assessed during the physical examination. A team approach, coordinated by a trusted family physician, can bring much relief to patients with this frustrating clinical problem.

References
1. Ryder RM. Chronic pelvic pain. *Am Fam Physician* 1996;54(7):2225–2232.
2. Stiege JF, Stout AL, Somkuti SG. Chronic pelvic pain in women: toward an integrative model. *Obstet Gynecol Surv* 1993;48:95–110.
3. Chan PD, Winkle CR, eds. *Gynecology and obstetrics, 1999–2000.* Laguna Hills, CA: Current Clinical Strategies Publishers; 1999:23–25.

11.4 Dysmenorrhea

Albert A. Meyer

I. **Approach.** Dysmenorrhea can be defined as a complaint of pain experienced during or immediately before menstruation. Up to 90% of women experience this symptom for some part in their lives (1). Risk factors include the concomitant presence of prolonged, heavy, and irregular periods. Pregnancy history and dietary factors do not seem to correlate with this symptom.

II. **History (2)**
A. It is extremely important to **distinguish primary from secondary dysmenorrhea.**
B. **Primary dysmenorrhea** starts at the onset of menarche, and is thought to be the result of prostaglandin-2α, which produces uterine ischemia. It can be treated with antiprostaglandins and oral contraceptives.
C. **Secondary dysmenorrhea** starts later in a woman's ovulatory life and may be caused by endometriosis or pelvic pathology.
D. **If abnormal bleeding** is associated with either type of dysmenorrhea, it is important to elicit symptoms of pregnancy, such as missed or late menses, breast tenderness, nausea, or urinary frequency (Chapter 11.5).

E. **If severe pain develops** during the first part of the menstrual cycle, ascertain the history of a new sexual partner, abnormal vaginal discharge, or dyspareunia. These symptoms could point toward pelvic inflammatory disease (PID) (Chapter 11.3).

F. **Pain that develops during menses**, but not related to pregnancy or infection, can also be caused by tumor. In younger women, secondary dysmenorrhea sufficiently severe to affect daily functioning or relationships suggests endometriosis. This condition can affect as many as 10% of women. Deep dyspareunia and sacral backache with menses are common symptoms. Premenstrual tenesmus or diarrhea correlates with endometriosis of the rectosigmoid area, whereas cyclic hematuria or dysuria may indicate bladder endometriosis.

G. **Infertility** is often a consequence of endometriosis.

III. **Physical examination.** As with all menstrual complaints, a thorough physical examination is an essential part of making a diagnosis.

A. **The general condition of the patient needs to be assessed**. Are the vital signs stable or is the patient showing signs of systemic illness such as fever, which can indicate pelvic infection. Hypotension and pallor can indicate a ruptured ectopic pregnancy.

B. **A general physical assessment** with attention to the back, sacrum, spine abdomen, and bladder is important.

C. **A thorough pelvic examination is key.** The external genitalia may show signs of cyanosis, as is seen with pregnancy, or abnormal discharge, as is seen with infection. Palpate the vaginal area for nodules which may present on the anterior cul-de-sac or on the posterior vaginal fornix on bimanual examination; they could indicate endometriosis. Cervical motion tenderness and cervical leukorrhea may be present in PID. Uterine tenderness is often present and uterine displacement and fixation may be noted. Ovarian enlargement or adnexa fixation, which correlates with endometriosis or adnexal mass from neoplastic or infectious cause, may be found. Nodules may also be palpated along the uterosacral ligaments on rectovaginal examination.

IV. **Laboratory testing (3)**

A. **A complete blood count** looking for anemia or leucocytosis is helpful.

B. **If abnormal bleeding is associated with the dysmenorrhea**, thyroid testing and a qualitative serum pregnancy test are indicated.

C. **Urine analysis** looking for hematuria should be obtained. With any indication of infection, a urine culture is often helpful.

D. **A pelvic ultrasound** may be helpful if any masses seem apparent on pelvic examination.

E. **The definitive diagnosis of endometriosis** can only be positively diagnosed with laporoscopy.

V. **Diagnostic assessment (1).** Difficult menstrual periods occur at some point for most women during their reproductive years. If it is recurrent and significantly interferes with daily activity or relationships, it warrants treatment. Primary dysmenorrhea not associated with abnormal bleeding can often be treated successfully with nonsteroidal agents or oral contraceptives. If it does not respond to these agents or if it is associated with abnormal bleeding, further diagnostic testing is indicated. Secondary dysmenorrhea, either with or without abnormal bleeding, may point to a pelvic tumor, infection, or pregnancy. Further testing is essential in this setting.

References

1. Jamieson DJ, Steege JF. The prevalence of dysmenorrhea, dyspareunia, pelvic pain and irritable bowel syndrome in primary care practices. *Obstet Gynecol* 1996;87: 55–58.
2. Apgar BS. Dysmenorrhea and dysfunctional uterine bleeding. *Prim Care* 1997; 24(1):161–179.
3. Chan PD, Winkle CR. *Gynecology and obstetrics 1999–2000*. Laguna Hills, CA: Current Clinical Strategies Publishers, 1999:25–26.

11.5 Menorrhagia

Albert A. Meyer

I. **Approach.** Menorrhagia, defined as excessive bleeding from the uterus, is a common gynecologic complaint. Each year, 200,000 American women undergo hysterectomy for the treatment of menorrhagia. Approximately 20% of women consult their doctor during their lives about this problem. Of women, 15% will have at least one endometrial sampling and 10% of all American women will have had a hysterectomy by age 50 years. Although it is caused by anovulatory cycles in most cases, menorrhagia can be related to pregnancy, infection, cancer, and thyroid disease. When unrelated to any uterine or systemic disease, it is referred to as dysfunctional uterine bleeding (1).

II. **History (2)**
   A. **A menstrual and reproductive history is necessary.** First, assess the first day of the last menstrual period and the first day of the previous menstrual period; the regularity, duration, frequency, and intermenstrual flow; and the number of pads or tampons per period.
   B. **Pregnancy should always be considered and diagnosed,** if present. Complications of pregnancy (e.g., spontaneous abortion, ectopic pregnancy, abruptio placentae, and placenta previa) need to be considered if pregnancy is diagnosed.
   C. **Weight loss or gain, excessive exercise, anxiety or stress disorders, as well as symptoms of systemic disease** (e.g., coagulopathy; thyroid, renal, and hepatic disease), must be considered when taking the history.
   D. **A key question.** Is the patient having ovulatory or anovulatory cycles? Do molimenal symptoms (e.g., edema, abdominal bloating, pelvic cramping, and breast fullness) precede menses that follow an ovulatory cycle. If these symptoms are not present and the patient has irregular, heavy periods, the patient is anovulatory and has dysfunctional uterine bleeding.
   E. **How old is the patient?**
      1. Menarche to 16 years. Without molimenal symptoms and with irregularity, the problem in the young woman is most probably anovulatory. Whereas some irregularity is normal, it is not normal to soak 25 to 30 tampons or pads per day. In this setting, pregnancy remains a consideration if the patient is sexually active. Fever and pelvic pain can indicate pelvic inflammatory disease (PID). Easy bruising suggests a coagulopathy and neurologic symptoms (e.g., blurred vision, visual field defects, and headache) point to a pituitary lesion.
      2. Age 16 to 40 years. Anovulation is a less common cause of abnormal bleeding; up to 8% of problems are caused by pregnancy and contraception complications in this age group. Endometriosis, endometrial hyperplasia, and endometrial polyps increase in frequency as a woman ages. PID and endocrinopathies also occur in this age group.
      3. Age 40 years and above. Abnormal bleeding in this age group should arouse suspicion of cancer, until proved otherwise. Of women in this age group, 90% who have abnormal bleeding are anovulatory. Menopausal symptoms, use of estrogens, and personal or family history of malignancy are important to elicit.

III. **Physical examination**
   A. **Assess vital signs and the patient's general appearance.** Signs of impending shock (e.g., hypotension and tachycardia) are likely related to pregnancy, particularly in the younger age group, but they can be related to trauma, sepsis, or cancer.

    B. **Pallor** not associated with hypovolemia can be found with chronic blood loss associated with anovulatory cycles, leiomyoma, blood dyscrasia, or malignancy (Chapter 16.1).

    C. **Fever, leukocytosis, and pelvic tenderness** are usually found in acute PID (Chapter 2.6).

    D. **Pelvic masses** found on physical examination point toward abscess, ectopic pregnancy, or malignancy.

    E. **Signs of thyroid disease** (e.g., rapid or slow pulse, reflex changes, hair changes, and thyromegaly) can be associated with menstrual abnormalities.

    F. **Excessive bruising** can indicate nutritional deficiency, eating disorder, trauma, abuse, medication overuse, or coagulopathy (Chapter 15.3).

IV. Testing

    A. **A baseline complete blood count and serum pregnancy test** are essential in most pre- and perimenopausal women.

    B. **A bleeding disorder** should be excluded with a platelet count, a prothrombin time, a partial thromboplastin time, and a bleeding time.

    C. **Screening** for sexually transmitted diseases and thyroid dysfunction, particularly in those of childbearing age, is important.

    D. **Any nonpregnant woman with irregular bleeding and a pelvic mass** requires evaluation with ultrasound, computed tomography (CT), or laparoscopy.

    E. **Endometrial sampling** is recommended before initiating hormone therapy in women aged more than 30 years or in those older than 20 years with prolonged bleeding. Long-term estrogen stimulation in anovulatory patients can result in endometrial hyperplasia, which can result in endometrial carcinoma. This procedure is best done on the first day of menses to avoid an unexpected pregnancy. In the perimenopausal or postmenopausal woman, amenorrhea preceding abnormal bleeding suggests endometrial carcinoma. It is useful to obtain a transvaginal ultrasound prior to the endometrial biopsy because biopsy is often unnecessary if the endometrial stripe is less than 5 mm thick.

V. Diagnostic assessment (3). Menorrhagia is defined as excessive menstrual flow. The definition of excessive varies widely among patients but "different" and "worrisome" to the patient appear to be important historical features. When excessive bleeding is regular, pregnancy and systemic illness must be excluded. Of menorrhagia, 90% of cases have no obvious cause and it is thought to be anovulatory or dysfunctional. Dysfunctional bleeding is usually not preceded by premenstrual (molimenal) symptoms. It is seen most frequently at the extremes of the reproductive years, after menarche and before the onset of menopause. Pregnancy must always be excluded as a cause in women of childbearing age. Excessive estrogen stimulation that occurs during anovulatory cycles can lead to endometrial hyperplasia and to carcinoma. Endometrial biopsy is indicated for most nonpregnant women with prolonged, irregular bleeding. Abnormal bleeding following amenorrhea in menopause is endometrial carcinoma until proved otherwise. Any pelvic mass occurring in the context of menorrhagia ought to be evaluated with ultrasound, CT, or magnetic resonance imaging. If confusion still exists, laparoscopy or hysteroscopy with saline infusion may be indicated.

References

1. Rosenfield J. Treatment of menorrhagia due to dysfunctional uterine bleeding. *Am Fam Physician* 1996;53:165–172.
2. Smith CB. Pinpointing the cause of abnormal uterine bleeding. *Women's Health in Primary Care* 1998;1(10):835–844.
3. Nelson AL. A practical approach to dysfunctional uterine bleeding. *Fam Prac Recertification* 1997;19(8):14–39.

11.6 Nipple Discharge

Joyce A. Copeland

I. **Approach.** The evaluation of a nipple discharge in the nonpregnant female patient helps determine if the cause is physiologic, pathologic, or is a "pseudodischarge," and to assess the risk of malignancy.

II. **History**

A. **Presentation.** How old is the patient? When and how was the discharge first discovered? Discharges that have been apparent for longer periods of time are more likely to be benign. The risk of cancer increases with advancing age.

B. **Discharge characteristics.** What is the color and consistency of the discharge? Is the discharge spontaneous or associated with manipulation or sexual activity only? Is the discharge unilateral or bilateral, uniductal or multiductal? What part of the nipple is affected?

1. A bloody, red discharge or a discharge that has the appearance of old blood is suggestive of, but not specific to, breast cancer.

2. A spontaneous, unilateral, uniductal discharge raises the level of suspicion for cancer. This does not exclude cancer from the differential diagnosis in the multiductal presentation.

C. **Pain.** Cyclic pain suggests a physiologic cause. Continuous pain and burning may indicate pathology related to inflammation (e.g., ductal ectasia or infection).

D. **Reproductive history.** What is the patient's menstrual history? Has she had a recent pregnancy or abortion? Amenorrhea or irregular menses in a premenopausal woman with a nipple discharge suggests the need to evaluate the patient for pregnancy, hypothyroidism, or a disruption of the hypothalamic-pituitary axis (Chapters 11.1 and 11.5).

E. **Medical history.** Is there a history of significant chest wall trauma? Is there a recent history of herpes zoster infection? Does she have a history of atopic dermatitis? Does the patient have a history of breast cancer or breast surgery?

1. Chest wall trauma (e.g., a thoracotomy) and herpes zoster infection have been reported to cause nipple discharge.

2. Any systemic disease that affects the hypothalamic-pituitary axis or alters the clearance of prolactin can result in hyperprolactinemia. Visual disturbance or headache can be associated with the presence of a pituitary adenoma.

F. **Medication.** Is the patient taking any medications? Offending agents include:

1. Phenothiazines, haloperidol, and numerous other antipsychotics
2. Tricyclic antidepressants, benzodiazepines, selective serotonin reuptake inhibitors
3. Metoclopramide, cimetidine
4. Reserpine, methyldopa, digitalis, verapamil
5. Oral contraceptives, estrogens, progestins
6. Heroin, marijuana, amphetamines, cocaine
7. Isoniazid, danazol

G. **Activity and lifestyle.** Is the patient a jogger or does she participate in aerobic exercise? Does she smoke; if so, how much? Has the patient deliberately manipulated or traumatized the nipple? Friction of clothing on the nipple can create discharge, bleeding, and tenderness, which can result in bleeding, crusting, or traumatic erosions. Smoking increases the risk of cancer and ductal ectasia.

H. **Family history.** Is there a family history of breast cancer?

I. **Review of symptoms.** A review of systems for thyroid, renal, liver, adrenal, or pituitary disease should be included in the query. Ask about visual disturbances or headache, which can be associated with a pituitary adenoma.

III. **Physical examination**

A. **Clinical breast examination** (Chapter 11.2)

1. **Inspection**. Observe the skin of the breast for crusting or a rash on the nipple or areolar region. Document the color of any discharge. Look for evidence of nipple retraction. Locate the site of the discharge on the nipples. Magnification can assist localization. Look for chest wall scars, evidence of viral infections (e.g., herpes zoster or simplex), and signs of eczema or inflammation.
2. **Palpation.** Feel the skin surface for warmth in the presence of erythema. Palpate both breasts for evidence of a mass or tenderness. Palpate regional nodes for evidence of lymphadenopathy (Chapters 11.2 and 15.2).
3. **Compression.** Compress the nipple and areolar area of both breasts with the thumb and index finger in an effort to elicit a discharge. Perform this examination in several directions. Note the location of any discharge and the number of ducts involved, as well as whether the discharge is unilateral or bilateral.

   B. **Other examination components.** Palpate the thyroid and liver if history indicates the need. Perform a neurologic examination, including visual fields, in patients with visual disturbance or headache.

IV. **Testing**
   A. **Clinical laboratory.** Order blood tests looking for evidence of thyroid, renal, and liver diseases or establishing a prolactin level, based on clinical history.
   B. **Discharge.** Test for occult blood if blood is not readily apparent. The specificity and sensitivity of cytology limits its effectiveness and is not necessary.
   C. **Imaging.** Mammography is indicated to look for nonpalpable masses or calcifications. Ductography may help distinguish the location of ductal pathology in a localized discharge but is not a substitute for exploration of the ductal system.
   D. **Ductal exploration.** The patient who does not have a good physiologic explanation for her discharge should be referred for surgical exploration or biopsy.

V. **Diagnostic assessment (1,2)**
   A. **Categories of risk.** The four categories of risk described by Arnold and Neiheisel include lactation, physiologic, pathologic, and false discharge (1).
1. **Physiologic** discharges are usually bilateral, multiductal, painless, and associated with either stimulation of the nipple or medications. Color may be white, yellow, gray, or green, and the consistency is usually milky. Occasionally, blood is present.
2. **Pathologic** discharges are usually unilateral, uniductal, and spontaneous. Color is variable and blood or purulence may be apparent. Cancer, benign tumors, infections, and systemic disease are pathologic causes of discharges of this type.
3. **Pseudodischarge.** A false discharge is often associated with staining on clothing or crusting on the nipple. This is different from the "droplets" of a true discharge. Eczema, viral infections (herpes zoster or simplex), or Paget's disease can cause a pseudodischarge.

   B. **Specific disorders of interest**
1. **Intraductal papilloma** is the most common cause of benign pathologic discharges.
2. **Ductal ectasia** is the result of a progression of ductal stagnation and resultant inflammatory process. The incidence of this disorder is higher in smokers and is most prominent in those aged 40 to 60 years. Induration and noncyclic burning pain are characteristic of this disorder.
3. **Paget's disease** involves the skin of the nipple and areola. It is usually associated with ductal carcinoma. Send any areolar lesion that does not respond to antibiotics or topical treatment for biopsy to exclude this disorder.

References
1. Arnold G, Neiheisel M. A comprehensive approach to evaluating nipple discharge. *Nurse Pract* 1997;22(7):96–108.
2. Andolsek K, Copeland J. Conditions of the breast. In: Taylor RB, ed. *Family medicine: principles and practice*, 5th ed. New York: Springer-Verlag, 1998.

11.7 Pap Smear Abnormality

Stephen Schmidt and Kathryn M. Andolsek

Worldwide, cervical cancer is one of the most common malignancies; 16,000 cases are diagnosed and 4,800 deaths occur annually in the United States (1). An American woman's lifetime risk of cervical cancer is 0.83%; her risk of dying 0.27%. A 40% decrease in incidence and mortality appear to result from increased screening and early treatment. Pap smears are one of the few interventions awarded an "A" recommendation from the US Preventive Services Task Force, although no randomized trials support its efficacy. In addition to cancer, 5% of the 50 million yearly pap smears performed in the United States reveal low grade abnormalities (2).

I. **Approach**. Management of the abnormal pap smear must be individualized.
   A. The Bethesda System was developed in 1988 and revised in 1991 by the National Cancer Institute to provide uniform terminology for cervical cytopathology reports (2). Knowledge of the natural history of each abnormality is crucial and is summarized in Table 11.1 (3).
   B. **Special concerns: frequency of screening, patient reliability, and prevalence of disease**. All women who are at least aged 18 years or sexually active (1,4,5) should be screened. The frequency of screening after the initial smear is controversial. Many experts agree that after three annual normal results, the screening interval can be increased to 3 years in low risk patients (1). Some countries and professional organizations recommend discontinuing pap smear screening in older women (age 65) without previous dysplasia. Central to both this decision and the management of abnormal results is the reliability of the patient for follow-up. Aggressive management is recommended for women felt to be less likely to follow-up (2) or with risk factors that increase the prevalence of cancer.
   C. **New technologies.** The sensitivity of traditional pap smear screening may be as low as 50%. Three new devices recently approved by the Food and Drug Administration (ThinPrep, Papnet, and AutoPap) were designed to reduce the rate of false–negative findings. Although these devices improve sensitivity, it is not clear they improve specificity. Further research is needed to determine their appropriate role. They are not useful in the evaluation of a woman with an abnormal pap smear by traditional screening (4).
II. **History.** Gynecologic history, which is essential in determining a patient's risk, should be shared with the cytopathologist. Risk factors include early age at first intercourse or pregnancy, immunosuppression of any cause, human immunodeficiency virus infection, human papilloma virus (HPV), smoking, multiple sexual partners, and a history of lower genital tract neoplasia (5).
III. **Physical examination.** The cervix usually appears normal to the naked eye. Gross cervical abnormalities should prompt further evaluation. When present,

Table 11.1 Summary of pap smear abnormalities

Pap abnormality	Regress at 24 months (%)	Progress to HGSIL at 24 months (%)	Progress to invasive cancer at 24 months (%)
ASCUS	68	7	0.25
LGSIL	47	20	0.15
HGSIL	35	N/A	1.4

ASCUS, atypical squamous cells of uncertain significance; LGSIL, low-grade squamous intraepithelial lesion; HGSIL, high-grade squamous intraepithelial lesion.

discharge should be gently removed prior to the pap smear. Tests for sexually transmitted diseases, when indicated, should be obtained after the pap smear. If the cervix appears normal, vaginitis can be treated and the smear obtained after resolution of the discharge (5).

IV. **Testing.** Evaluation of an abnormal pap smear may involve further testing or an attempt to diagnose and establish the extent of the lesion.

    A. **Repeat pap smear.** Low grade lesions can be followed with serial testing. Although false–negative finding rates of 20% to 45% have been reported, rates as low as 10% have been reported, using conization specimens as the reference (1). Repeat testing at frequent intervals minimizes this risk.

    B. **Cervicography.** Photographic evaluation of the cervix may have a sensitivity comparable to a pap smear, but it has much lower specificity (50%). A 10% to 15% rate of unsatisfactory cervicograms further limits the utility of this test (1). Current recommendations limit its use to experienced physicians who understand its limitations (2).

    C. **Human papillomavirus typing.** HPV types 16, 18, 45, and 56 are strongly correlated with cervical cancer. Screening for HPV and HPV typing have been studied to identify high risk individuals. The positive predictive value of HPV screening is less than 10% (1), limiting its clinical usefulness. The role of typing as an adjunctive triage strategy remains under investigation.

V. **Diagnostic assessment**

    A. **Reactive changes associated with inflammation.** Infectious causes (e.g., *Candida* sp., *Trichomonas vaginalis, Gardnerella vaginalis,* herpes simplex virus, or *Chlamydia trachomatis*) are common. The pathologist may be able to identify an offending organism or typical cytologic changes. However, the clinician must provide clinical correlation regarding symptoms and the need for treatment. No data support empiric therapy. The pap smear should be repeated in 3 to 6 months, regardless of cause or treatment (5).

    B. **Atypical squamous cells of uncertain significance (ASCUS).** Multiple options are currently recommended based on the clinical setting and the patient's risk. In a reliable patient, ASCUS can be followed with repeat cytology every 4 to 6 months for 2 years or until three consecutive, adequate, and negative smears are obtained. Recurrent ASCUS should be evaluated with colposcopy and biopsy (2,5). If the patient is postmenopausal or inflammation is present, a repeat pap smear after estrogen vaginal cream or appropriate antibiotic therapy can be considered (2). Close communication with the cytopathologist can clarify whether this process favors reactive or neoplastic changes and the relative incidence of neoplasia. ASCUS favoring a neoplastic process should be managed as a low grade squamous intraepithelial lesion (2).

    C. **Low grade squamous intraepithelial lesion** frequently reverts to normal. In the appropriate clinical setting with a reliable patient, cytology every 4 to 6 months until three consecutive, adequate, and negative smears is appropriate. However, because of the high rate of false–negative cytology findings, further evaluation with colposcopy, including biopsy and endocervical curettage (ECC) (2,5), is appropriate. Unreliable or high risk patients should undergo more aggressive evaluation. After the entire lesion and transformation zone are visualized, the histologically confirmed lesion can be ablated, excised, or observed (5).

    D. **High grade squamous intraepithelial lesion.** This category includes cancer *in situ* and moderate to severe dysplasia. Evaluation should include colposcopy, biopsy, and ECC. After identifying the entire lesion, excise or ablate the entire transformation zone (2,5).

    E. **Cancer.** Cytology suggestive of invasive cancer should be evaluated with biopsy and referral to a physician experienced in the management of this disease.

    F. **Atypical glandular cells.** Atypical glandular cells of undetermined significance (AGUS, AGCUS) should be subclassified according to favoring reactive process or neoplasia and by origin (endocervical or endometrial) (2). Endocervical atypia can be followed with colposcopy and ECC (5). If a neoplastic process is suspected, many believe that the best evaluation is diagnostic conization (2,5). Endometrial atypia should be evaluated by biopsy, hysteroscopy, or dilation and curretage (2,5).

References

1. US Preventive Services Task Force. Screening for cervical cancer. *Guide to clinical preventive services*, 2nd ed. Baltimore: Williams & Wilkins, 1996:105–117.
2. Kurman, RJ, Henson, DE, Herbst, AL, et al. Interim guidelines for management of abnormal cervical cytology. *JAMA* 1994;271:1866–1869.
3. Melnikow J, Nuovo J, Willan AR, et al. Natural history of cervical squamous intraepithelial lesions: a metaanalysis. *Obstet Gynecol* 1998;92:727–733.
4. Evaluation of cervical cytology. Summary, evidence report/technology assessment. No. 5. Rockville, MD: AHCPR, January 1999; http://www.ahcpr.gov/clinic/cervsumm.htm
5. American College of Obstetricians and Gynecologists. Cervical cytology: evaluation and management of abnormalities. *Technical Bulletin* No. 183. Washington, DC: American College of Obstetricians and Gynecologists, 1993.

11.8 Postmenopausal Bleeding

Victoria S. Kaprielian

Postmenopausal bleeding is defined as vaginal bleeding that occurs in a woman who has had no menses for a year or more. This is a common outpatient problem, estimated to account for approximately 5% of gynecologic office visits.

I. **Approach.** Any vaginal bleeding in a postmenopausal woman not on hormone replacement therapy (HRT) requires a diagnosis, as malignant causes are found in 10% to 20% of cases. Endometrial cancer is the primary concern; other malignancy may occasionally be implicated. Nonmalignant causes include endometrial atrophy [up to 82% of cases (1)], endometrial hyperplasia or polyps, cervical polyps, infections, and lacerations. Women on cyclic HRT are expected to have uterine bleeding; bleeding at unexpected times or in excessive amounts requires investigation.

II. **History**
   A. **Pattern of bleeding.** Although the amount of bleeding is not helpful in identifying malignancy, it should be assessed to determine the likelihood of significant anemia or hypovolemia that may require intervention. Timing of bleeding may suggest its cause.
      1. Specific relationship to medication courses or cycles suggests drug-induced bleeding.
      2. Postcoital bleeding suggests an atrophic cause or cervical polyp.
      3. Association with bowel movements or urination suggests a nongenital source.
   B. **Current medications.** Any hormonal therapy, including estrogen, progesterone, tamoxifen, thyroid replacement, or corticosteroids, should be quantified and recorded.
      1. Acyclic bleeding is common in the first 3 to 4 months on continuous estrogen–progestin therapy, and usually does not indicate pathology. Bleeding that is excessive, persists after months of therapy, or occurs after amenorrhea has been established on these regimens should be evaluated.
      2. The rate of endometrial cancer in women on tamoxifen or unopposed estrogen is six to seven times the rate for untreated women. The frequency of endometrial polyps is also increased.
      3. Exogenous corticosteroids and incorrect dosage of thyroid replacement can lead to menstrual irregularities and postmenopausal bleeding.

C. **Past medical history.** Nulliparity, early menarche, late menopause, and history of chronic anovulation are risk factors for endometrial hyperplasia and carcinoma. Obesity, hypertension, diabetes, and liver disease are commonly associated with estrogen excess, and can also increase risk (1). Past use of oral contraceptives is associated with decreased risk.

D. **Family history.** A strong family history of endometrial or colon cancer is a risk factor for endometrial cancer.

III. **Physical examination**

A. **Vital signs.** Blood pressure and pulse can indicate the degree and acuity of blood loss; orthostatic changes can be evidence of significant volume depletion. Fever suggests infection as a potential cause (Chapter 2.6).

B. **Abdomen.** Tenderness or guarding suggests an infectious or inflammatory cause. Palpation for suprapubic masses is necessary as part of the evaluation for malignant causes.

C. **Pelvis.** Examine external genitalia, vagina, and cervix for lesions or lacerations that could be the source of bleeding. The uterus and ovaries must be palpated to assess for enlargement, masses, and tenderness.

D. **Rectum.** Rectal examination and anoscopy may be warranted to rule out hemorrhoids or other intestinal source of bleeding (Chapter 9.11).

IV. **Testing**

A. **Office laboratory testing.** Urinalysis, stool guaiac testing, or both can be useful to look for nongenital sources of blood. A complete blood count may be helpful in assessing the degree of blood loss and likelihood of infection. Testing for gonorrhea and chlamydia may be warranted when tenderness or fever is present.

B. **Pap smear.** Many sources recommend a pap smear as part of the evaluation, although its diagnostic yield in these cases is low. Cervical lesions or friability raise the possibility of a cervical bleeding source. Endometrial cells found on the pap smear of a postmenopausal woman not on HRT warrants further evaluation of the endometrium.

C. **Biopsy**

1. Visible lesions of the vulva, vagina, or cervix should be sent for biopsy.

2. In the absence of a clear nonuterine source of bleeding, endometrial biopsy is usually recommended. This office test can cost-effectively identify endometrial hyperplasia and carcinoma, with a sensitivity of 85% to 95% (3), and it is lower in cost and risk than other procedures (2).

3. Traditional wisdom required dilation and curettage (D&C) for diagnosis if endometrial biopsy was negative. Recent evidence indicates this is unlikely to be of benefit (despite higher risk and cost), except in cases where other procedures are not possible (2–5).

4. If bleeding continues after normal biopsy, consider repeat biopsy or assessment by another method (5).

D. **Diagnostic imaging**

1. Palpable adnexal abnormalities should be evaluated by ultrasound or other imaging as appropriate.

2. Transvaginal ultrasound (TVUS) is gaining popularity as an alternative or adjunct to endometrial biopsy. A clearly identifiable endometrial stripe less than 4 or 5 mm in thickness is highly unlikely to contain hyperplasia or carcinoma, and biopsy may not be necessary (2,4). Fluid in the endometrial cavity has been associated with carcinoma, and its presence warrants further investigation (5). TVUS should not be used in place of biopsy in women on tamoxifen, as the drug is known to cause misleading ultrasound findings (3,5).

3. Hysteroscopy is becoming the "gold standard" against which other methods of endometrial assessment are compared (4,5). Flexible hysteroscopy allows direct visualization of the endometrium in the office setting, and can be used for directed biopsy and removal of small polyps. Rigid hysteroscopy allows greater intervention, but requires greater anesthesia.

4. Sonohysterography (ultrasound evaluation after instillation of fluid into the endometrial cavity) appears to offer promise as another alternative that provides additional information on the uterine architecture (3,5). This is the subject of ongoing study, especially in comparison with hysteroscopy, which provides similar information and may allow simultaneous biopsy of identified lesions.

V. **Diagnostic assessment.** Initial clinical evaluation may identify a nonuterine source. Postcoital spotting in conjunction with vaginal atrophy or cervical friability suggests cervical or vaginal mucosal bleeding. Gross hematuria or visibly bleeding hemorrhoids suggest that the bleeding source is not genital. If no other source is identified, however, the key to diagnosis is imaging and tissue sampling of the endometrium. A thin endometrial stripe in a woman in a low-risk category suggests endometrial atrophy. Findings on biopsy can include atrophy, proliferative changes, various degrees of hyperplasia (simple, complex, and atypical, in increasing order of risk), or carcinoma. If neither biopsy nor TVUS provides sufficient information, hysteroscopy is the recommended next step. D&C should be reserved for cases in which other methods are unsuccessful or unavailable.

References

1. Shelly MS. Endometrial biopsy. *Am Fam Physician* 1997;55(5):1731–1736.
2. Feldman S, Berkowitz RS, Tosteson ANA. Cost-effectiveness of strategies to evaluate post-menopausal bleeding. *Obstet Gynecol* 1993;81(6):968–975.
3. O'Connell LP, Fries MH, Zeringue E, Brehm W. Triage of abnormal postmenopausal bleeding: a comparison of endometrial biopsy and transvaginal sonohysterography versus fractional curettage with hysteroscopy. *Am J Obstet Gynecol* 1998;178(5):956–961.
4. Emanuel MH, Verdel MJ, Wamsteker K, Lammes FB. A prospective comparison of transvaginal ultrasonography and diagnostic hysteroscopy in evaluation of patients with abnormal uterine bleeding: clinical implications. *Am J Obstet Gynecol* 1995;172(2):547–552.
5. Good AE. Diagnostic options for assessment of postmenopausal bleeding. *Mayo Clin Proc* 1997;72:345–349.

11.9 Vaginal Discharge

Albert A. Meyer

Vaginal symptoms, especially discharge, are responsible for 10% of all physician visits by women. Each year, approximately 12 million women in the United States are treated for vaginitis (1).

I. **Approach.** An irritation or inflammation of the vagina with or without discharge occurs in all age groups and has a variety of causes. Of vaginitis, 90% occurs in women of reproductive age; it is caused by one of three types of infections: an overgrowth of yeast, usually *Candida albicans*; sexually transmitted *Trichomonas vaginitis*; or an excessive growth of anerobic microorganisms [bacterial vaginosis (BV)].

Many women with a vaginal complaint, itching, soreness, dysuria, or discharge, self-medicate with over-the-counter (OTC) preparations before seeking medical attention. Because many OTC preparations help symptomatically, the diagnosis can be clouded. The OTC products should be avoided for 3 days prior to the office visit.

A key element in the evaluation of a woman with a vaginal complaint is the awareness that many factors other than the three aforementioned infections can cause vaginitis. These include medications, repeated douching, foreign bodies, systemic illness, and sexually transmitted disease.

II. History (2)

A. What is the specific vaginal complaint? Is it soreness, discharge, odor, itching, or dyspareunia? Vaginal soreness correlates with vulvovaginal candidiasis, allergy, contact dermatitis, or atrophy. Yeast, BV, atrophy, and trauma produce significant dyspareunia.

B. What is the characteristic of the discharge? Is the discharge heavy or light, thick or thin? Does it have an odor? Most women have some physiologic discharge that changes during the menstrual cycle with hormonal flux. BV and *T. vaginitis* produce malodorous discharge of variable amount. Yeast produces a thick discharge that usually has no odor.

C. What is the sexual history (3)? Is there a new sexual partner in the last year? How does the patient protect herself from sexually transmitted disease? In taking this part of the history, it is key to convey necessary information concerning sexually transmitted disease transmission, both to allay anxiety and to modify behavior, when appropriate.

D. What is the menstrual history? Ask when was the last period? Are you pregnant? What is your method of contraception? Yeast often overgrows in the vagina premenstrually. Trichomoniasis and BV during pregnancy are associated with premature labor, premature delivery, and septic abortion. Yeast vaginitis is more common during pregnancy and when taking oral contraceptives.

E. Are you taking any medications? Have you tried any medications for your vaginal problem?

Antibiotics, contraceptive preparations, hormones, vaginal medications, and other OCT preparations often alter the vaginal ecosystem and allow infection to be introduced or normal vaginal flora to become unbalanced. Foreign bodies (e.g., tampons, diaphragms, or condoms) can create vaginal irritations, inflammation, and infections.

F. If the problem is vaginal irritation, have any substances been used that cause allergic reaction or chemical irritation? Do you douche?

These might include deodorant soaps, feminine hygiene sprays, scented douches, laundry detergent, bath oils, dyed toilet tissue, synthetic clothing, or hot tub or swimming pool chemicals.

At times, only elimination of all possible offending agents, skin testing, or both permit identification of the allergies or irritants.

G. If no obvious infectious, traumatic, or chemical agent is identified, could the vaginal complaint be related to a systemic illness [e.g., diabetes mellitus or human immunodeficiency virus (HIV) infection] or with a life change?

Idiopathic vulvovaginal ulceration can be associated with HIV disease.

Atrophic vaginitis secondary to hormone depletion can cause significant dyspareunia, swelling, and discharge. Collagen-vascular disease, pemphigus, and Bechet's syndrome can manifest in vaginal symptoms.

III. Physical examination (4).

A general physical examination should be performed if systemic illness is suspected. Record vital signs, including temperature, blood pressure, and pulse.

In most cases, a genital examination with the patient in the lithotomy position is adequate.

The external genitalia is carefully inspected for evidence of trauma, blisters, lymph nodes excoriations, swelling, erythema, ulcerations, tenderness or pain.

The amount, color, texture, odor, and location of the discharge should be noted. A complete pelvic examination should be performed with particular attention given to the cervix for evidence of friability or inflammation and a cervical motion test which may indicate pelvic inflammatory disease.

IV. Testing (5)

A. Vaginal fluid pH. Immersing pH paper in the vaginal discharge or the lateral wall of the vagina will give the vaginal pH.

A pH greater than 4.5 indicates BV or *T. vaginalis*.

B. Saline wet mount. Obtain a drop of vaginal discharge from the posterior fornix; place it on a slide with a drop of saline and apply a cover slip.

1. Clue cells, which are bacteria-coated, stippled epithelial cells, are characteristic of BV.
2. Trichomonads, which are mobile, oval flagellated parasites, confirm the presence of trichomoniasis.

C. Potassium hydroxide (KOH) preparation. Place a second drop of vaginal secretions on a slide containing a drop of KOH; "a positive whiff test" indicates the presence of BV. Threadlike hyphae and budding yeast observed microscopically are characteristic of a candidal infection.

D. Cultures for gonorrhea and chlamydia are not routinely indicated, but should be taken with a history of a new sexual partner, purulent cervical discharge, or cervical motion tenderness.

V. **Diagnostic assessment.** BV causes 40% to 50% of vaginitis, followed by candidiasis (20% to 25%) and trichomoniasis (15% to 20%). Together, these infections account for more than 90% of vaginitis diagnoses.

When evaluating a woman with a vaginal complaint, be sure to hear her true concern. Evaluate and treat appropriately those with acute symptoms (e.g., pain or swelling) and be careful to understand the effect of pretreatment with OTC preparations in the presumptive diagnosis. It is wise to be mindful of the possibility of sexually transmitted diseases with any vaginal complaint and to test appropriately for these diseases. If a vaginitis, presumably infectious, does not respond to initial therapy, consider other causes including trauma, herpes, menopause, contact dermatitis, toxic shock syndrome, steroid-responsive inflammatory vaginitis, and collagen-vascular or other systemic disease.

References

1. Lash DJ, Garcia TA. Diagnosis and treatment of vaginitis. *The Female Patient* 1998;23:25–41.
2. Carr PL, Majeroni BA, Robinson JC, Talarico LD. Vaginitis: solid diagnosis means effective treatment. *Patient Care* 1999;33(2):86–106.
3. Miller KE. Sexually transmitted diseases. *Prim Care* 1997;24(1):179–193.
4. Chan PD, Winkle CR, eds. *Gynecology and obstetrics' 1999–2000 edition.* Laguna Hills, CA: Current Clinical Strategies Publishers, 1999:73–79.
5. Sabel JD. Vaginitis. *N Engl J Med* 1997;337:1896–1903.

12. MUSCULOSKELETAL PROBLEMS

ELISE M. COLETTA

12.1 Arthralgia

Meredith A. Goodwin

Arthralgia is a general term that describes pain in one or more joints, with or without joint inflammation. The source can be local or systemic. Pain location, onset, duration, and associated symptoms are important data in determining the cause of arthralgia (1).

I. **Approach.** Joint pain can be categorized by pattern of involvement (Table 12.1).
II. **History**
   A. **Demographics.** The patient's age is sometimes helpful in determining the cause of arthralgia. Systemic lupus erythematosus (SLE) commonly presents between the second and fourth decades of life. Rheumatoid arthritis (RA) is more common between the fourth and sixth decades; osteoarthritis (OA) peaks in the seventh and eighth decades. Infectious causes, as well as trauma, have no particular age association. Younger, female patients are more likely to have RA or SLE, whereas postmenopausal women are affected by gout and OA of the knee and hand. Male patients more likely have gout, ankylosing spondylitis, and OA of the hip. Race is helpful in some disorders: SLE is more common in African-Americans.
   B. **Affected joints.** The new onset of monarticular symptoms can be seen in trauma, infection, crystal-induced disease, periarticular problems, and degenerative and inflammatory arthritic processes. Early OA can present in one joint, most commonly the knee, or in any joint damaged by antecedent trauma. Recurrent pain in one joint can indicate OA flare, gout or pseudo-gout attack, SLE, sarcoidosis, or a periarticular problem. Gout presents in the first metatarsal phalangeal joint in 50% of cases (Chapter 12.6).
   Multiple joint involvement, especially with other associated symptoms, is characteristic of a systemic process. Symmetric involvement of the metacarpal-phalangeal, proximal interphalangeal joints (PIPs), wrist, and feet is common in RA; involvement of the knees or hips is unusual (1). OA favors the PIPs, distal interphalangeal, carpal-metacarpal joint of the thumb, hips, knees, ankles, feet, and spinal column (1), but involvement is not necessarily symmetric. Erosive OA can affect multiple joints of the hands. SLE often affects the hand and wrists.
   C. **Pain characteristics.** Additional history includes the exact location of the pain (around vs. inside the joint), the time course (episodic or intermittent vs. constant pain), and the presence and onset of joint swelling or warmth. Joints that are stiff in the morning and hurt at rest are seen in RA. RA pain waxes and wanes throughout the day and night, and is unrelated to activity. OA pain is associated with use and improves with rest.
   D. **Family history.** RA, SLE, gout, ankylosing spondylitis, and OA of the fingers all have a familial component. SLE is also found in families with other autoimmune diseases.
   E. **Lifestyle factors.** Dietary history is important in gout, as a diet high in purine foods (liver, sweetbreads, kidneys, red meat, sardines, and anchovies) can precipitate an attack in susceptible individuals. Certain underlying diseases, sexual practices, alcoholism, and intravenous drug use are risk factors for septic arthritis.
   F. **Associated symptoms.** Other complaints are often helpful in narrowing the differential diagnosis. Fatigue that does not improve with rest can be seen in RA, SLE, and infectious arthralgia. Rash can be seen in arthralgia resulting from a variety of infectious and inflammatory causes. Urticaria is common in the acute serum sickness syndrome. A history of a tick bite or targetlike rash may indicate arthritis from Lyme disease. Vaginal discharge, pelvic pain, or

Table 12.1 Causes of arthralgia

Monarticular or polyarticular	Polyarticular	Monarticular

Degenerative arthritis
  Osteoarthritis, hemochromatosis,
  acromegaly, thyroid disease
Inflammatory arthritis
  Rheumatoid arthritis, systemic
  lupus erythematosus, psoriatic
  arthritis, sickle cell disease,
  Lyme disease, hemophilia,
  inflammatory bowel disease,
  Reiter's syndrome, sarcoidosis,
  ankylosing spondylitis,
  immunodeficiency
Crystal-induced arthritis
  Gout, pseudogout
Septic arthritis
  Any bacterial pathogen,
  mycobacteria, fungi
	Vaccine related
	  Rubella
	Infection related
	  Viral (rubella, hepatitis B), mycoplasma
	Acute serum sickness syndrome
	Medication side effect
	Metabolic bone disease
	  Osteomalacia
	Overuse syndromes
		Periarticular process
		  Bursitis, tendinitis
		Trauma-induced disease
		  Fracture, joint dislocation, meniscal
		  damage
		Prosthetic joint problem
		  Loosening of prosthetic components

urethritis symptoms or discharge should raise the possibility of an infectious cause or Reiter's disease. Fever is likely with infectious, and some inflammatory, causes of arthralgia.

G. **Past medical history.** Other known medical illnesses are also important as they may be associated with inflammatory or degenerative causes of arthralgia (Table 12.1). Childhood joint disease predisposes to early onset degenerative disease.

New medications, including diuretics, chemotherapeutic agents, antituberculosis drugs, and low-dose aspirin, can precipitate gout. Other medications and vaccination reactions can cause polyarticular arthralgias.

III. **Physical examination**

A. **Joint examination.** Inspect the joint for evidence of trauma, breaks in the skin, swelling, erythema, deformity (e.g., bony changes, tophi), and asymmetry with contralateral joints. Palpate the joint and surrounding tissues for warmth, tenderness, effusion, edema, and crepitus. Perform joint range of motion (ROM). Pain with active, but not passive ROM is more consistent with a periarticular problem.

B. **Examination of other systems.** Conjunctivitis, oral lesions, urethritis, genital or extremity ulcers, rash, tophi, and nail pitting can indicate a more systemic problem. Rheumatic disease can affect other organs (e.g., pleural effusion, splenomegaly, Raynaud's phenomenon).

IV. **Testing**

A. **Laboratory tests.** Perform arthrocentesis of an isolated, acutely inflamed joint and examine synovial fluid for cell count and differential, crystals, Gram's stain, and culture (2). Suspected cases of gonococcal disease warrant culture of the pharynx, urethra, cervix, and rectum to increase the likelihood of a positive culture. Potentially useful blood tests include an erythrocyte sedimentation rate (ESR), antinuclear antibody, rheumatoid factor, syphilis, Lyme disease and other serologies, blood culture, uric acid, thyroid-stimulating hormone, calcium, liver function tests, blood urea nitrogen, and creatinine (2). The ESR is often elevated with inflammatory or infectious conditions, and can be mildly increased in primary generalized OA (Chapter 16.3).

B. **Diagnostic imaging.** Perform an x-ray study with a history of significant trauma or focal bone pain (2). In adults, x-ray findings of degenerative changes are more prevalent than symptomatic disease at all ages. Soft tissue swelling and erosive changes can be seen with rheumatic disease. Disruption of joint integrity is most clearly seen on magnetic resonance imaging (MRI). Radiographs and MRI are more helpful in the evaluation of trauma than in other situations, but can be used to follow the progression of a chronic process. Plain radiographs of the chest looking for lung nodules, infiltrates, interstitial processes, and cardiac enlargement may be helpful if rheumatic disease is suspected.

V. **Diagnostic assessment.** Arthralgia has many causes. Trauma and infection are the most serious problems in the acute setting where the history and physical examination will be the key to the diagnosis. Chronic or recurrent mon- or polyarticular arthralgia more likely indicates an arthritic process; further testing may be needed to narrow the differential diagnosis. Arthralgia without physical findings may suggest an overuse syndrome, viral infection, vaccine or other medication side effect, or metabolic bone disease (2). Keep in mind that arthralgia can be caused by disease in the surrounding soft tissue structures.

References

1. Johnson BE. Adult rheumatic disease. *AAFP home study self assessment*. Kansas City: American Academy of Family Physicians July, 1997.
2. American College of Rheumatology Ad Hoc Committee on Clinical Guidelines. Guidelines for the initial evaluation of the adult patient with acute musculoskeletal symptoms. In: Kelley WN, Ruddy S, Harris ED, Jr, Sledge CB, eds. *Textbook of rheumatology*, 5th ed. Philadelphia: WB Saunders, 1997.

12.2 Calf Pain

Alicia J. Curtin

Calf pain, a common complaint that has many causes, can pose a challenge diagnostically.

I. **Approach. Assess potential risk factors and the chronology of events.**
Common causes of calf pain are listed in Table 12.2.
   A. **Special concerns.** The aim is to establish or eliminate the most concerning diagnoses, and select those patients who require further workup. Medically urgent diagnoses include deep venous thrombosis (DVT), compartment syndrome, cellulitis, and pyomyositis. Accurate assessment is important in order to treat the patient promptly and appropriately and prevent complications.

II. **History**
   A. **Pain characteristics.** What is the pattern of onset, quality, location, duration, and intensity of the pain? What, if anything, helps relieve the pain? A report of a sensation of being "clubbed in the back of the leg" or "shot in the calf," along with an audible pop or snap sound, suggests an acute Achilles tendon rupture (ATR) (1). Cramping calf pain may indicate a metabolic disturbance or a denervating disease. Numbness and burning pain or an electric-shock sensation, may indicate a neurological process. A "creeping and crawling" sensation deep within the muscles of the legs and thighs that is somewhat relieved with movement of the extremity is suggestive of restless leg syndrome (RLS).
   B. **Preceding events.** Was the pain preceded by any specific activity or trauma? Any recent prolonged inactivity? Unilateral calf pain after a period of immobility, especially in the presence of risk factors (e.g., lower extremity venous disease, oral contraceptive use), is DVT until proved otherwise. If the patient presents with a history of direct trauma to the calf, a compartment syndrome or intramuscular hematoma should be suspected. Pain occurring at night and disrupting sleep is suggestive of RLS or arterial disease.
   C. **Associated symptoms.** Coexisting symptoms can help to differentiate the cause of the pain. Any fever or back or knee pain should be noted. Ask about leg swelling, bruising, weakness, tingling, or other changes in sensation.
   D. **Pertinent medical history.** Does the patient smoke? Is there a history of any form of arthritis, or a Baker's cyst? Any recent hip, knee, gynecologic, or lower abdominal surgery? Is the patient pregnant or postpartum? Pertinent medical illnesses include peripheral vascular disease, varicosities, malignancy, hematologic disorders, and diabetes. Acquired immune deficiency syndrome has been associated with a syndrome of calf pain, swelling, and tenderness along with cutaneous hyperesthesia to light touch. The syndrome is believed to be caused by hyperalgesic thrombophlebitis (2).
   E. **Family history.** A family history of DVT or inherited causes of hypercoagulability increase the risk for DVT (3).

III. **Physical examination (PE)**
   A. **Initial PE.** Is the patient febrile? Inspect the patient's back and check the curvature of the spine. Examine both legs from the groin and buttocks down for size, symmetry, skin color, pigmentation, hair distribution, and venous pattern. Note any skin lesions. Palpate lower extremity pulses and check for edema. Assess capillary refill. Note the temperature of the leg, especially over the area of pain. Palpate the calf for localized tenderness or a cord, which can indicate a superficial or deep thrombophlebitis. Feel for any increased firmness of the calf muscles. Palpate for masses, swelling, or tenderness in the lower back and entire leg. Check the mobility and flexibility of the spine and note if movement provokes any distal pain or weakness. Examine the knee and ankle joints on the affected side. Assess joint range of motion (ROM) and

Table 12.2 Causes of calf pain

MUSCULOSKELETAL

Achilles tendon rupture, muscle strain or tear, fracture, intramuscular hematoma, compartment syndrome, ruptured Baker's cyst, localized myositis, referred pain from the knee or lumbar spine

METABOLIC

Hypothyroidism, thyrotoxic myopathy, uremia, dehydration, hyponatremia, hypomagnesemia, hyperkalemia, hypercalcemia

NEUROLOGIC

Amyotrophic lateral sclerosis, lumbar spinal stenosis, peripheral neuropathy, restless leg syndrome

VASCULAR

Arterial insufficiency, deep venous thrombosis

INFECTIOUS

Cellulitis, pyomyositis

muscle strength. Check lower extremity reflexes and perform a good peripheral sensory examination.

- **B. Additional PE**. If evaluation suggests arterial insufficiency, assess for postural color changes by elevating the patient's leg 60°. If ATR is suspected, perform a Thompson test. With the patient prone, squeeze the calf muscle just distal to its maximal girth. Plantar flexion of the foot is the normal result, indicating an intact Achilles tendon. A positive Homan or Lowenberg sign is suggestive of DVT. However, these signs are neither sensitive or specific for the diagnosis (4,5).

IV. Testing

- **A. Blood tests.** No laboratory tests are necessary unless the history or PE suggests an infectious process or a metabolic disorder. In these cases, obtain a complete blood count (CBC) with differential, creatine phosphokinase (CPK), blood urea nitrogen, creatinine, electrolytes, calcium, magnesium, and thyroid-stimulating hormone.
- **B. Diagnostic imaging**. Radiographs are useful if fracture or bony injury is suspected. Duplex ultrasound is used to evaluate for DVT, but can also detect masses, popliteal cysts, or incomplete rupture of the Achilles tendon (5). The definitive radiographic test for both symptomatic and asymptomatic DVT is venography. Sensitivity and specificity are greater than 90%; however, the test is invasive and costly compared with duplex ultrasound (4,5). In symptomatic cases, the sensitivity and specificity of duplex ultrasound is also very good, as long as a negative test is followed up with a repeat study in 5 to 7 days if clinical suspicion remains high (4,5). Magnetic resonance imaging has comparable sensitivity and sensitivity to venography and gives more information regarding surrounding soft tissue structures when the clinical assessment is not straightforward (4).

V. Diagnostic assessment. The diagnosis of DVT is unreliably made without objective testing. Of patients presenting with suspected DVT, 75% will actually have a nonthrombotic cause of leg pain (4). The patient with acute calf pain that develops after athletic activity, a tender calf muscle, and pain and decreased muscle strength with passive ankle or knee ROM likely has a muscle tear or sprain. Acute calf pain, with posterior ankle swelling and an abnormal Thompson test, is characteristic of ATR. Claudication-type calf pain, possibly bilateral, with decreased peripheral pulses and decreased capillary refill, suggests arterial disease. The pseudoclaudication of lumbar spinal stenosis is provoked by ambulation or posture change (e.g., standing straight at the waist). A ruptured

Baker's cyst typically produces calf pain along with erythema and diffuse swelling of the calf and ankle. A clinical history of calf pain and fever, with an open wound or a well-demarcated area of erythema, is suggestive of cellulitis. Calf pain, gastrocnemius weakness, swelling, and increased CPK levels are suggestive of localized myositis. An additional symptom of fever, with calf erythema and an abnormal CBC, may indicate pyomyositis. An intramuscular hematoma or compartment syndrome will often present with pain out of proportion to the physical signs, which can include increased firmness of the calf muscles and localized ecchymosis and swelling.

References

1. Schuberth J. Achilles tendon trauma. In: Scurran B, ed. *Foot and ankle trauma*, 2nd ed. New York: Churchill Livingston, 1996.
2. Banerjee A. The assessment of acute calf pain. *Postgrad Med J* 1997;73:86–88.
3. Harris J, Abramson N. Evaluation of recurrent thrombosis and hypercoagulability. *Am Fam Physician* 1997;56:1591–1596.
4. Weinmann EE, Salzman EW. Deep vein thrombosis. *N Engl J Med* 1994;331: 1630–1641.
5. Anand S. Does this patient have deep vein thrombosis? *JAMA* 1998;279:1094–1099.

12.3 Hip Pain

Meredith A. Goodwin and Elise M. Coletta

I. **Approach.** The evaluation of hip pathology is challenging for several reasons. Compared with other joints, the hip is relatively inaccessible to palpation and evaluation. Hip pathology can cause referred pain to the groin, buttock, thigh, or knee. Pain located in the hip area can have a lower back source (Chapter 12.5). In addition, hip pain can be referred from pelvic, intraabdominal, or retroperitoneal pathology (Table 12.3).

II. **History**
   A. **Pain characteristics.** What is the exact location of the pain? Pain arising from the lumbar spine is perceived in the buttock and, less commonly, in the

Table 12.3 Differential diagnosis of hip pain

Intraarticular	Periarticular	Referred
Osteoarthritis	Muscle contusion	Lumbosacral disease
Rheumatoid arthritis	Muscle strain	Hernia
Gout or pseudogout	Trochanteric bursitis	Lymphadenitis or lymph-adenopathy
Tumor (primary or metastatic)	Ischial bursitis	Deep venous thrombosis of groin or thigh
Synovitis	Iliopsoas bursitis	
Septic joint	Iliotibial band syndrome	Retroperitoneal disease (e.g., renal calculus)
Dislocation of joint	Leg length discrepancy	Pelvic disease (e.g., tumor)
Aseptic necrosis of femoral head		Intraabdominal disease (e.g., tumor)
Osteomyelitis		
Loosening of prosthetic components		

groin and anterior thigh. This must be differentiated from radicular pain arising from the spine. True hip pain more often localizes to the anterior midgroin or midthigh area. Lateral hip or thigh pain most likely represents trochanteric bursitis (1). How is the pain described? A "snapping" type discomfort is most commonly caused by iliotibial band syndrome. Constant pain can indicate infection or cancer.

  B. Involved joints. Hip osteoarthritis (OA) can have a monarticular onset, or other joints may be involved. Of hip OA patients, 20% will develop bilateral involvement.

  C. Precipitating factors. Has there been a recent fall or other trauma? In an elderly or an osteoporotic patient, hip fracture can occur after a very minor incident. A contusion over the greater trochanter can lead to persistent bursitis; a contusion over the iliac crest, to a tear of the muscle aponeurosis. Has there been any preceding athletic or overuse activity that could cause muscle strain? Ischial bursitis usually develops after prolonged sitting.

  D. Other symptoms. Bacterial involvement of the hip joint can be accompanied by fever and shaking chills (2). Other symptoms may be present in cancer, pelvic, intraabdominal, or retroperitoneal pathology. Sciatica commonly accompanies trochanteric bursitis.

  E. Past medical history. Any prior hip problems or hip surgery? A patient with a hip replacement may develop loosening of prosthetic components, which can be a source of pain, or can seed the joint during a recent infection or invasive procedure. Aseptic necrosis of the femoral head is more likely in patients with sickle cell disease. Previous occult hip fracture or delayed treatment, can also lead to aseptic necrosis. Patients receiving long-term steroids may manifest constant hip pain. Congenital or developmental defects are found in 80% of patients with hip OA.

III. Physical examination

  A. General. If referred pain is suspected, evaluate the appropriate organ system. Palpate the groin and thigh for hernias, lymph nodes, and vascular cords. Assess gait. An unwillingness to bear weight suggests fracture, even with a negative preliminary x-ray finding. Check the neurovascular status of the distal extremity after any traumatic episode.

  B. Musculoskeletal. Observe the involved extremity. In femoral neck fractures, the involved leg may appear slightly shortened and externally rotated. Intertrochanteric fractures can cause the involved leg to be internally rotated and shortened. Evaluate the spine, including the straight leg raise test, if spinal pathology is being considered. Compression of the patient's pelvis with the patient side lying may localize pain to the sacroiliac joint. Check for leg length discrepancy by measuring each extremity from the anterior superior iliac spine (ASIS) to the medial malleolus; for hip joint shortening, measure from the ASIS to the greater trochanter.

  Palpate the greater trochanter, ischial tuberosity, and surrounding muscle groups for tenderness. The hip joint is not easily palpated; palpable warmth is produced only when intensely inflamed. Document joint range of motion. Nondisplaced or impacted fractures may not be painful, except at extremes of motion. Pain in all directions suggests intraarticular disease. Pain arising from the hip is typically elicited at the extreme ranges of motion, as well as with motion against resistance. With the patient supine, bend the uninvolved leg at the knee and hip and bring it toward the chest. Watch the opposite hip for flexion (Thomas test), indicating a flexion contracture of that hip. Loss of internal rotation occurs early in OA, followed by the loss of extension, adduction, and flexion. Pain and an inability to fully abduct or extend the hip can also be seen in rheumatoid arthritis (RA). Trochanteric bursitis may present with pain on external rotation only. Muscle strain (e.g., a "groin pull") will produce pain on passive stretch or resisted contraction of the involved muscles only. In iliotibial band syndrome, the "snapping" of the band may be audible and palpable as the hip is flexed and extended. Document any muscle weakness or muscle atrophy.

IV. Testing

  A. Radiographs. A suspected hip fracture requires anteroposterior and lateral or "frog leg" hip films. A fracture of the femoral neck can be difficult to visualize. In trauma cases, lateral oblique films are needed to evaluate the acetabulum. Radiologic changes of OA are ubiquitous in older patients and do not rule out other causes of hip pain. Radiographs of a septic hip joint often reveal a "moth-eaten" appearance of the subchondral bone on both sides of the joint (2).

  B. Clinical laboratory. The sedimentation rate and white blood cell count are normal in synovitis; leukocytosis and an elevated erythrocyte sedimentation rate may be seen with a septic joint. If a septic joint is suspected, synovial fluid aspiration must be done promptly, as a delay of a few hours increases the chance of substantial joint damage. Joint fluid should be examined for glucose, protein, crystals, Gram's stain, culture, cell count, and differential. Fluoroscopic guidance is needed to confidently localize the joint space.

V. Diagnostic assessment

  A. Intraarticular disease. A deep, aching discomfort that is increased with weightbearing is characteristic of OA. In the later stages, hip OA can lead to rest or night pain. Femoral neck fractures occur most commonly in patients aged more than 50 years; intratrochanteric fractures occur at even older ages. Dislocation of the hip is rarely seen; it is most often associated with severe trauma.

  Joint fluid analysis will assist in distinguishing a septic joint from a transient synovitis or crystal-induced arthropathy. Septic arthritis can lead to severe joint destruction within 2 to 3 weeks. Involvement of the hip joint in gout or pseudogout is rare. The femoral neck is a common site for metastatic cancer, which may lead to a pathologic fracture.

  B. Referred pain. Lumbosacral disease is the most common cause of hip pain in a postadolescent, nonelderly individual (3).

References

1. Shbeeb MI, Matteson EL. Trochanteric bursitis. *Mayo Clin Proc* 1996;71:565–569.
2. Medsger TA, Jr. Diagnosis and treatment of arthritis. *Emerg Med* 1999;31:13–28.
3. Birnbaum JS. *The musculoskeletal manual.* Philadelphia: WB Saunders, 1986.

12.4 Knee Pain

Charles B. Eaton

Knee pain is a very common condition, ranking number seven in the National Ambulatory Care survey. It has been suggested that 90% of knee pain in patients can be diagnosed after an appropriate history and knee examination.

I. Approach. Key clinical questions include: What is the possibility of internal derangement or fracture? Does this patient need an imaging study? Are the history, physical examination, and time spent with the patient sufficient to make the most cost-effective diagnosis and treatment plan? Does this patient need specialist referral?

  A. Causes of knee pain. Dividing the onset of knee pain according to the time course of symptoms (acute—minutes to hours; subacute—hours to days; or intermittent and chronic—weeks to months) helps to differentiate the common causes of knee pain. (Table 12.4). In addition, referred knee pain can develop from hip or back problems.

Table 12.4 Causes of knee pain differentiated by time course of symptoms

Acute	Subacute or intermittent	Chronic
Fracture	Patellar tendinitis	Degenerative arthritis
Tibial plateau; supra-	Pes anserine bursitis	Rheumatoid arthritis
condylar, intra-	Patellofemoral syndrome	Tumor
condylar, patella	Infrapatellar tendinitis	
Dislocation	Gout or pseudogout	
Meniscal tear	Reiter's syndrome	
Medial or lateral	Septic arthritis	
Ligamentous sprain	Osgood-Schlatter's disease	
or tear	Osteochondritis dissecans	
Patellar tendon rupture	Degenerative meniscal tear	
Popliteal aneurysm	Plica syndrome	
	Iliotibial band syndrome	

II. History

A. **Age and etiology.** The patient's age is an important factor in determining the likelihood of certain knee problems. Because of stronger ligaments, avulsion fracture (anterior intercondylar eminence of the tibia, tibia tubercle) is more common in younger age groups, whereas ligamentous rupture occurs in older persons. Patellar dislocations and apophysitis are more likely in growing adolescents.

B. **Trauma.** Understanding the mechanism of injury and estimating the acceleration or deceleration and torsional forces across the knee joint, predict the likelihood of occult fractures and internal derangement. Patients describing a popping sensation during a rotational or twisting injury, followed by an immediate swelling, usually have internal derangement of either meniscal or ligamentous components, or both. Locking of the knee suggests a "bucklehandle" meniscal tear obstructing normal hingejoint activity of the femoraltibial joint.

C. **Alleviating or exacerbating factors.** Patellofemoral syndrome (PFS) or chrondromalacia patella is associated with anterior knee pain that worsens going up or down stairs or with prolonged sitting. Morning stiffness that improves with mild activity, but worsens as the day progresses, is typical of degenerative arthritis (osteoarthritis). The stiffness of rheumatoid arthritis (RA) generally does not improve with activity. Patients with multiple joint pains should be questioned about fever or skin rash to rule out infectious or inflammatory joint disease.

III. Physical examination.

Both knees, as well as the hip, ankle, and foot on the affected side, should be examined. The knees are inspected for symmetry, signs of quadriceps or calf wasting, and any obvious swellings, discoloration, or pallor. Thigh, knee, calf circumference, and leg length are measured to document any asymmetry. Measurement of the quadriceps or Q angle (normal <15°) is important to evaluate anterior knee pain. Inability to perform full knee flexion and extension will highlight any effusion. Neurovascular supply should also be evaluated.

In nonacute circumstances, the suprapatellar bursa is milked to determine if effusion is present. The patellar apprehension test may detect patellar dislocation; the patellar grind test is used to detect PFS. Evaluation of patellofemoral tracking within the femoral groove also helps make the latter diagnosis as the patella will track laterally in PFS, leading to the characteristic "jockey cap" patella. The knee should be carefully palpated for tenderness of the patellotibial insertion (Osgood-Schlatter's disease), the body of the infrapatellar tendon (tendinitis), the insertion of the tendon on the patella (Sinding-Larsen-Johannson disease), medial and lateral joint line (potential meniscal pathology), pes anserine bursa (bursitis), or iliotibial band insertion. Plica, a painful, thickened band of exuberant synovium, can also be diagnosed by palpitation of the medial and lateral joint lines.

Ligamentous testing is done next. Test the posterior cruciate ligament through the posterior drawer sign. Use the Lachman test for the anterior cruciate ligament, or, in obese patients, the anterior drawer sign. The medial collateral ligament is tested in zero and 15° of flexion by applying a valgus stress to the knee. The lateral collateral ligament is tested similarly using a varus stress. McMurray's test may detect a meniscal tear. A duck walk test can also be used to look for a posterior meniscal tear. The patient's gait is observed, specifically looking for forefoot varus and heel valgus, Morton's foot deformity, and femoral anteversion, all of which can accentuate valgus stress on the knee and lead to a painful overuse syndrome.

IV. **Testing.** Most diagnoses can be made without an x-ray study or expensive diagnostic test.

   A. **Ottawa rules**. For acute injuries, the Ottawa knee rules are highly sensitive, but less specific, in determining the need for a plain knee x-ray study in adults (1). This decision rule has not been tested in children. The Ottawa rules recommend an x-ray study if any of the following are found: age 55 years or older, tenderness at the head of the fibula, isolated patellar tenderness, inability to flex the knee to 90°, or inability to bear weight immediately after the trauma (1).

   B. **Radiographs and procedures.** Testing depends on the diagnosis suspected, medicolegal requirements, and response to therapy. Knee films are important when surgical treatment of degenerative arthritis is considered, or if chondrocalcinosis, gout, RA, osteomyelitis, or osteochondritis dissecans should be ruled out. Magnetic resonance imaging (MRI) of the knee is a sensitive and specific test for detecting meniscal or ligament injury; however, it is no better than a consistent history, a positive McMurray's or Lachman's test, and medial joint line tenderness (2). MRI is indicated when a patient has a good history for internal derangement and a normal clinical examination, or fails to improve despite adequate conservative therapy. A bone scan is warranted when a stress fracture or cancer is suspected. Computed tomography may define bony pathology and, with arthrography, detect meniscal and ligamentous pathology when an MRI is contraindicated. Duplex ultrasound will rule out a deep venous thrombosis or detect a Baker's cyst. Arthrocentesis can be used to diagnose gout, pseudogout, or septic arthritis, and to relieve pain and allow corticosteroid instillation. Arthroscopy is helpful when internal derangement is suspected and the probability of arthroscopic treatment is high.

V. **Diagnostic assessment.** Clinical information may trigger further immediate diagnostic workup. Hemarthrosis could indicate internal derangement or fracture. Knee pain and a limp in a child with a normal knee examination suggests hip disease (Legg-Calvé-Perthes, slipped femoral capital epiphysis). Bony swelling and night pain suggest tumor; fever and joint swelling, infectious or inflammatory arthritis. A knee effusion with rash suggests gonorrhea, Reiter's syndrome, or collagen vascular disease.

Of nontraumatic anterior knee pain, 70% is related to patellofemoral syndrome. Meniscal tears can develop in older patients without a trauma history. Knee pain in a growing adolescent is jumper's knee (patellar tendinitis) or traction apophysitis until proved otherwise.

References

1. Steil IG. Derivation of a decision rule for the use of radiography in acute knee injuries. *Ann Emerg Med* 1995;26:405–413.
2. Gelb HJ, Glasgow SG, Sapega AA, Torg JS. Magnetic resonance imaging of knee disorders. Clinical value and cost-effectiveness in a sports medicine practice. *Am J Sports Med* 1996;24:99–103.

12.5 Low Back Pain

Stephen Davis

I. **Approach.** Low back pain is a common problem with many causes. The differential diagnosis can be grouped into three over-lapping categories: urgent ("red flag") diagnoses, structural (musculoskeletal) problems, and medical causes (Table 12.5).

II. **History.** The history should include evaluation for "red flag" conditions.

   A. **Pain characteristics.** Assess the nature of the pain, along with the onset and duration of the symptom. Is there any radiating pain, leg weakness, or paresthesia? Pseudoclaudication is suggestive of spinal stenosis. Pain radiating below the knee is more likely to be a true radiculopathy (1). Nerve root compression is highly unlikely without sciatic pain (1). Was the onset after a traumatic event? A seemingly insignificant episode (e.g., a minor fall) may be a "red flag" for fracture in an elderly patient. Are there alleviating or exacerbating factors? Does the pain limit the patient physically or socially? Is there a history of previous back problems or back surgery?

   B. **Review of systems.** Look for associated symptoms that can indicate a "red flag" condition or an underlying medical cause. Gastrointestinal and genitourinary symptoms are particularly important, especially incontinence (Chapter 10.10).

   C. **Psychosocial information.** Has the patient initiated any new activities? If work-related, assess typical job tasks. Investigate whether the back pain could have any relationship, sexual, or mood implications. Sexual activity can be severely affected simply because of pain, but sexual dysfunction can also result from neurologic abnormalities associated with the cause of the back pain. Back pain is associated with depression and poor sleep patterns. Drug-seeking behavior may be exhibited along with a complaint of back pain. Addiction may have resulted from former or on-going treatment of the pain. Legal issues can complicate the diagnosis and treatment of back pain. Ask the patient whether litigation involving the back pain is under consideration.

III. **Physical examination.** Evaluation should be both general and specific. It is prudent to leave the potentially most painful parts of the examination to the end.

Table 12.5 Causes of low back pain

Musculoskeletal	Medical[a]
Lumbar muscle strain	Infection
Lumbar or sacral nerve root compression	Osteomyelitis, discitis, epidural abscess
Disc herniation, cauda equina syndrome,[a] sciatica, spinal stenosis	Hematologic
	Multiple myeloma, myelodysplasia, cancer (primary or metastatic)
Vertebral fracture or subluxation[a]	Benign tumors
Arthritic conditions	Aortic aneurysm
Osteoarthritis, rheumatologic conditions	Retroperitoneal pathology
	Pyelonephritis, renal calculus, cancer
Sacroiliac joint sprain or degenerative disease	Abdominal pathology
	Perforated viscus, pancreatitis

[a] Urgent or life-threatening.

A. **General.** Examination includes auscultation of the heart and assessment of peripheral pulses and blood pressure. Abdominal examination should focus on possible causes of back pain (Table 12.5). Assess gait.

B. **Neurologic.** The lower extremity examination includes motor strength, deep tendon reflexes, sensation, proprioception, and certain functional maneuvers (Table 12.6). Romberg and Babinski reflexes should also be assessed. Rectal examination should assess sphincter tone, which can be compromised in sacral root dysfunction. In the primary care setting, most clinically significant disc herniations will be detected by the following limited examination: dorsiflexion of the great toe and ankle, Achilles reflex, light touch sensation of the medial (L_4), dorsal (L_5), and lateral (S_1) aspect of the foot, and the straight leg raise (SLR) test (1).

C. **Musculoskeletal.** Assess range of motion of the spine and lower extremities. Perform the SLR test passively with the patient supine. Note the angle of leg elevation precipitating pain. A positive test for sciatica is buttock pain radiating to the posterior thigh, and perhaps to the lower leg and foot. Sciatica, with pain and resistance on internal rotation of the hip, can indicate piriformis muscle spasm or strain. The SLR test is usually negative in spinal stenosis (2). Percussion of the spine and upper pelvis helps to identify areas of localized tenderness, as in fracture, metastatic disease, and some rheumatologic conditions. Palpate standard trigger points looking for fibromyalgia. Check for paraspinal muscle spasm. Measure thigh and calf circumferences to look for muscular atrophy.

IV. **Testing**

A. **Clinical laboratory tests.** Testing will be guided by the differential diagnosis as determined by the history and physical examination. If the back pain is felt to be of musculoskeletal origin, no test may be indicated. A urinalysis can help rule out hematuria or infection, if the pain is thought to be urologic or as a result of trauma. If the history suggests a medical problem, the considered diagnoses will determine the laboratory work. Extensive medical workup may be needed for a primary or metastatic malignancy. A calcium level should always be measured to identify a potentially lethal hypercalcemia. Rheumatologic studies may be indicated if a connective tissue disease (e.g., ankylosing spondylitis or rheumatoid arthritis) is suspected. If the pain is thought to be secondary to an urgent or life-threatening condition, have pertinent tests done expeditiously.

B. **Diagnostic imaging.** In the absence of "red flags," lumbar spine films are not indicated for musculoskeletal sounding low back pain of less than 1 month duration (1). Neurologic emergencies (e.g., major spine trauma, cauda equina syndrome) require magnetic resonance imaging (MRI) studies. It is usually unproductive to order an MRI for straightforward lumbar muscular strain or for initial evaluation of simple disc herniation, as the prevalence rate of nonsignificant abnormal findings is high. A bone scan may be helpful when tumor, infection, or occult fracture is suspected. Electromyography may be useful to assess for nerve root dysfunction when symptoms are questionable.

Table 12.6 Neurologic findings seen with disc herniation

Disc pain/numbness	Motor weakness	Functional maneuver	Reflex
L_3-L_4/anteromedial thigh and knee	Quadriceps	Deep knee bends	↓Patellar
L_4-L_5/lateral leg, first three toes	Dorsiflexion of foot or great toe	Heel walking	
L_5-S_1/posterior leg, lateral heel	Plantar flexion of foot or great toe	Toe walking	↓Achilles

V. Diagnostic assessment. The most common cause of low back pain in the outpatient setting is musculoskeletal strain. Although temporarily very debilitating, muscle strain can be conservatively treated and usually has few long-term complications. Variations from this basic presentation must be recognized to identify more structurally significant or medically threatening problems. Clues to these other diagnoses, which are found in the history, are reinforced by abnormalities in the physical examination; they are found less often by diagnostic testing.

The following "red flags" suggest possible urgent diagnoses. A history of recent trauma or motor vehicle accident can signify a vertebral fracture or subluxation. Fever can indicate an infection of the spine or pyelonephritis (Chapter 2.6). Recent genitourinary instrumentation or other invasive procedure can precede this presentation. Weight loss, other constitutional symptoms, or pain at rest (or at night) may suggest cancer (Chapter 2.13). Neurologic abnormalities can signify nerve dysfunction or cord compression. Urinary or fecal incontinence or retention, saddle area perineal numbness, or anal sphincter incompetence suggests cauda equina syndrome. A sudden tearing sensation in the back with associated hypotension can be caused by a rupturing abdominal aortic aneurysm.

References

1. Bigos SJ. Acute low back problems in adults. *Clinical Practice Guideline*. No. 14. AHCPR Publication No. 95-0642. Rockville, MD: Agency for Health Care Policy and Research, Public Health Service, US Department of Health and Human Services; December 1994.
2. Alvarez JA, Hardy Jr. RH. Lumbar spine stenosis: a common cause of back and leg pain. *Am Fam Physician* 1998;57:1825–1834.

12.6 Monarticular Joint Pain

Margaret A. Tryforos

I. Approach. Evaluation of monarticular joint pain should differentiate inflammatory from degenerative conditions and clarify whether immediate treatment is needed to prevent permanent joint damage. Distinction must be made between peri- and intraarticular disease. Consideration of an underlying systemic disease is also important. The differential diagnosis of monarticular joint pain is shown in Table 12.7.

II. History

   A. Timing of the pain. What is the onset and duration of the pain? Was there a specific inciting incident or trauma? When does the pain occur? Pain wakening the patient from sleep may suggest a malignancy. Is pain present at rest? Does movement or weightbearing exacerbate the symptom? Any associated joint stiffness?

   B. Location of the pain. Localization to the joint is typical in osteoarthritis (OA). Exceptions are hip OA, where pain can localize to the groin or thigh, and OA of the spine, where pain can localize to the buttocks. Radiation of the pain may suggest periarticular or neuropathic problems.

   C. Associated symptoms. Fever, night sweats, or weight loss may suggest an infectious cause or an underlying systemic illness. Rash can occur with infectious or inflammatory arthritides.

   D. Medical history. Many medical problems can be associated with an inflammatory or a degenerative arthritis (Table 12.7). Knowledge of prior joint surgery or prosthesis placement is important. A history of childhood joint disease (e.g., slipped capital epiphysis) or bone disease (e.g., osteochondritis dissecans) can predispose to early onset degenerative joint disease.

Table 12.7 Differential diagnosis of monarticular joint pain

DEGENERATIVE ARTHRITIS
Osteoarthritis, arthritis secondary to other disease (e.g., hemochromatosis, myxedema)

INFLAMMATORY ARTHRITIS
Rheumatoid arthritis, systemic lupus erythematosus, psoriatic arthritis, sickle cell disease, Lyme disease, hemophilia, inflammatory bowel disease, Reiter's syndrome, sarcoidosis, ankylosing spondylitis, immunodeficiency

CRYSTAL-INDUCED ARTHRITIS
Gout, pseudogout

TRAUMA-INDUCED DISEASE
Fracture, joint dislocation, meniscal damage

SEPTIC ARTHRITIS
Bacterial, mycobacterial, mycotic, viral pathogens

PROSTHETIC JOINT PROBLEMS
Loosening of prosthetic components

TUMOR

    E. **Social history**. The patient's support system is especially important if severe functional impairment is present. The employment or recreational history may indicate a risk of repetitive joint trauma. Sexual risk factors and a history of alcohol or intravenous (IV) drug abuse are important.

    F. **Medications**. What medication or treatment has been used and what was the response? A history of systemic steroid use can lead to osteonecrosis of the femoral head.

III. **Physical examination**. Is discomfort apparent? Is fever present? Assess the patient's gait and note if a mobility aide is used. Inspect the joint for surgical or traumatic scars, muscle atrophy, deformity, joint swelling, and erythema. Palpate for warmth, tenderness, and effusion. Evaluate joint range of motion (ROM). If active ROM is full and normal, evaluation of passive ROM is unnecessary. Pain with active, but not passive ROM suggests a periarticular process. Depending on the joint involved, palpate the relevant periarticular structures and perform the appropriate provocative maneuvers. Examine for rash.

IV. **Testing.** No studies are routinely indicated for all cases of monarticular joint pain.

    A. **Imaging studies.** Radiographs may be warranted if evaluation suggests degenerative joint disease, but they are not necessarily indicated at initial presentation. Radiographic findings of OA, which are more prevalent than symptomatic disease, can be found in 85% of patients aged 65 years (1). Radiographic study is clearly indicated if the pain is chronic, or if there is a history of recent trauma, night pain, or childhood joint disease. In cases of acute inflammatory arthritis, radiographs will likely reveal soft tissue swelling and not provide diagnostic certainty, but could exclude other diseases. Bone scans are not helpful, as they will be positive in all forms of arthropathy. Computed tomography or magnetic resonance imaging scans are not indicated in the routine initial evaluation of monarticular joint pain.

    B. **Laboratory testing.** In the presence of an inflamed joint, a complete blood count and erythrocyte sedimentation rate (ESR) may help distinguish a septic or inflammatory condition from crystal-induced arthritis. Rheumatoid factor or antinuclear antibody may be positive in inflammatory arthritis (Chapters 16.3 and 17.3). Serologic testing for syphilis should be done when gonococcal infection is suspected. Serum uric acid, Lyme titers, and human immunodeficiency virus testing may be warranted. The uric acid level may be normal during an acute gouty attack.

C. **Joint aspiration.** Fluid analysis is necessary in all cases of suspected septic arthritis, and for the definitive diagnosis of presumed crystal-induced arthropathy at initial presentation. Fluid should be analyzed for cell count and crystals and sent for Gram's stain, culture, and sensitivity. Patients with immune compromise or tuberculosis require culture for mycobacteria and opportunistic organisms. In suspected septic arthritis, Gram's stain and culture of the blood, skin lesions, cervix, urethra, pharynx, and rectum may be indicated.

V. **Diagnostic assessment.** The history and physical examination usually determine whether the cause of joint pain is inflammatory or degenerative. Occasionally, an acute, inflammatory appearing monarthritis, with a mildly elevated ESR, can be the initial presentation of degenerative disease. OA typically presents with a slow, insidious progression of symptoms over months to years. The pain is achy, brought on by joint use, and relieved by rest. Short-lived (<30 minutes) stiffness may be apparent in the morning and after inactivity.

Gouty arthritis is seen most frequently in men aged more than 30 years. Of patients, 50% present classically with inflammation in the first metatarsal joint of the foot. In women, upper extremity joint involvement predominates. Synovial fluid analysis will reveal monosodium urate crystals or calcium pyrophosphate crystals in the case of pseudogout. Synovial white blood cell (WBC) count suggests inflammation (3,000–50,000 cells/µL). Synovial fluid should be cultured, even if crystals are identified, as bacterial infection can coexist. When in doubt, a diagnostic or therapeutic trial of colchicine can be considered.

Infectious arthritis should be considered with any inflamed joint. Risk factors include an immunocompromised state, a damaged or prosthetic joint, sexual promiscuity, and alcohol or intravenous drug abuse. Onset is usually rapid, over hours to days. Gonococcal arthritis can present with a few days of migratory polyarthralgias. In septic arthritis, the joints commonly affected are the knees, hips, and shoulders. Severe joint pain, swelling, and limited ROM suggest the diagnosis, especially if high fever is present. An elevated WBC count, with a left shift, is present in more than 50% of cases. Definitive diagnosis is dependent on arthrocentesis. Synovial fluid WBC count of greater than 50,000 is supportive of infection. A negative Gram's stain finding does not rule out infection. Gonococcal arthritis can present with a lower synovial fluid WBC count and the synovial fluid culture is positive in only 25% of cases (2).

Lyme arthritis has an acute, oligoarticular onset and especially affects large joints, most commonly the knee. Symptoms tend to be episodic and are associated with marked swelling, often disproportionate to the amount of pain. Presentation can be weeks to months after the initial infection, and the patient may be unable to give a history of tick bite or the erythema chronicum migrans rash (3). Serology and Western blot testing for Lyme disease should be positive.

References

1. Baker DG, Schumacher HR. Acute monoarthritis. *N Engl J Med* 1993;329:1013–1020.
2. Zimmerman B, Lally EV, Liu NYN. Infectious agents and the musculoskeletal system. In: Noble J, ed. *Textbook of primary care*, 2nd ed. St. Louis: Mosby, 1996.
3. Sigal LH. Musculoskeletal manifestations of Lyme arthritis. *Rheum Dis Clin North Am* 1998;24:323–351.

12.7 Neck Pain

Elise M. Coletta and Meredith A. Goodwin

I. **Approach.** The differential diagnosis for neck pain can be thought of by pattern of onset (Table 12.8). Disease, which can originate in the neck, can be felt there or elsewhere. The neck is also a site of referred pain.

Table 12.8 Potential causes of neck pain by site and mode of onset

Source	Acute or subacute onset	Insidious onset
Spinal cord	Acute contusion or hemorrhage Acute cord compression Epidural abscess or hematoma Meningitis	Tumor
Intervertebral disc	Acute herniation	Chronic degeneration
Vertebra	Fracture Dislocation Osteomyelitis	Spondylosis Degenerative: osteoarthritis of facet joints Inflammatory: rheumatoid arthritis Tumor: primary or metastatic
Supportive tissues of spine	Ligamentous tear Ligamentous sprain Muscular strain or spasm Torticollis	Polymyalgia rheumatica Temporal arteritis Fibromyalgia Polymyositis or dermatomyositis
Other neck structures	Pharyngitis, lymphadenitis	Thyroid cancer
Referred	Myocardial infarction, aortic dissection	Apical lung tumor, temporomandibular joint dysfunction

II. History

- **A. General.** Patient age and occupation are important. An individual's job can involve awkward or prolonged body positioning (1). Some of the conditions listed in Table 12.8 can present with fever or with constitutional or other musculoskeletal symptoms. More diagnosis-specific symptoms may be present (e.g., chest pain with a myocardial infarction).
- **B. Pain characteristics.** What is the character, location, frequency, and duration of pain? Tumors of the cervical spine can present with unremitting neck pain that is worse at night. Referred neck pain from intrathoracic pathology is more often located anteriorly.
- **C. Precipitating factors.** Any prior history of neck problems? Has there been any preceding neck trauma or change in work or avocational activities? A history of collision trauma may warrant consideration of concurrent head injury. Is there any relationship of the pain to a particular neck position or movement? Careful questioning may be needed to uncover this latter information, but it is crucial to determining the mechanism of pain production. Have there been any emotional stressors?
- **D. Associated symptoms.** Is headache present? Any paresthesia, dyskinesia, or weakness of the trunk or upper or lower extremities? Bladder dysfunction can occur with a central spinal cord injury. What is the distribution of any radicular pain? An increase in radicular symptoms with coughing or sneezing suggests nerve root impingement (2).

III. Physical examination

- **A. General.** After any cervical spine injury, order an x-ray study first to rule out an unstable injury. Assess gait, which can be impaired with a cervical myelopathy. Notice neck posture (3). Torticollis can occur secondary to trauma, muscle strain, vertebral subluxation, viral infection or from a psychogenic cause. Examine other head and neck structures (e.g., lymph nodes) and the temporomandibular joints (1). Look for meningeal signs, if appropriate.
- **B. Musculoskeletal examination.** Palpate for muscle tenderness or spasm in the neck and head. Tender trigger points may be found in fibromyalgia. Assess active and passive range of motion (ROM) of the neck and shoulders. ROM is not affected with referred sources of pain. Decreased passive ROM may be seen in rheumatoid arthritis (RA), ankylosing spondylitis (AS), disseminated idiopathic skeletal hyperostosis (DISH), compression fractures, and cervical spondylosis. Active contraction or stretching of strained muscles or ligaments will precipitate pain.
- **C. Neurologic examination.** Include the examination of cranial nerves, motor function, tone, and reflexes of the upper and lower extremities. Look for muscle atrophy. Check pinprick and light touch sensation in the upper extremities, looking for a dermatomal pattern of loss. Evaluate cerebellar, vibration, and position sense in the legs. The exact level of nerve root involvement *cannot* be precisely known from the physical examination because of overlapping innervation (2) (Table 12.9). A Spurling's test (extension and rotation of the head and neck while applying downward pressure to the top of the head) that precipitates radicular symptoms is very suggestive of nerve root pathology (1).

IV. Testing

- **A. Clinical laboratory testing.** A complete blood count and erythrocyte sedimentation rate are warranted for suspected infection or neoplasm. A positive rheumatoid factor (RF) is found in more than two-thirds of patients with RA, but is also found in 10% to 20% of all elderly individuals. RF and antinuclear antibody are absent in AS. Creatine phosphokinase is elevated in myositis and, possibly, muscle trauma (Chapters 16.3 and 17.3).
- **B. Diagnostic radiology.** Cervical spine films are mandatory after any spine trauma (3). A cross-table lateral film is used to rule out an unstable fracture or dislocation (2). The lateral view must include all seven cervical vertebrae as well as the C7-T1 interspace (3). Cervical spine films are also useful for a vertebral compression fracture, cancer, and rheumatologic disorders. Cortical

Table 12.9 Neurologic changes with nerve root compression

Root	Referred pain	Paresthesia	Motor weakness	Reflex
C5	Shoulder or upper arm	Shoulder	Shoulder abduction or external rotation	↓Biceps
C6	Radial aspect of forearm	Thumb	Elbow flexion, wrist extension	↓Biceps
C7	Dorsal aspect of forearm	Index or middle finger	Elbow extension, wrist flexion	↓Triceps
C8	Ulnar aspect of forearm	Ring or little finger	Finger intrinsics	No change

erosion of the vertebral body indicates an inflammatory process. Increased width of the prevertebral soft tissues can suggest a prevertebral hematoma. Degenerative changes in the vertebral joints, also called spondylosis, are very common with aging and do not correlate well with symptomatology (1,2). Computed tomography scans are excellent for definitive delineation of bony fracture anatomy, when necessary. Magnetic resonance imaging (MRI) is the most effective means to evaluate the soft tissues of the neck. An MRI will distinguish between neoplasm and degenerative disorders of the vertebrae, and visualize ligamentous injury, occult disc herniation, hematoma, or edema around the spinal cord. MRI may identify abnormalities that have no clinical significance (1).

C. **Other.** An electromyogram (EMG) can delineate the site of a particular nerve lesion or clarify the diagnosis when symptoms and physical examination are discordant (1). An EMG may be negative in nerve damage of less than 3 weeks' duration (1,2).

V. **Diagnostic assessment**

A. **Spondylosis.** Degenerative changes can encroach on the spinal canal or intervertebral foramina. Consider spondylosis-related symptoms in patients aged more than 40 years. Symptoms affect men twice as often as women. Common symptoms include a unilateral or bilateral occipital headache that is worse in the morning and radiates to the frontal region, upper chest, and shoulders.

B. **Radiculopathy or myelopathy.** Radicular pain usually involves the proximal arm with more distal paresthesias (Table 12.9) (Chapter 4.6). Cervical myelopathy presents with upper extremity nerve root symptoms and long tract signs in the legs. Spasticity may be the most prominent neurologic change. Long tract signs in the legs occur uncommonly without root signs (2). Symptoms can be precipitated by neck movement. Myelopathy is more typically secondary to spondylosis rather than disc herniation.

C. **Rheumatologic.** Axial involvement with RA may be limited to the upper cervical spine; atlantoaxial subluxation can present as occipital pain. Subluxation can cause cord compression. DISH has a characteristic appearance on x-ray film. It is the most common rheumatologic process affecting the cervical spine, but rarely causes symptoms (1). AS also affects the cervical spine. Gout and pseudogout usually do not.

References

1. Swezey RI. Chronic neck pain. *Rheum Dis Clin North Am* 1996;22:411–437.
2. Cailliet R. *Neck and arm pain*. Philadelphia: FA Davis, 1989.
3. Graber MA, Kathol M. Cervical spine radiographs in the trauma patient. *Am Fam Physician* 1999;59:331–342.

12.8 Polymyalgia

Arnold Goldberg

Polymyalgia or diffuse painful muscles (myalgia) does not always imply muscular disease. Chronic aches, pains, or stiffness in multiple areas of the body are increasingly common complaints among patients.

I. **Approach.** Differential diagnosis is best approached by dividing the various causes of polymyalgia into those with muscular weakness and those without (Table 12.10).

II. **History.** Is the onset insidious or acute? What body areas are involved? Is there associated joint pain? Does the patient complain of weakness? Is fever or prominent fatigue present (Chapters 2.5 and 2.6)? Is the patient's sleep disturbed? Is depression an overriding symptom? Look for precipitating events. Is there domestic abuse? Could there be any potential emotional or financial gain from the symptoms? Are there any symptoms suggestive of the diseases mentioned in Table 12.10? Take a careful medication, travel, occupational, and family history.

III. **Physical examination**
   A. **Musculoskeletal.** Inspect for muscle atrophy. Palpate for muscle tenderness. Is any tenderness diffuse or focal in nature? Evaluate joint range of motion and gait.
   B. **Neurologic.** Assess muscle strength and cranial nerve function.
   C. **Other.** Palpate for scalp tenderness and tender areas or nodules localized to the temporal or occipital arteries. Look for rash.

IV. **Testing.** For the workup, costs are increasingly relevant. Initial testing can be divided into pathways.
   A. **With objective muscle weakness.** Electromyography (EMG), a complete blood count (CBC), erythrocyte sedimentation rate (ESR), creatine phosphokinase (CPK), potassium, calcium, phosphorous, magnesium, and thyroid-stimulating hormone (TSH) are warranted. If CPK is elevated or a myopathic picture appears on EMG, consider a muscle biopsy in cases of moderately weak, but not atrophic, muscle and no history of recent muscle trauma.
   B. **Without objective muscle weakness.** Obtain a CBC, electrolytes, TSH, CPK, and ESR. If normal, evaluate, as needed, for other disorders listed in Table 12.10.

V. **Diagnostic assessment**
   A. **Polymalgia rheumatica (PMR).** Typical onset is from age 50 years to more than 90 years. Symptoms can begin abruptly or insidiously. Fatigue, anorexia, weight loss, and low grade fever are common. Patients with PMR complain of aching and stiffness in the morning. "Jelling" of the joints after inactivity, in two of the three proximal (hips, shoulders, neck) areas of the extremities and torso for 1 month or longer is diagnostic of PMR. On examination will be found diffuse, proximal muscle tenderness without weakness. Temporal arteritis (TA) is associated with PMR in 16% to 20% of cases. In TA, scalp tenderness and diffuse or focal tender areas or nodules are localized to the temporal or occipital arteries. Headache is present in two-thirds of patients (Chapter 2.7). Visual symptoms and claudication of the jaw, tongue, or entire swallowing mechanism are common. The visual deficit is usually permanent.
   B. **Fibromyalgia** is a chronic, widespread pain syndrome without overt muscular pathology. The pain typically waxes and wanes in intensity. The core symptom is widespread musculoskeletal pain with multiple tender points on both sides of the body, above and below the waist. Classically, tenderness is found in more than 11 of 18 trigger point sites with the application of 4 kg of palpation pressure (1,2). Other point areas can be tender and fibromyalgia can still be diagnosed in patients with fewer than 11 classic trigger points. Other symptoms are stiffness, skin tenderness, postexertion pain, poor sleep pattern, and, at times, fatigue. Patients are more sensitive to pain throughout their body

Table 12.10 Causes of polymyalgia

Polymyalgia without muscular weakness	Polymyalgia with muscle weakness
Acute viral infections	Vasculitis
Vaccine-related (e.g., influenza)	Paraneoplastic syndrome
Fibromyalgia	Eosinophilia myalgia syndrome
Polymyalgia rheumatica	Sarcoidosis
Chronic fatigue syndrome	Inflammatory
Psychogenic rheumatism	Polymyositis, dermatomyositis, inclusion body myositis
Muscle trauma from vigorous activity	Neuromuscular: myasthenia gravis, Eaton–Lambert syndrome, genetic muscular
Lyme disease	dystrophies, spinal muscular atrophy, amyotrophic lateral sclerosis, myotonic dystrophy,
Thyroid disease	familial periodic paralysis
Arthritis of adjacent joints	Electrolyte disorders
Electrolyte disorders	Hypo- or hypercalcemia (-kalemia, -natremia), hypomagnesemia
Rheumatologic disorders	Endocrine
Rheumatoid arthritis	Hypo- or hyperthyroidism, Cushing's disease, Addison's disease
Systemic lupus erythematosus	Metabolic
Deconditioning	Disorders of carbohydrate and lipid metabolism, carnitine deficiency, mitochondrial
Muscle overuse	myopathies, disorders of purine metabolism
	Toxic myopathies
	Alcohol, chloroquine, cocaine, colchicine, corticosteroids, D-penicillamine, ipecac,
	lovastatin, zidovudine, dilantin, ketoconazole
	Infectious
	Viral (Ebstein–Barr, human immunodeficiency virus, coxsackie, influenza), bacterial
	(staphylococcus, clostridium), rickettsial (Rocky Mountain spotted fever), parasitic
	(toxoplasmosis, trichinosis, schistosomiasis), protozoan (toxoplasmosis)

leading to many associated symptoms including headache, crampy abdominal pain, vertigo, vulvodynia, nondermatomal paresthesias, and premenstrual syndrome symptoms as well as other somatic complaints (1). Fibromyalgia patients have a higher incidence of psychiatric illnesses such as depression, but the debate continues to whether this is the cause or effect of the chronic pain and ensuing disability. Chronic fatigue syndrome (CFS) has characteristics similar to fibromyalgia. Persisting, debilitating fatigue and postexertion malaise are the paramount symptoms. Myalgias, low grade fevers, pharyngitis, adenopathy, and cognitive impairment are common occurrences (3). At least 25% to 40% of patients with misdiagnosed Lyme disease have fibromyalgia or CFS (Chapter 2.5).

C. **Psychogenic rheumatism**, typically, has a histrionic presentation where the fatigue symptom is very prominent (4). Neurologic and musculoskeletal examination are often inconsistent on repetition.

D. **Rheumatic disorders.** Soft tissue pain can be secondary to well-established rheumatoid arthritis or systemic lupus erythematosus. Sjögren's syndrome may be the exception, as myalgia symptoms can antecede the full presentation of the syndrome.

E. **Inflammatory disorders.** Causes of polymyalgia symptoms and muscle weakness include polymyositis, dermatomyositis, and inclusion body myositis (IBM). Proximal limb or neck weakness is the most prominent symptom. Fewer than 50% of patients have associated muscle pain. Other symptoms include difficulty climbing stairs, getting into or out of a car, rising from a chair, combing hair, and lifting objects (4). There may be a history of falls (4). On examination, muscle atrophy is more typical of myositis. Muscle weakness is symmetric and diffuse. Unlike PMR, the hip, shoulder, and neck are infrequently tender to palpation. Gait is slow and waddling. Joint contractures may be present. Facial and ocular weakness almost never occur, which separates myositis from myasthenia gravis and some inherited myopathies. In IBM, more distal muscle involvement is seen. Weakness is usually bilateral and greater in the legs. In dermatomyositis, cutaneous manifestations can precede, follow, or develop together with muscle weakness. Cutaneous findings include Grotton's papules, a heliotropic rash on the upper eyelids, and rash on the neck (V sign), shoulders, and upper back (shawl sign) (4).

F. **Other.** The other illnesses mentioned in Table 12.10 have polymyalgia as a finding that is secondary to their underlying illness; however, myalgia may be the first symptom described.

References

1. Clauw DJ. Fibromyalgia. More than just a musculoskeletal disease. *Am Fam Physician* 1995;52:843–851.
2. Wolfe F, Smythe HA, Yunus MB, et al. The American College of Rheumatology 1990 criteria for the classification of fibromyalgia: report of the multicenter criteria committee. *Arthritis Rheum* 1990;33:160–172.
3. Meenan RF. *The evaluation of arthralgia.* American Academy of Family Physicians 46th Annual Scientific Assembly, 1994.
4. Olsen NJ, Wortmann RL. Inflammatory and metabolic diseases of muscle. In: Schumacher HR Jr, ed. *Primer on rheumatic diseases*, 11th ed. Atlanta: Arthritis Foundation, 1997.

12.9 Shoulder Pain

Gowri Anandarajah

Shoulder pain is the second most frequent orthopedic complaint seen in the primary care setting (1). The joint's complex anatomy, versatile range of motion, and central location make accurate diagnosis a challenge.

I. **Approach.** The major categories of shoulder pain are summarized in Table 12.11 (1).

II. **History**

    A. **Characteristics of the pain.** What is the onset, location, radiation, severity, and duration of the pain? Is there any instability, weakness, stiffness, or locking? Are there exacerbating or alleviating maneuvers? Has there been any associated trauma? What was the mechanism of injury? Any associated neurologic or systemic symptoms? Is there a history of prior shoulder problems? Are other joints involved?

III. **Physical examination.** Observe the shoulder for symmetry, motion, and signs of injury. Palpate all bony structures [including the acromioclavicular (AC) joint and bicipital groove]; check cervical spine range of motion (ROM) and the neurovascular status of the affected arm. If fracture is suspected, obtain an x-ray study. If finding on the x-ray is negative, proceed with passive and active ROM testing of the shoulder. Assess muscle strength and perform provocative tests for specific suspected pathology (Table 12.12) (1).

IV. **Testing**

    A. **Laboratory tests.** A complete blood count (CBC) and analysis of synovial or bursal aspirate for cell count, Gram's stain, and culture are obtained for suspected infectious arthritis or bursitis. Obtain an erythrocyte sedimentation rate (ESR), rheumatoid factor, antinuclear antibody, and aspirate for crystals for inflammatory arthritis.

    B. **Radiographic study.** Routine shoulder views are obtained for a history of acute trauma or chronic injury not responsive to conservative management. Special axillary or scapular Y views are needed if posterior dislocation is suspected. Views with and without weights may better assess for AC joint separation.

    C. **Diagnostic injection.** Anesthetic infiltration of the involved area may relieve symptoms and establish the diagnosis. Injection sites include the subacromial and intraarticular spaces, AC joint, and biceps tendon sheath (2).

    D. **Other imaging studies.** Computed tomography (CT) scan, magnetic resonance imaging (MRI), ultrasound, arthrography, fluoroscopy, and bone scan can be used when diagnosis is unclear or surgery is considered. MRI is superior for soft tissue pathology. Arthrography is useful for rotator cuff tears if MRI is unavailable or the patient is claustrophobic. A CT scan is useful to evaluate bony structures. Ultrasonography can identify moderate and full-

Table 12.11 Major causes of shoulder pain

Extrinsic	Intrinsic
Cervical spine disease	Non traumatic
Muscular sprains or strains	Inflammatory arthritis, infectious arthritis or bursitis, tumors
Thoracic outlet syndrome	
Diaphragmatic irritation (e.g., gallbladder disease)	Acute traumatic
	Fractures, contusions, shoulder (acromioclavicular or sternoclavicular) separation, glenohumeral instability, rotator cuff tears
Cardiac disease	
Intrathoracic disease (e.g., lung tumor)	
Dissecting aortic aneurysm	Chronic traumatic (due to repetitive injury)
Abdominal or pelvic pathology	
Systemic illness	Impingement syndrome (e.g., subacromial bursitis, tendinitis, rotator cuff injury), chronic glenohumeral instability, adhesive capsulitis or frozen shoulder

Table 12.12 Provocative tests in the evaluation of shoulder pain

Pathology	Maneuver	Technique/positive test response
AC pathology	Cross-chest adduction	Patient reaches across chest to touch opposite shoulder. Push down on elbow against patient's resistance./Pain in AC area
Biceps tendon pathology	Speed	Forward flex arm to 60° with thumb up. Apply downward force to distal forearm./Pain or weakness
	Yergeson	Flex elbow to 90° with thumb up. Have patient supinate arm and flex elbow against resistance./Pain or popping sensation
Glenohumeral instability	Anterior apprehension	Patient supine with shoulder in 90° of abduction. Apply slight anteriorly directed force to proximal humerus while externally rotating arm./Apprehension signs. Follow with relocation test.
	Relocation	Same position as above. Apply posteriorly directed force on proximal humerus while externally rotating shoulder./Decrease in apprehension signs
	Posterior apprehension	Patient supine. Forward flex shoulder to 90°, flex elbow to 90°, and internally rotate arm. Apply posterior force axially along the humerus./Apprehension signs or excessive movement of humeral head
	Sulcus sign	Arm in neutral. Pull down on wrist while observing infraacromial area for soft tissue dimpling./Greater degree of dimpling on affected side
Impingement syndrome	Neer	Internally rotate arm with elbow extended, then forward flex arm to 180°./Pain
	Hawkins	Place shoulder at 90° forward flexion and 45° to 90° internal rotation. Attempt to further internally rotate shoulder./Pain
Rotator cuff tear	Drop arm	Lower fully abducted arm slowly./Arm will suddenly drop at approximately 90° of abduction.
Thoracic outlet syndrome	Adson	Patient stands with arms at sides. Record radial pulse and then, while still palpating pulse, extend and externally rotate arm. Have patient hold a deep breath and turn the head toward the affected side./Decreased pulse or reproduction of symptoms.
Cervical root irritation	Spurling	Seat patient. Extend and rotate neck toward affected side and apply downward pressure to superior aspect of head./Reproduction of symptoms

AC, acromioclavicular.

thickness tears, but accuracy is operator-dependent. Bone scan can identify areas of bone remodeling (e.g., metastatic tumors, nonunion of fractures). Fluoroscopy allows dynamic assessment of fracture stability and can detect loose bodies or impingement (1).

V. Diagnostic assessment (3,4)

A. Nonshoulder origin. Painless ROM without localized tenderness suggests referred pain. Muscular sprain or strain presents with pain on active, but not passive, ROM and muscle tenderness or spasm; cervical disc herniation with radicular symptoms, neurologic findings, and an abnormal CT or MRI scan. Thoracic outlet symptoms include pain and numbness in the shoulder or arm (especially with head turning) and a positive Adson test.

B. Shoulder origin, nontraumatic. Both inflammatory and infectious arthritis may present with a joint effusion and inflammatory signs on examination. Serologic testing may be positive in the former; joint aspirate analysis and culture will help differentiate the two. An x-ray study or bone scan can help to rule out osteomyelitis. Tumor presents with localized pain and a positive imaging study.

C. Shoulder origin, acute traumatic

1. Fractures and contusions have point tenderness on examination. An associated pneumothorax should be ruled out with a clavicular fracture. Scapular fractures are infrequent, and usually occur with other severe thoracic injury. Contusions present with point tenderness on examination, but have no evidence of ligament injury and an x-ray study is negative.

2. Shoulder separation is more common at the AC joint. An AC dislocation may occur secondary to a fall on an outstretched hand or the lateral shoulder. Pain and swelling are seen at the joint, and a crossover test is positive. An x-ray study can be negative. Sternoclavicular separation is usually associated with other severe injuries.

3. Glenohumeral instability can develop with trauma. In anterior dislocation, the patient uses the other hand to hold the injured arm in abduction and external rotation. Visually, the acromion will be prominent. In the less-common posterior dislocation, the arm is held across the chest. Only an axillary or scapular x-ray view may show the displaced head.

D. Shoulder origin, chronic traumatic

1. An AC joint sprain is usually caused by overuse, degenerative joint disease, or incorrect weightlifting. On examination, tenderness is found over the AC joint.

2. Chronic glenohumeral instability occurs when recurrent trauma causes small labral or capsular tears. The patient presents with chronic or subacute pain and may report that the shoulder "pops" in and out. On examination, mild instability signs may be seen (Table 12.12).

3. Impingement syndrome is a common cause of shoulder pain.

   a. Rotator cuff tendinitis most often involves the supraspinatus tendon and is secondary to overuse of the joint. It presents with diffuse pain in the anterior or lateral shoulder. The patient cannot sleep on the affected side. The shoulder is tender in the upper deltoid region or below the acromion. Seen are decreased ROM and pain, especially between 70° and 120° abduction; impingement signs are positive. The x-ray study is normal or shows calcific tendinitis or a prominent acromial spur.

   b. Subacromial bursitis is usually secondary to tendinitis and presents with the same findings. Inflammatory, infectious, or crystalline causes may need to be ruled out by joint fluid aspiration.

   c. A rotator cuff tear develops with overuse or trauma in the presence of an underlying abnormality. On examination, supraspinatus weakness and positive impingement signs may be seen.

   d. Bicipital tendinitis is another overuse injury. Pain in the anterior shoulder radiates to the biceps and forearm. Examination findings include limited abduction, positive impingement signs, biceps tendon tenderness, and pain on resisted elbow flexion or wrist supination.

4. Adhesive capsulitis presents with chronic pain and stiffness, often following a period of prolonged immobility. It is especially common in elders. Decreased active *and* passive ROM occurs in all planes.

References

1. Howard TM, O'Connor FG. The injured shoulder: primary care assessment. *Arch Fam Med* 1997;6:376–384.
2. Larson HM, O'Connor FG, Nirschl RP. Shoulder pain: the role of diagnostic injections. *Am Fam Phys* 1996;53:1637–1643.
3. Glockner SM. Shoulder pain: a diagnostic dilemma. *Am Fam Phys* 1995;51:1677–1687.
4. Diagneault J, Cooney LM. Shoulder pain in older people. *J Am Geriatr Soc* 1998;46: 1144–1151.

13. DERMATOLOGIC PROBLEMS

MICHAEL L. O'DELL

13.1 Alopecia

Cynthia M. Moore-Sledge

Alopecia, or hair loss, is a common disorder that occurs in all age groups. Aplasia cutis and congenital triangular alopecia occur in infancy. Alopecia areata typically occurs in adolescents and young adults. Androgenic alopecia (triangular frontal recession) occurs in middle-aged men and women (1). Postmenopausal alopecia occurs in elderly patients. Of the numerous causes of alopecia, 90% of cases result from androgenic alopecia or chronic telogen effluvium. Because self-esteem and identity are linked to physical appearance, the evaluation of alopecia should be approached by the physician with thoughtfulness and concern.

I. **Approach.** Based on the pattern of hair loss, alopecia is categorized as generalized or localized. Based on scalp changes, alopecia can also be categorized as scarring or nonscarring.
   A. **Generalized alopecia** causes include acute anagen and telogen effluvium, chronic telogen effluvium, loose anagen syndrome, and postpartum alopecia. It can also be radiotherapy-induced, cytotoxin-induced (chemotherapy, heavy metals), drug-induced (analgesics, anticoagulants, antiepileptics, central nervous system drugs, psychotropics, cardiovascular drugs, and oral contraceptives), and can result from use of immunosuppressants. Syphilis causes diffuse, patchy alopecia.
   B. **Localized alopecia** causes include androgenic alopecia of the male variety, alopecia areata, trichotillomania (hair pulling), traction alopecia, discoid lupus, hirsutism, lichen planopilaris, pseudopelade, tinea capitis, sarcoidosis, follicular mucinosis, human immunodeficiency virus (HIV), metastatic adenocarcinoma, sclerosing basal cell carcinoma, bacterial infection, burns, herpes zoster, squamous cell carcinoma, and aplasia cutis.
   C. **Scarring alopecia** causes include discoid lupus erythematosus, scleroderma, lichen planopilaris, aplasia cutis congenita, dissecting cellulitis, kerion, metastatic carcinoma, lymphoma, sarcoidosis, prolonged pressure, and cicatricial pemphigus.
II. **History.** Important questions to ask: What are the patient's normal grooming habits? When was hair loss initially noted? Was hair loss gradual or abrupt in onset? Is the pattern of hair loss localized or generalized? Are there other family members with a similar pattern of hair loss? Has there been recent psychological or physical stress? Was there exposure to radiation therapy, cytotoxic chemotherapy, or chemicals, including heavy metals?
   A. Androgenic alopecia and chronic telogen effluvium are insidious in onset. Alopecia caused by radiation therapy, cytotoxic chemicals, heavy metals, or severe stress occurs almost immediately.
   B. Androgenic alopecia can be localized (male pattern) or diffuse (female pattern). Diffuse hair loss is common in postpartum, radiation therapy- or chemotherapy-induced alopecia and in telogen anagen effluvium and loose anagen syndrome.
      Patchy hair loss occurs with bacterial and fungal infections, discoid lupus, alopecia areata, trichotillomania, HIV, and traction alopecia.
   C. Androgenic alopecia and alopecia areata have a familial predisposition.
   D. Hair loss can be related to stressors such as childbirth or severe illness.
   E. Chemotherapy and radiation therapy induce the rapid development of alopecia.
   F. Excessive brushing or shampooing can cause hair loss. Damage to both the hair and scalp can result from the use of chemicals, tight braids, thermal heat, or rubber bands (2,3).

III. Physical examination. Carefully assess the scalp, hair on all body parts, and other body areas for rashes or signs of virilization. Signs of virilization include acne, hypertrichosis, clitoromegaly, frontotemporal balding, and deepening of the voice. Discoid lupus presents as scarred, patchy alopecia of the scalp and can cause loss of facial hair. Trichotillomania can involve the eyebrows and eyelashes. Frontotemporal balding is common in male pattern androgenic alopecia, whereas diffuse hair loss occurs in the female variety; both are associated with normal skin on the scalp. Tinea capitis and psoriatic alopecia should be considered with scalp flaking. "Moth eaten" areas on the scalp suggest sarcoidosis, syphilis, or discoid lupus.

The texture, length, or thickness of individual hairs may suggest the cause of alopecia. Shorter, fine hairs may be found in areas of thinning in androgenic alopecia. Trichotillomania and tinea capitis result in short broken hairs. "Black dots" occur in the lesions of tinea capitis, whereas "exclamation point" hairs occur with alopecia areata (4). Long eyelashes and straightening of scalp hair suggest infection with HIV.

Hair in loose anagen syndrome is easily removed with gentle pulling. The hair in traction alopecia and trichotillomania is firmly rooted in the scalp.

Both lichen planopilaris and discoid lupus may have associated lesions on other parts of the body, a finding that may be useful in diagnosis.

IV. Testing

  A. Laboratory tests should be based on clinical findings. Androgenic alopecia, with normal skin on the scalp of male patients, requires no further evaluation.

   1. Female patients with diffuse hair loss should be evaluated with complete blood count, serum ferritin, and thyroid stimulating hormone to rule out infection, iron deficiency anemia, and thyroid abnormality. Screening tests for ovarian, adrenal, and pituitary or hypothalamic disorders include dehydroepiandrosterone sulfate, total testosterone, testosterone-estradiol binding globulin, and prolactin.

   2. Tests ordered in patients with virilization are 17-hydroxyprogesterone, luteinizing hormone, follicle-stimulating hormone, and ovarian ultrasound.

   3. Repeat testosterone, corticotropin stimulation tests, computed tomography of the adrenals, urinary free cortisol, dexamethasone suppression tests, adrenal or ovarian vein catheterization, and surgical exploration may be indicated if screening tests are abnormal.

   4. Patient with scarred, "moth eaten" scalp lesions should have antinuclear antibodies and syphilis serology checked to rule out systemic lupus and syphilis.

   5. Patients with flaking of the scalp should have potassium hydroxide examination of scalp scrapings and hair for fungal elements. Scalp scrapings or scalp hairs can be cultured for fungus or bacteria.

   6. Bacterial cultures of any drainage should be obtained.

   7. The gentle hair pull test is done to assess pluckability. Fewer than four hairs should be obtained per pull. Large numbers of hairs are easily plucked in loose anagen syndrome.

   8. The forcible hair pluck test and trichogram assess the stages (anagen, catagen or telogen) of hairs obtained by forceful pulling of hairs with rubber-tipped forceps. These tests are best performed by the dermatologist. If a biopsy is to be done, these tests are not necessary.

  B. Scalp biopsy taken with a 4-mm punch of the active area of a lesion is useful in establishing a diagnosis when the findings are equivocal; in diagnosing scarring alopecias (discoid lupus, sarcoid, lichen planopilaris, pseudopelade) or infiltrating alopecias (scleroderma, metastatic adenocarcinoma); and in distinguishing alopecias that can be similar in appearance (lichen planopilaris, pseudopelade, discoid lupus, or scleroderma). Hair samples are studied to assess follicular structure and number, the stages of the sampled hair and its structure and number. The tissue can be studied using direct immunofluorescence for evidence of an autoimmune or infectious cause (2,3).

V. Diagnostic assessment. Most cases of alopecia are caused by androgenic alopecia and chronic telogen effluvium. Early diagnosis and intervention can be critical in the remaining cases, if caused by metastatic adenocarcinoma, squamous cell carcinoma, melanoma, HIV, syphilis, systemic lupus, adrenal carcinoma, or a thyroid disorder. Permanent hair loss may be prevented by early institution of therapy when alopecia is caused by fungal infection or an infiltrative, scarring processes. If the offending agent is a drug (e.g., oral contraceptives, beta-blockers, antidepressants, or neuroleptics), hair loss can be reversible if the drug is stopped early in the process.

References
1. Van Neste DJ, Rushton DH. Hair problems in women. *Clin Dermatol* 1997;15: 113–125.
2. Habif TP. *Clinical dermatology: a color guide to diagnosis and therapy*, 3rd ed. St. Louis: Mosby-Yearbook, 1996.
3. Sullivan JR, Kossard S. Acquired scalp alopecia. Part I: A review. *Aust J Dermatol* 1998;38:2207–2221.
4. Nielsen TA, Reichel M. Alopecia: diagnosis and management. *Am Fam Physician* 1995;51(6):1513–1522.

13.2 Erythema Multiforme

Melissa B. Black

I. Approach. Erythema multiforme (EM) is a clinical syndrome, not a diagnosis. It is thought to be a hypersensitivity reaction to an antigenic stimulus, commonly a drug or infection. It occurs in males more often than in females; and 50% of cases occur in those aged less than 20 years, with most of the remaining cases occurring in those aged 20 to 30 years (1). The spectrum of symptoms allow categorization into:

　　A. EM minor— an eruption usually with little to no mucous membrane involvement or systemic symptoms and causing little or no complications.

　　B. EM major
　　　　1. Stevens–Johnson syndrome presents with bullae or vesicles with more systemic symptoms. Significant complications, including keratitis and visual impairment or damage to upper airways, can occur with this syndrome.
　　　　2. Toxic epidermal necrolysis (TEN) is a life-threatening condition with widespread cutaneous damage with a prognosis similar to that of a second degree burn. Death can occur in up to 50% of cases (2).

II. History
　　A. Were there any prodromal symptoms?
　　　　1. Prodromal symptoms occur in one-third of cases, usually in the form of an upper respiratory illness (3).
　　　　2. A prodrome is unusual in EM minor, but fever, malaise, and myalgias can precede the more severe varieties (Chapters 2.6 and 13.6).
　　B. Characteristics of the rash
　　　　1. What was the time course of onset and the duration of lesions?
　　　　　　a. An acute onset with enlargement of papules over 24 to 48 hours is typical of EM. New lesions can develop over 10 days or more with a usual duration of 1 to 6 weeks from onset to healing (3). Be aware of late onset lesions as they may also be a recurrence.
　　　　2. Where are the lesions?
　　　　　　a. EM lesions usually start on the hands and feet, including palms and soles, and can spread proximally to become generalized.

      b. The mouth and lips are involved up to 99% of the time. More extensive mucosal involvement is seen in the more severe cases. Mouth lesions are usually tender.

      c. The rash is symmetric.

  3. Skin symptoms

      a. Are the lesions painful or pruritic? Oral lesions are usually tender. The patient may complain of itching, swelling, and tenderness of the hands and feet.

C. Recent exposures

  1. Has the patient been exposed to any drugs 1 to 3 weeks prior to onset (4)? These most often include sulfonamides, penicillin, anticonvulsants, and nonsteroidal antiinflammatory drugs. Drugs often lead to extensive mucosal erosions with large bullae.

  2. Has the patient recently been ill?

      a. The percent of EM cases precipitated by herpes simplex virus (HSV) is likely greater than 50% (3). HSV usually presents as EM minor, and it is recurrent in one-third of cases.

      b. Another well-documented factor is infection with mycoplasma pneumonia (2). In this case, EM generally presents in bullous form or as Stevens–Johnson syndrome (Chapter 13.8).

      c. Other bacterial and viral causes have been suggested, including tuberculosis (TB), β-hemolytic streptococci, staphylococcal infections, and the bacillus Calmette-Guérin vaccine.

      d. Other factors such as radiation therapy, collagen vascular diseases, pregnancy, and carcinomas have been implicated.

III. Physical examination

A. Description of lesions

  1. The rash begins as a round erythematous papule, which enlarges up to 1 to 2 cm over 24 to 48 hours. The periphery of the lesion is erythematous and raised or edematous. The center becomes more cyanotic looking and can be white/yellow or gray. This is the pathognomonic "target lesion," but it may not be present in all cases. If a blister forms in the middle, the term "iris lesion" is more appropriate.

  2. Lesions are generally symmetrical, with acral to central spread including extensor surfaces, face, palms, and soles. Mucosal lesions indicate a more severe type; bullae with sloughing in large sheets suggests TEN.

B. Systemic signs

  1. Systemic signs are present in the more serious Stevens–Johnson syndrome and TEN.

  2. Systemic signs include high fever, involvement of eyes with corneal ulceration, pulmonary findings, widespread cutaneous involvement, or pneumonia, indicating higher morbidity and mortality.

IV. Testing

A. Biopsy. The history and physical examination will be most helpful in making the diagnosis; however, biopsy of an early lesion helps to confirm it and exclude others. The differential diagnosis would include urticaria, vasculitis, fixed drug eruptions, and bullous pemphigoid.

B. Other tests. If underlying infection is suspected, laboratory tests including a complete blood count, throat culture, antistreptolysin-O titer, slide test for infectious mononucleosis, and hepatitis screen may be indicated. A chest x-ray study may be needed if *Mycoplasma pneumoniae*, histoplasmosis, coccidiomycosis, or TB is suspected. Skin tests or serum complement fixation titers for infectious agents may be needed.

V. Diagnostic assessment

A. If the history and physical examination are consistent with the diagnosis of EM, a symmetric, fixed, discrete, round, erythematous rash is seen, which lasts 1 to 6 weeks from onset to healing, which is self-limited, acute, or episodic in nature. If biopsy supports the diagnosis, then the clinical criteria for EM have been met.

B. Cause. Then, determine the most likely cause in order to remove the antigenic stimulus, whether this means stopping a drug, treating an infection, or invoking preventative measures such as avoiding a drug or providing prophylaxis for recurrent HSV.

C. Determining which subtype of EM is present helps dictate treatment and anticipate prognosis.

References

1. Fitzpatrick TB, Johnson RA, Polano MK, Suurmond D, Wolff K. *Color atlas and synopsis of clinical dermatology*, 2nd ed. New York: McGraw-Hill, 1992:474–477.
2. Goldberg GN. Erythema multiforme controversies and recent advances. *Adv Dermatol* 1987;2:73–90.
3. Huff JC. Erythema multiforme. In: Sams WM, Lynch PJ, eds. *Principles and practice of dermatology*, 2nd ed. New York: Churchill Livingstone, 1996:483–490.
4. Stampien TM, Schwartz RA. Erythema multiforme. *Am Fam Physician* 1992;46(4): 1171–1176.

13.3 Maculopapular Rash

Michael L. O'Dell

I. **Approach.** Rashes are commonly described in a defined set of ways. Macules are skin lesions that are flat and discolored, and up to 1 cm in diameter. Papules are also up to 1 cm, but they are elevated, solid, and well circumscribed. Often, a patient presents with a rash that is a mixture of these two elements, hence the term "maculopapular." The term maculopapular is subject to disagreement among various diagnosticians (1).

A. **Maculopapular rashes** can be accompanied by fever, in which case they are generally associated with an infection, particularly a viral infection (Chapter 13.6). Rashes not accompanied by fever often result from allergic reactions, but infection remains common. Rarely, a maculopapular rash is a systemic sign of an underlying malignancy. Table 13.1 contains a partial listing of common causes of maculopapular rash.

B. **Serious infectious illnesses,** such as meningococcemia, disseminated gonorrhea, and Rocky Mountain spotted fever (RMSF) can present with acute onset of maculopapular rash and fever, often prior to more classic signs (2). The early wheal and flare response of anaphylaxis occasionally presents early in the course with a maculopapular rash, often with palmar or pharygeal itching.

II. **History**

A. **Seek a history of preceding illness, concurrent fever, or ingestion of medications**. A travel history and exposure history are useful.

B. **Have the lesions spread?** Are they painful, itching, or simply bothersome cosmetically? Have any been on the palms or soles?

C. **Are other signs present?** Joint swelling can indicate gonococcemia. Headache and confusion can indicate meningococcemia. Difficult breathing can indicate impending collapse from anaphylaxis.

III. **Physical examination**

A. **Carefully examine the lesions and their distribution.**

1. A rash that is on the face and spreading to the trunk is characteristic of measles or rubella. Many viral illnesses have a predilection for the trunk.

2. A maculopapular rash occurring on the palms initially should prompt concern about syphilis. RMSF rash also occurs on the palms; usually, however, this rash is not raised until 3 or so days into the course of illness and it is accompanied by purpura on the ankles and wrists. Disseminated gonorrhea lesions are usually on the fingers and quickly become pustular.

Table 13.1 Common causes of a maculopapular rash

Underlying cause of rash	Viral	Bacterial and other treatable infectious causes	Allergic and drug-induced	Other
Common examples	Measles Rubella Echovirus Enterovirus Primary human immuno-deficiency virus-1 Dengue fever Adenovirus Epstein-Barr virus infection	Meningo-coccemia Gonococcemia Secondary syphilis Rickettsial diseases (Rocky Mountain spotted fever and others) Lyme disease Mycoplasma	Urticarial reactions Drug-induced reactions Radiocontrast-induced reactions	Myelogenous leukemia Graft-versus-host reactions Still's disease Erythema multi-forme Systemic lupus erythematosus Dermatomyo-sitis

Meningococcemia can spread widely, but can present as a macule with central petechiae, which progressively becomes nodular.

B. Conduct a general physical examination. Areas of particular concern are:

  1. Head, eyes, ears, nose, and throat. Although measles is becoming rare, the presence of Koplik's spots is pathognomic for the illness. A common location for ticks is in the scalp hair, and the discovery of a tick lends support to the diagnosis of RMSF. Rarely, meningococcemia will be a complication of sinusitis, and often it develops following complaints of pharyngitis. Mucous membrane swelling may indicate early anaphylaxis.
  2. Lung examination. Wheezing on examination, especially in a patient who has recently received medications or contrast dye, can indicate anaphylaxis.
  3. Genital examination. Purulent urethral drainage or evidence of pelvic inflammatory disease supports consideration of gonorrhea (Chapter 10.9). A chancre would support a diagnosis of syphilis, although palmar lesions often occur well after healing of the initial chancre.
  4. Joint examination. Evidence of joint swelling supports a diagnosis of meningococcemia or gonococcemia. A maculopapular rash may be seen in juvenile rheumatoid arthritis as well.
  5. Neurologic examination. Evidence of meningitis supports a diagnosis of meningococcemia. Patients with RMSF may also have meningeal signs.

IV. Testing. Tests are generally selected according to the most likely cause of the rash, with a complete blood count (CBC) being the most commonly ordered test.

A. A CBC is often useful. Increased neutrophils may indicate a bacterial infection; especially when immature neutrophils are present. The CBC is not a sensitive indicator for these infections, however. A relatively normal white blood count does not exclude serious infections (3). Lymphocytosis may indicate a viral infection. Increased eosinophils are occasionally seen with allergic reactions. Myelogenous leukemias generally present with abnormalities on CBC.

B. Other testing should be performed on the basis of the most likely causes of the rash.

  1. Consider syphilis testing in all cases, especially in those patients with palmar rashes.

2. Consider a smear and culture of any pustules, especially if meningococcemia or gonococcemia is suspected.
3. Cerebrospinal fluid examination is useful if meningococcemia is suspected; it is usually negative in RMSF, despite headache, back stiffness, and other signs.

V. **Diagnostic assessment.** Although no one key is seen to diagnosing a maculopapular rash, history is the most important key (4). The presence or absence of a fever aids in narrowing the diagnostic field to infectious versus noninfectious causes. The age of the patient aids in determining whether the rash is likely the result of a common viral childhood illness versus an illness more often associated with adults (e.g., syphilis). The exposure history helps in ruling in or out diseases common in selected geographic areas (e.g., RMSF on the United States east coast or dengue fever in Central America). Nevertheless, a careful and thorough physical examination is required as well as judicious use of laboratory testing.

References

1. Schwarzenberger K. The essentials of the complete skin examination. *Med Clin North Am* 1998;82(5):981–999.
2. Granier S. Recognizing meningococcal disease in primary care: qualitative study of how general practitioners process clinical and contextual information. *BMJ* 1998; 316(7127):276–279.
3. Kuppermann N. Clinical and hematological features do not reliably identify children with unsuspected meningococcal disease. *Pediatrics* 1999;103(2):E20.
4. Schlossberg D. Fever and rash. *Infect Dis Clin North Am* 1996;10(1):101–110.

13.4 Pigmentation Disorders

Michael L. O'Dell

Patients often present complaining of lighter or darker patches of skin. These complaints represent a range of minor to quite serious illnesses.

I. **Approach.** Classify the complaint into a hyperpigmentation disorder or a hypopigmentation disorder (1).
   A. **Disorders of hyperpigmentation** include pityriasis versicolor, *café au lait* macule, melasma, acanthosis nigricans, Becker's melanosis, drug eruptions, and postinflammatory hyperpigmentation.
   B. **Disorders of hypopigmentation** include vitiligo, pityriasis alba, ash leaf macules, and postinflammatory hypopigmentation.

II. **History**
   A. **Onset**
      1. Hyperpigmented lesions. An upper back or chest rash following exposure to a humid and warm climate is typical for young adults with pityriasis versicolor. *Café au lait* macules are present at birth and regress with time. Melasma occurs in women with pregnancy, institution of oral contraceptives, liver dysfunction, or phenytoin use. *Acanthosis nigricans* becomes noticeable with weight gain. Becker's melanosis occurs after severe sun exposure in teenagers and young adults. Drug-induced hyperpigmentation is associated with many drugs, especially minocycline and zidovudine. Fixed hyperpigmenting drug reactions are common with exposures to phenolphthalein, barbiturates, phenacetin, salicylates, tetracyclines, and sulfonamides. Inflammation of the skin caused by nearly any agent can result in hyperpigmentation.
      2. Hypopigmented lesions. Vitiligo, which generally starts between ages 10 and 30 years, can be associated with stress, illness, and personal crises.

Pityriasis alba occurs in young children and is generally associated with eczema. Ash leaf macules, which are rare, are found in patients with tuberous sclerosis. Inflamed skin can depigment following inflammation.

B. Duration. Most pigment disorders are generally long-lasting.

C. Exacerbating factors

  1. Hyperpigmented disorders. Pityriasis versicolor worsens with continued exposure to heat and humidity and with malnutrition. Melasma worsens with pregnancy and continued exposure to medications or deterioration of liver function. *Acanthosis nigricans* worsens with weight gain and can increase with the use of insulin, nicotinic acid, glucocorticoids, or estrogens. Drug-induced hyperpigmentation and eruptions worsen with each exposure to the offending agent. With continued inflammation, postinflammatory hyperpigmentation worsens.

  2. Hypopigmented disorders. Vitiligo can worsen with stress, illness, and personal crises, and with skin trauma. Pityriasis alba can worsen from use of drying agents (e.g., soap) or by sunlight.

D. Relieving factors

  1. Hyperpigmented disorders. *Café au lait* macules regress with age. Melasma can improve, but rarely vanishes, after delivery or removal of the offending agent. *Acanthosis nigricans* improves with weight loss and removal of offending medications. Fixed drug reactions can fade after removal of the agent, but often remain. Minocycline-induced hyperpigmentation is often permanent. Inflammatory changes often fade slowly over several months.

  2. Hypopigmented disorders. Vitiligo rarely spontaneously repigments and it is generally progressive. Pityriasis alba improves with age and moisturizing of the affected skin.

E. Associated symptoms

  1. Hyperpigmented disorders. Pityriasis versicolor is often itchy. *Café au lait* spots can be a marker for neurofibromatosis with associated neurologic symptoms, especially if six or more of the macules are present. Melasma *per se*, is asymptomatic, as is *acanthosis nigricans. Acanthosis nigricans* is often associated with diabetes and may even be a marker for diabetes (2). It can be associated with underlying malignancy as well. Becker's melanosis may be slightly itchy. Fixed drug reactions can be painful or itchy. Other drug-induced hyperpigmentation is usually asymptomatic. On resolution of inflammation, postinflammatory lesions are usually asymptomatic.

  2. Hypopigmented disorders. The lesions of vitiligo are usually asymptomatic, but depression is commonly associated with vitiligo (3). Lesions of pityriasis alba can be slightly itchy or burning. Ash leaf macules are often associated with tuberous sclerosis and its associated neurologic symptoms.

III. Physical examination

A. Hyperpigmented disorders, lesion description. Pityriasis versicolor begins as a reddish macule, generally on the upper back, appearing darker than surrounding skin during winter and lighter than tanned skin during summer. *Café au lait* macules are 0.2 to 10 cm, uniform, well demarcated, brown areas found on sun-protected sites of the trunk and extremities. Melasma generally is most prominent on the malar eminence and other sun-exposed areas. *Acanthosis nigricans* is thickened plaques in a symmetric pattern in the axillae, neck, groin, and folds of the breast and groin. *Acanthosis nigricans* neck lesions often appear as dirty or unwashed skin. Mecke's melanosis is a hyperpigmented macule of varied size, generally solitary and with thick and darkened hair. Acneiform eruptions are often present in the center of the lesion. Minocycline-induced hyperpigmentation can occur in old scars, on the lower extremities and forearms, or diffusely in sun-exposed areas. Fixed drug eruptions occur in the same place with each exposure; initially, they can be vesicobullous, and then resolve as a hyperpigmented patch.

Postinflammatory hyperpigmentation is generally light brown to black discoloration in an area of previous inflammation.
B. **Hypopigmented disorders, lesion description.** Vitiligo appears as depigmented macules with scalloped edges, initially generally on the face, hands, wrists, axillae, umbilicus, and genitalia. The macules often coalesce with time into larger areas of depigmentation. Pityriasis alba appears as a small macule, failing to tan, that is pale pink to light brown with irregular borders on the midforehead, malar ridge, periorbital area, or perioral area. Ash leaf macules are hypopigmented lesions appearing with one end rounded and the other pointed (*lance ovate*) resembling an ash tree leaf. They can occur in normal children; if accompanied by acnelike lesions, however, they are particularly suspicious, as markers for tuberous sclerosis.
C. **Ophthalmologic examination** is important for patients with vitiligo, as pigmentation abnormalities of the choroid and retina can lead to poor visual acuity or blindness.
D. **Lung examination of children** with pityriasis alba is useful, because atopy and asthma often coexist.
E. **A complete physical examination**, searching for underlying malignancy is necessary in patients with rapid onset of *acanthosis nigricans*, especially if it occurs without weight loss or in the absence of diabetes.
F. **Neurologic examination** is necessary in persons with *café au lait* macules or ash leaf spots.

IV. **Testing**
A. **Hyperpigmented disorders.** Skin scraping of pityriasis versicolor may reveal the characteristic "spaghetti and meatballs" appearance of *Malassezia furfur*, the causative organism. Wood's light illumination often reveals a yellow-gold luminescence. More than six *café au lait* macules should prompt an evaluation for neurofibromatosis (1). Evaluate the patient with unexplained *acanthosis nigricans* for possible diabetes or underlying tumor, especially gastrointestinal adenocarcinomas.
B. **Hypopigmented disorders.** Vitiligo can be associated with diabetes, adrenal insufficiency, or pernicious anemia, and patients with signs of these illnesses should be evaluated appropriately. Have patients with ash leaf macules screened for tuberous sclerosis.

V. **Diagnostic assessment.** Patients with pigmentary disorders are best initially classified into disorders of excessive pigmentation or hypopigmentation. History is useful in eliciting inciting factors, especially drug-induced or inflammation-induced changes. Characteristic appearances of the lesions further define the illness. Biopsy of lesions is generally not necessary, although selected lesions may require further testing for underlying diseases.

References

1. Kim NY, Pandya AG. Pigmentary diseases. *Med Clin North Am* 1998;82(5): 1185–1207.
2. Stuart CA. Ananthosis nigricans as a risk factor for non-insulin dependent diabetes mellitus. *Clin Pediatr* 1998;37(2):73–79.
3. Agarwal G. Vitiligo: an under-estimated problem. *Fam Pract* 1998;15(Suppl):S19–S23.

13.5 Pruritus

Beverly A. VonderPool

I. **Approach.** Pruritus, a sense of the need to scratch, is an unpleasant cutaneous sensation that has numerous causes. A practical approach is to look for causes with the highest probability first; generally, pruritus is caused by a primary skin disorder instead of a systemic disorder. The itching can be localized or generalized, mild or sufficiently severe to impair sleep. Pruritus can be classified as primary (nonspecific or specific) or secondary to a systemic disease. The main disorders include (1):

A. **Primary skin disorders with nonspecific or inconspicuous eruption** include aquagenic pruritus, atopic dermatitis, bullous pemphigoid, contact dermatitis, dermatitis herpetiformis, fiberglass dermatitis, insect bites, miliaria (prickly heat), pediculosis (lice), scabies, urticaria (hives), and xerosis (dry skin).

B. **Primary skin disorders with specific or apparent eruptions** include drug reactions, folliculitis, fungal infections, lichen planus, lichen simplex chronicus, mycosis fungoides, pemphigus foliaceus, pityriasis rosea, pruritic urticarial papules and plaques of pregnancy, psoriasis, and sunburn.

C. **Pruritus associated with systemic disease** includes acquired immune deficiency syndrome (AIDS), biliary disease caused by drugs, pregnancy or cirrhosis, chronic renal failure, hyperthyroid disease, lymphoreticular disorders (Hodgkin's and non-Hodgkin's lymphoma), psychiatric disease, and visceral malignancy.

D. **Most common causes and concerns.** Xerosis (dry skin) is the most common cause of generalized pruritus in both the young and the old (2,3). Chronic renal failure is the systemic disorder most commonly associated with secondary pruritus. Although malignancy is of concern in the patient with chronic pruritus, associated malignancy occurs in less than 1% of patients referred to a dermatologist (1,4).

II. **History.** The history frequently suggests whether the pruritus is primary or secondary, and often provides clues to its cause. In taking the history, ascertain the location and duration of the pruritus, exacerbating and alleviating factors, and the patient's medications, occupation, travel, bathing habits, and family history of atopy or cancer. Also ask about possible pregnancy, diabetes mellitus, chronic renal failure, or hepatic disorders. Onset or worsening of the itching in winter would suggest xerosis. The presence of itching in family members or a household pet raises concern that the cause is an infection from a scabies or a nonscabies mite. Pruritus during or after bathing is characteristic of aquatic pruritus. Exposure to chemicals, new soaps, or detergents could cause allergic or irritant dermatitis. The review of systems often reveals other medical disorders that can be associated with pruritus (section **I.C.**).

III. **Physical examination** The physical examination includes a thorough examination of the skin in adequate lighting. Direct special attention to skin areas not easily observed or reached by the patient. Such areas may reveal a primary skin disorder or evidence of a systemic disease because some disorders present in particular areas. For example, scabies involves the interdigital webs, volar wrists, and genitalia, whereas atopic dermatitis occurs in the antecubital or popliteal fossae. Pityriasis rosea typically has a "herald patch" on the trunk. Fungal infections tend to occur in warm, dark, moist body surfaces (e.g., genitalia, feet, and inguinal folds).

Be able to recognize the classic signs of common skin disorders. Dematographism and wheals typically indicate uticaria (hives) (Chapter 13.7). Flat-topped polygonal papules with delicate white lines ("Wickham's straiae") are characteristic of lichen planus. Silver plaques on an erythematous base with a positive Auspitz sign (punctuate bleeding of the scale after blunt scraping) are characteristic of psoriasis. The application of lateral pressure on superficial, crusting lesions resulting in dislodging the epidermis, referred to as Nikolsky's sign, indicates pemphigus foliaceus. The differential diagnosis of lymphadenopathy includes mycosis fungoides (Chapter 15.1). Pustular or lesions over hair follicles is a sign of folliculitis. Pay attention to new unscratched lesions because chronically excoriated skin from any cause has similar secondary changes. If lesions are present in unreachable areas, a systemic disease should be considered. In addition to the skin, examine other organ systems for organomegaly, lymphadenopathy, goiter, pregnancy, and signs of anemia or psychiatric disorders.

IV. Diagnostic tests. If the history and physical examination do not reveal the diagnosis, certain tests can be helpful. For primary skin disorders the testing should include a wet preparation, the addition of potassium hydroxide (KOH), microscopic examination of scrapings, and as a last resort, skin biopsy. If a systemic disorder is suspected, include the following in the evaluation: a complete blood count with differential; tests for liver, renal, and thyroid function; stool for occult blood; human immunodeficiency (HIV) screen; serologic test for syphilis; and a chest radiograph. If the history and physical examination suggest other systemic diagnoses, additional recommended tests to consider include urinalysis, serum iron studies, stool for ova and parasites, serum glucose, and serum electrophoresis.

V. Diagnostic assessment. The diagnostic approach should initially be limited to the history and physical examination because most patients have a primary skin disorder (section **I.A., I.B.**). If the diagnosis is still unclear, 2 weeks of empirical treatment for the most common cause of pruritus (xerosis) is recommended. This includes less-frequent baths, use of lukewarm water and a mild soap, "pat" drying after a bath, immediate application of a lubricant, and avoidance of irritating fabrics (e.g., wool) (5). Further diagnostic tests for systemic disorder can be considered to rule out the more obscure diagnoses listed above. Because malignancy can present several years after pruritus, follow-up is important. Sometimes, no cause is found. Remember, a diagnosis of psychogenic pruritis is a diagnosis of exclusion. The relationship between the psyche and organic disease is unclear. Depression, anxiety, and other psychiatric disorders can be secondary instead of the primary illness. It is important to follow up with appropriate psychiatric or dermatologic consultation as needed.

References

1. Greco PJ, Ende J. Pruritus: a practical approach. *J Gen Intern Med* 1992;7:172–181.
2. Leshaw SM. Itching in active patients. *Phy and Sports Med* 1998;26(1):47–53.
3. Beacham BE. Common dermatoses in the elderly. *Am Fam Physician* 1993;47(6): 1445–1450.
4. Lober CW. Should the patient with generalized pruritus be evaluated for malignancy? [Editorial]. *J Am Acad Dermatol* 1988;2(Part 1):350–352.
5. Phillips WG. Pruritus. What to do when the itching won't stop. *Postgrad Med* 1992; 92(7):34–53.

13.6 Rash Accompanied by Fever

Michael L. O'Dell

Fever with an accompanying rash represents a diagnostic challenge for even the most experienced of clinicians, as this combination of signs can represent trivial or life-threatening illnesses.

I. Approach. A useful way of approaching the differential diagnosis is to differentiate between the various entities that cause fever and illness by the types of rash they commonly cause. Various febrile diseases can present by more than one type of rash; however, this grouping allows the clinician to look at fewer causes rather than the entire spectrum of possible causes (1).

    A. Petechial rashes (Chapter 15.3) are commonly associated with:

        1. Treatable infections, including endocarditis, meningococcemia, gonococcemia, septicemia from any bacteria, and rickettsial infections, especially Rocky Mountain spotted fever (RMSF) (2).

        2. Infectious causes not necessitating acute treatment, include enteroviruses, dengue fever, hepatitis B, rubella, and Epstein-Barr virus (EBV).

3. Noninfectious causes, including urticaria, include thrombocytopenia, scurvy, Henoch-Schönlein purpura, hypersensitivity vasculitis, acute rheumatic fever, and systemic lupus erythematosus (SLE).

B. **Maculopapular rashes** (Chapter 13.3) are commonly associated with:
   1. Treatable infections, including typhoid, secondary syphilis, meningococcemia, gonococcemia, mycoplasmal infection, Lyme disease, psittacosis, rickettsial infections (especially RMSF).
   2. Infectious causes not subject to acute treatment, including enterovirus, parvovirus B-19, human herpesvirus-6 (HHV-6), rubeola, rubella, adenovirus, Epstein–Barr virus (EBV), and primary human immunodeficiency virus-1 (HIV-1),
   3. Noninfectious causes, including allergy, erythema multiforme (Chapter 13.2), SLE, dermatomyositis, serum sickness, and juvenile rheumatoid arthritis.

C. **Vesiculobullous rashes** (Chapter 13.8) are commonly associated with:
   1. Treatable infections, including staphylococcal large vesicle impetigo and toxic shock syndrome, gonococcemia, rickettsial pox, varicella zoster, herpes simplex virus, *Vibrio vulnificus* sepsis, and folliculitis.
   2. Infectious causes not requiring acute treatment, including enterovirus, parvovirus B-19, and HIV, although none of these three commonly present in this manner.
   3. Noninfectious causes, including eczema vaccinatum and erythema multiforme bullosum.

D. **Diffuse erythematous rashes** are commonly associated with:
   1. Treatable infections, including streptococcal scarlet fever, toxic shock syndrome, ehrlichiosis (3), *Streptococcus viridans* (in chemotherapy patients), *Corynebacterium haemolyticum* pharyngitis, and Kawasaki's disease.
   2. Infectious causes requiring acute treatment, including enteroviral infections.
   3. Noninfectious causes of erythema are only rarely associated with fever.

E. **Urticaria rashes** are commonly associated with:
   1. Treatable infections, including mycoplasma infections and Lyme disease.
   2. Infectious causes not requiring acute treatment, including enteroviral infections, adenoviral infections, EBV, HIV, and hepatitis.
   3. Noninfectious causes of urticaria are only rarely associated with fever.

II. **History.** History is quite important and should include standard items, such as onset, duration, aggravating factors, relieving factors, and associated symptoms. Additionally, other factors to consider, include:

A. **Exposure history.** Are any other family members or close contacts ill? Is there a history of exposure to brackish water, mosquitoes, foreign travel, and so forth?

B. **Are there any underlying illnesses** or a significant possibility of immunologic compromise (e.g., undiagnosed HIV infection)?

III. **Physical examination**

A. **Examine the lesions and their distribution** carefully. Classify the rash as petechial, maculopapular, vesiculobullous, erythematous, or urticarial. Note the distribution of the rash. For instance, rubella and rubeola generally begin on the face and spread to the trunk, whereas RMSF petechiae tend to occur on the ankles and wrists first.

B. **Conduct a general physical examination**. Areas of particular concern are:
   1. Head, eyes, ears, nose, and throat. The presence of Koplik's spots is pathognomic for rubeola. The discovery of a tick lends support to the diagnosis of RMSF. Sinusitis may represent a source for meningococcemia. Pharyngitis in a young adult with diffuse erythema may be caused by *C. haemolyticum*. Mucous membrane swelling may indicate early anaphylaxis.
   2. Lung examination. Expiratory wheezing, especially in a patient who has recently received medications or contrast dye, can indicate anaphylaxis. Evidence of pneumonia is consistent with psittacosis and mycoplasma.

3. Cardiac examination. Cardiovascular collapse is associated with meningo-coccemia and other sepsis. A new murmur (Chapters 7.6 and 7.7) may indicate subacute bacterial endocarditis in a patient with subungual or scleral petechiae.

4. Genital examination. Purulent urethral drainage or evidence of pelvic inflammatory disease supports consideration of gonorrhea. A chancre would support a diagnosis of syphilis, although palmar lesions often occur well after healing of the initial chancre.

5. Joint examination and extremities. A petechial rash near the ankles and wrists is suggestive of RMSF. Evidence of joint swelling supports a diagnosis of meningococcemia or gonococcemia. A maculopapular rash may be seen in juvenile rheumatoid arthritis and other rheumatologic conditions as well.

6. Neurologic examination. Evidence of meningitis supports a diagnosis of meningococcemia. Patients with RMSF may also have meningeal signs.

IV. **Testing** should be directed by illnesses suspected, with life-threatening illnesses being tested for on reasonable suspicion. A complete blood count is generally useful, although life-threatening sepsis often presents without significant elevation of white blood count. In general, a blood culture should be obtained in all patients with petechial rashes and in those with signs of cardiovascular collapse.

V. **Diagnostic assessment.** Based on history and physical examination, the likelihood of various illnesses can be assessed. Patients who appear toxic should be treated as septic until initial laboratory and culture results can be evaluated (4).

References

1. Schlossberg D. Fever and rash. *Infect Dis Clin North Am* 1996;10(1):101–110.
2. Drolet BA, Baselga E, Esterly NB. Painful, purpuric plaques in a child with fever. *Arch Dermatol* 1997;133(12):1500–1501.
3. Anonymous. Fever, nausea, and rash in a 37-year-old man [clinical conference]. *Am J Med* 1998;104(6):596–601.
4. Dellinger RP. Current therapy for sepsis. *Infect Dis Clin North Am* 1999;13(2): 495–509.

13.7 Urticaria

Rachelle L. Cassity

Urticaria (hives) is a common condition. The lesions appear well circumscribed. Typically, they are first erythematous and subsequently develop a central wheal. They usually clear within 3 to 4 hours, and the skin appears normal. It is estimated that at least 15% to 20% of the population will suffer one episode of hives during their lifetime. Urticaria occurs most frequently between the ages of 20 and 40 years, and more commonly in women than men.

I. **Approach.** Urticaria can be divided into two subcategories: acute and chronic. Acute urticaria is defined as intermittent or daily attacks that occur over a period of less than 6 weeks. If a urticaria attack lasts more than 6 weeks, it is classified as chronic (1).

A. **Urticaria can also be classified as immunologic, nonimmunologic, or idiopathic.**

1. Immunologic urticaria includes IgE-mediated hypersensitivity, complement-mediated hypersensitivity, and physical and contact urticaria.

2. Nonimmunologic urticaria includes mast cell release, physical agents, and contact urticaria.

3. Idiopathic

B. **Special concerns.** A severe urticarial reaction can be accompanied by angioedema and systemic symptoms. Also, urticarial vasculitis should be ruled out by skin biopsy if the lesions last longer than 24 hours.

II. **History**

A. **Characteristics.** Is the rash localized or systemic? Is it pruritic? What is the duration of symptoms? Does anything relieve the symptoms? Are there any specific triggers (2)?

1. Food and drugs are common causes of urticaria.
2. Certain systemic diseases can cause urticaria. Infections, connective tissue disorders, endocrine disorders, and neoplastic disorders are some examples.
3. Insect stings and bites are another common cause of urticaria.

B. **Symptom chronology.** When does it occur? How long does it last? Is it in association with physical trauma? Has the patient been on any medication that has helped relieve symptoms (e.g., antihistamines)?

C. **Family history.** Are there any members of the family who suffer from a connective tissue disorder? Do any complement disorders occur in the family, such as hereditary angioedema, which can be associated with urticaria? Also, is there a family history of atopy?

III. **Physical examination.** A complete physical is required to rule out infection or other systemic diseases. An urticarial wheal is usually well demarcated. It begins as an erythematous area, which then develops a white center. The size of the wheal can vary from 2 mm to well over 30 cm. The rash is usually pruritic, especially when it occurs on the palms of the hand and the soles of the feet. Most often, the wheal will disappear within 3 to 4 hours of onset. The accompanying angioedema can last for a couple of days. The skin will return to normal once the wheal is gone.

IV. **Testing**

A. **Laboratory tests.** Routine tests include (a) complete blood count to look for eosinophilia, neoplastic disorders, and occult infection; (b) thyroid studies (thyroxine and thyroid-stimulating hormone; (c) erythrocyte sedimentation rate to help rule out connective tissue disorders and occult infection, urine analysis with urine culture, chemical profile, stool cultures for parasites, liver function tests, and an antinuclear antibody test. Other tests can include immunoglobulins, prick testing, rheumatoid factor, cryoglobulins, serum complement, and skin biopsy. However, laboratory tests often do not provide answers beyond those obtained in the history (3).

B. **Diagnostic imaging.** Chest x-ray, sinus, and dental films may help to rule out cancer and infection.

V. **Diagnostic assessment.** It is important to rule out underlying conditions such as neoplastic disorders, endocrine disorders, connective tissue diseases, infections, and other disorders. The most significant factors in diagnosing acute urticaria are the history and physical examination. Facts must be obtained concerning food or drug ingestion, insect stings, current infections, or physical triggers such as cold or heat. Most acute urticarial reactions resolve spontaneously, but some continue and become chronic in nature. Of the chronic urticaria, a cause is found in only a few of these patients, with more than 75% of them having an idiopathic disorder (4).

References

1. Beltrani VS. Allergic dermatoses. *Med Clin North Am* 1998;82(5):1105–1133.
2. Greaves MW, Sabroe RA. ABC of allergies. Allergy and the skin. I—Urticaria. *BMJ* 1998;316(7138):1147–1150.
3. Kozel MM. The effectiveness of a history-based diagnostic approach in chronic urticaria and angioedema. *Arch Dermatol* 1998;134(12):1575–1580.
4. Greaves MW. Chronic urticaria [published erratum appears in *N Engl J Med* 1995; 333(16):1091]. *N Engl J Med* 1995;332(26):1767–1772.

13.8 Vesicular and Bullous Eruptions

Marcia J. Chesebro

I. Approach. The initial approach to the patient with fluid-filled lesions involves assessment of the severity of the illness: Does the patient look sick or toxic or does the patient appear generally well?

II. History

  A. Age. Newborns develop epidermolysis bullosa, pemphigus neonatorum, and syphilitic pemphigus. Children are more likely to have varicella (if unimmunized); primary herpes simplex; hand, foot, and mouth disease (HFM); and bullous impetigo. Recurrent herpes simplex, porphyria cutanea tarda (PCT), pemphigus vulgaris, dyshidrotic eczema, and dermatitis herpetiformis occur primarily in adults. Bullous pemphigoid and herpes zoster are more common in the elderly. Other vesiculobullous diseases that have no particular age predilection include allergic contact dermatitis, allergic vasculitis, erythema multiforme bullosum (EMB), toxic epidermal necrolysis (TEN), insect bites, and second-degree burns.

  B. Season. Varicella, HFM, and primary herpes simplex are often seen in epidemics after gatherings of children. Summer brings more bullous impetigo (from staphylococcal infection) and dyshidrotic eczema (increased sweating of hands and feet). Contact dermatitis caused by *Rhus* species can be seen in the spring, as people landscape their yards; in the summer, as people spend more time outdoors; and in the fall, as people rake leaves and cut firewood.

  C. Special precipitators. Recurrent herpes simplex can be precipitated by trauma, sunlight, wind, menses, dry skin, smoking, drinking alcohol, lack of sleep, and fever. PCT is precipitated by exposure to sunlight, ingestion of drugs metabolized in the liver, and by drinking alcohol (1). EMB can be caused by a viral or bacterial infection or by drug ingestion within 3 weeks preceding the eruption (Chapter 13.2). Allergic vasculitis is usually caused by drugs. Persons with contact dermatitis have been exposed to the allergen 12 to 48 hours before the rash appears.

  D. Pain or pruritus. Itching is very common with acute contact dermatitis, dyshidrotic eczema, varicella, dermatitis herpetiformis, and bullous pemphigoid (Chapter 13.5). Before the eruption of recurrent herpes simplex, the site may itch or tingle for a few hours or days; before herpes zoster erupts, the area may burn or mimic internal or visceral pain.

  E. Duration. Some diseases are chronic with exacerbations: dermatitis herpetiformis, dyshidrotic eczema, bullous pemphigoid, epidermolysis bullosa, and PCT. Some are episodically recurrent: acute contact dermatitis and herpes simplex. Some occur acutely without preceding episodes: EMB, varicella, bullous impetigo, herpes zoster, allergic vasculitis, HFM, TEN, and pemphigus vulgaris.

III. Physical

  A. Sick or toxic appearing

  1. In those who look sick, toxic, or ill, consider the possible diagnoses of EMB, pemphigus vulgaris, TEN, or primary herpes simplex. Rubbing normal skin in patients with pemphigus vulgaris may induce new blister formation or enlarge existing blisters (Nikolsky's sign).

  2. Patients with varicella and HFM may have low-grade fever and malaise. Patients with EMB, primary herpes simplex, or varicella may have preceding or concurrent fever and malaise.

  3. Oral lesions. The presence of oral lesions, either as vesicles or the secondary lesion of erosion or ulcer, tends to have more serious consequences because of decreased oral intake; consider EMB, pemphigus vulgaris, TEN, primary herpes simplex, varicella, and HFM.

B. Size of vesicles and bullae. The only distinction between vesicles and bullae is size: vesicles are less than 1 cm; bullae are more than 1 cm. The fluid in them can be clear, purulent, or hemorrhagic. Secondary lesions (e.g., erosions, ulcers, and crusts) evolve from vesicles and bullae. Most of the diseases in this section primarily will have either vesicles or bullae, but can have some of both. The primarily vesicular diseases are herpes simplex, varicella, herpes zoster, contact dermatitis, dyshidrotic eczema, hemorrhagic vasculitis, HFM, Kaposi's varicelliform eruption (KVE), and dermatitis herpetiformis; the bullous diseases are generally pemphigus vulgaris, bullous pemphigoid, bullous impetigo, PCT, EMB, TEN, and epidermolysis bullosa.

C. Appearance of the blisters
1. The bullae of bullous impetigo are thin, fragile, short-lived, and easily ruptured, leaving a thin, varnishlike crust with occasionally a delicate remnant of the blister roof at its rim.
2. Contact dermatitis may be mostly excoriations by the time the patient presents.
3. Varicella will have a variety of lesions—the newest ones vesicular ("dew drop on a rose petal"), the older ones becoming purulent, then crusting over.
4. The bullae of bullous pemphigoid are large and tense; those of pemphigus vulgaris are flaccid and easily ruptured, leaving large denuded, bleeding, and weeping erosions.
5. The lesions of PCT, dermatitis herpetiformis, and allergic vasculitis may be hemorrhagic, and secondarily crusted.
6. Umbilication. Always examine a fresh blister. Umbilication (a small dimple in the center) is characteristic of a viral cause—herpes simplex, herpes zoster, varicella, KVE, and molluscum contagiosum. EMB lesions, although not umbilicated, may have a depression in the center as part of the "bull's eye."

D. Location or distribution
1. Localized. If the lesions are found primarily on sun-exposed or usually uncovered areas, consider contact dermatitis, insect bites, and PCT (esp., the dorsum of the hands). Contact dermatitis is localized to the area of exposure and is frequently recognizable by its shape (linear streaks from contact with leaves, recognizable geometric patterns in reaction to shoe leather, belts, rings, necklaces, elastic bands, and so on). If the contactant is airborne or reacts with sunlight, the dermatitis will be on exposed surfaces (neck, arms, face, and so forth). The palms and soles are usually spared because of the skin thickness, unless the contactant is related to shoes, socks, or gloves. Allergic vasculitis occurs primarily distally—on the feet and lower legs—and under areas of pressure. HFM occurs in the mouth and on the hands and feet. Dermatitis herpetiformis occurs primarily on the shoulders, buttocks, elbows, and posterior upper back. Herpes zoster affects a sensory (cutaneous) dermatome and rarely crosses the midline. Bullous impetigo is frequent around the mouth, nose, and genital area. Dyshidrotic eczema involves the lateral aspects of the fingers, palms, and soles. KVE occurs at sites of preexisting dermatitis, especially areas of atopic dermatitis.
2. Some diseases begin in one area then become generalized. Varicella begins on the trunk or head, with successive crops erupting more distally. TEN begins in the oral cavity, groin, or axilla. Pemphigus vulgaris may begin in the oral cavity. Bullous pemphigoid occurs mostly in the flexor surfaces, axilla, and groin, but can be generalized. EMB involves the hands, feet, face, genitals, and mouth, but in severe cases is generalized.

IV. Testing
A. The Tzanck smear is used to diagnose viral dermatoses: herpes simplex, herpes zoster, KVE, and varicella. Select an early intact vesicle without infection or trauma; remove the blister top and scrape the floor lightly with a scalpel; smear the material on a clean glass slide; air dry and fix; stain

with Wright or Giemsa stain. A positive test is the presence of multi-nucleated giant cells (2).

B. Biopsy of the edge of the blister and subsequent immunofluorescent staining is helpful for diagnosing pemphigus vulgaris, bullous pemphigoid, and EMB (3).

V. Diagnostic assessment. The presence or absence of a toxic appearance guides the clinician initially. History that includes age, season of onset, special precipitators, whether the lesions are itchy, and the duration of lesions then further assists in classification. Finally, the appearance of the lesions and their distribution further reduce candidate illnesses. It is important to remember that significant and occasionally life-threatening illnesses present as vesiculobullous lesions.

References

1. Robin KL, Piette WW. Cutaneous manifestations of systemic diseases. *Med Clin North Am* 1998;82(6):1359–1379, vi–vii.
2. Brodell RT, Helms SE, Devine M. Office dermatologic testing: the Tzanck preparation. *Am Fam Physician* 1991;44(3):857–860.
3. Gellis SE. Bullous diseases of childhood. *Dermatol Clin* 1986;4(1):89–98.

14. ENDOCRINE AND METABOLIC PROBLEMS

RICHARD D. BLONDELL

14.1 Diabetes Mellitus

Michael Ostapchuk and Michael B. Foster

Diabetes mellitus (DM) is a group of metabolic diseases characterized by hyperglycemia resulting from defects in insulin secretion, insulin action, or both (1). There are two types of DM: type 1 and type 2. Approximately 7.8 million people in the United States have DM (2). Of these, 10% to 15% have type 1. The prevalence of type 1 DM is 1/400 individuals aged 18 years or less. Approximately 20% of those with type 1 DM present after 18 years of age.

I. **Approach.** The initial goal is to determine which type of diabetes the patient has.
   A. **Type 1 diabetes.** Type 1 DM is thought to be caused by a gradual autoimmune destruction of pancreatic beta cells (3). This leads to a critical deficiency in the production of insulin that often leaves the patient dependent on insulin throughout life. Type 1 DM has no seasonal variation and the gender-based differences are not clinically significant. The genetics of type 1 DM remains unclear. Early institution of insulin therapy may help to preserve pancreatic secretory reserve, which enhances the ability of the patient to maintain stable blood glucose control.
   B. **Type 2 diabetes.** In type 2 DM is found a combination of resistance to insulin action and an inadequate secretory response. Risk factors for type 2 DM include (a) a family history of type 2 DM, (b) prior gestational diabetes, (c) advanced age, (d) sedentary lifestyle, (e) upper body obesity, and (f) African-American, Hispanic, or native American ethnicity (1). These individuals often do not need insulin to survive. Because type 2 DM can go unrecognized, patients are at increased risk for developing microvascular and macrovascular complications.
II. **History.** The initial presentation of DM can vary. Either type may present with the insidious onset of the symptoms associated with hyperglycemia (polyuria, polydipsia, and polyphagia) or with the abrupt onset of an acute complication [diabetic ketoacidosis (in type 1 DM) or nonketotic hyperglycemic-hyperosmolar coma (in type 2 DM)].
   A. **Type 1 diabetes.** Patients with type 1 DM typically present before the age of 18 years. The symptoms heralding the disease emerge gradually as hyperglycemia appears and becomes more frequent and profound. Physiologic stress (e.g., an acute illness or trauma), which increases the requirement for insulin, can unmask the insulinopenia and give the impression that the problem is acute. Enuresis may be a clue for polyuria in a child who was previously toilet-trained. Lethargy, weakness, and weight loss are other common features.
   B. **Type 2 diabetes.** Patients with type 2 DM usually present after the age of 40 years. The diagnosis is often made in an asymptomatic patient as a result of routine blood tests that reveal an elevation of plasma glucose. Other patients may present with the symptoms of hyperglycemia. The patient may have a history of recurrent skin infections or persistent vulvovaginitis. Other common symptoms include altered sensations in the extremities, nocturia, erectile dysfunction, and visual disturbances (Chapters 4.6, 5.1, 10.3, and 10.4). The use of glucocorticoids, β-adrenergic agonists, or thiazides can precipitate the symptoms of type 2 DM.
III. **Physical examination.** Patients often present with similar physical findings in both type 1 and type 2 DM, owing to hyperglycemia. In the young child, failure to grow and gain weight can occur with type 1 DM. The child may be ill appearing, lethargic, and often have signs of dehydration (tachypnea, tachycardia, and low blood pressure). Ketone production will produce a fruity odor on the patient's breath. The patient with type 2 DM tends to be obese (especially

upper body obesity) and may appear fatigued and have muscle weakness or decreased vision. The neurologic examination may reveal painful feet and numbness. Monilial infections may be found in the vagina and pubic areas.

IV. **Testing**

A. **Type 1 diabetes.** Not all children with hyperglycemia have diabetes. Some children with a severe illness (e.g., severe dehydration from diarrhea or asthma treated with corticosteroids) may have elevated serum glucose and ketosis. If the diagnosis is uncertain, a low serum insulin level along with hyperglycemia supports the diagnosis of DM and excludes all other diagnoses. Elevated glycosylated hemoglobin provides a strong circumstantial case for the diagnosis of DM, but it is not used alone for the diagnosis. Performing a glucose tolerance test is rarely necessary. However, it is imperative to obtain insulin levels along with the blood glucose values when it is performed.

B. **Type 2 diabetes.** The American Diabetes Association (ADA) diagnostic criteria for type 2 DM are either (a) symptoms of diabetes and a casual plasma glucose level of 200 mg/dl or greater, (b) a fasting plasma glucose level of 126 mg/dl or greater, or (c) a plasma glucose level of 200 mg/dl or greater 2 hours after an oral glucose load (75 g). A "casual" plasma blood glucose level is obtained at any time of the day without regard to the time of the last meal, and a "fasting" level is obtained after a fast of at least 8 hours. If the only criterion is hyperglycemia, confirmation should be made on a different day (1).

V. **Diagnostic assessment.** The presence of polyuria, polydipsia, polyphagia, and weight loss along with hyperglycemia and ketosis are sufficient to establish the diagnosis of type 1 DM. This provides an ample basis for beginning insulin therapy. Hyperglycemia can also occur during a severe illness. Therefore, the diagnosis of type 1 DM is not always clear. Low insulin levels may be needed to make the diagnosis. The key to the diagnosis of type 2 DM is the detection of hyperglycemia. Patients with symptoms of diabetes should have testing according to the ADA recommendations. Once the diagnosis is made, formulate a treatment program with the patient.

References

1. American Diabetes Association. Report of the Expert Committee on the Diagnosis and Classification of Diabetes Mellitus. *Diabetes Care* 1997;20:1183–1197.
2. National Diabetes Data Group. *Diabetes in America*, 2nd ed. Bethesda, MD: National Institute of Diabetes and Digestive and Kidney Diseases, 1995. NIH publication 1468-1995.
3. Baker JR. Autoimmune endocrine disease. *JAMA* 1997;278:1931–1937.

14.2 Gynecomastia

Charles M. Kodner

Gynecomastia is the palpable enlargement of the breast tissue in men. Presentation occurs in three peak age groups, corresponding to the common physiologic causes of breast enlargement. After the neonatal period, the most common causes of gynecomastia are idiopathic (25%), puberty (25%), medications (10% to 20%), cirrhosis or malnutrition (8%), or primary hypogonadism (8%) (1). Klinefelter's syndrome increases the risk of breast cancer, but other causes do not.

I. **Approach.** Most patients with gynecomastia have a transient, physiologic imbalance between circulating estrogens and androgens. Gynecomastia that is persistent or symptomatic, or presents outside the expected age ranges, requires further diagnostic evaluation.

A. **Differentiation from pseudogynecomastia.** Physical findings are usually adequate to distinguish true breast tissue enlargement from breast enlargement from adipose tissue.

B. **Physiologic conditions causing normal, transient gynecomastia.**
   1. Neonatal period. Transplacental estrogen causes transient breast tissue enlargement in most newborns; this may be associated with nipple discharge; typically, it resolves over 3 to 4 weeks. No additional evaluation is necessary.
   2. Puberty. Hormonal changes and breast tissue proliferation during puberty cause transient gynecomastia in adolescent males; this may be asymmetric and it can be tender. The condition usually resolves within 1 year, but can persist for up to 2 years.
   3. Older adults. Many men (aged 50–80 years) have palpable breast tissue enlargement that is often physiologic, caused by a relative increase in body fat and increased aromatization of estrogen precursors, but medical disorders or medication effects should be considered (2).

II. **History.** Does the history suggest breast cancer or an underlying endocrine disorder? Are there immediately identifiable causes?
   A. **History.** Persistent or rapid breast tissue enlargement may necessitate further evaluation if no diagnosis is apparent. Mild pain or tenderness by itself does not indicate a concerning underlying cause.
   B. **Medications.** Substances that can cause gynecomastia include alcohol, marijuana, androgens, estrogens, digitoxin, cimetidine, spironolactone, ketoconazole, and antiandrogens (1).
   C. **Medical disorders.** Hyperthyroidism, renal failure, liver disease, starvation, or malnutrition can cause gynecomastia. Underlying cancers (lung, liver, kidney) can produce ectopic human chorionic gonadotropin (HCG), which stimulates aromatase activity.
   D. **Endocrine disorders.** Primary testicular failure and Klinefelter's syndrome can be associated with gynecomastia.

III. **Physical examination (PE).** True gynecomastia is confirmed with the PE. With the patient supine, the breast is grasped between thumb and forefinger and the digits are moved toward the nipple. A firm, rubbery, mobile, disk-shaped mass of tissue beneath the nipple indicates true breast tissue enlargement. A focused PE can help exclude cancer of the breast or testes and some medical or endocrine disorders (Chapter 11.2).
   A. **Pseudogynecomastia.** Adipose tissue deposition produces the soft and poorly defined breast enlargement of pseudogynecomastia.
   B. **Breast cancer.** A unilateral, eccentric mass that is hard or firm, fixed to underlying tissue or associated with overlying skin dimpling, nipple discharge, or retraction, or axillary lymphadenopathy may represent breast cancer.
   C. **Testicular examination.** Congenital anorchia is a rare cause of gynecomastia. Bilateral small testes suggest gonadal failure. Testicular atrophy can result from alcohol abuse, mumps, leprosy, or other granulomatous disorders. Asymmetry or a palpable mass suggests testicular cancer (Chapter 10.7).

IV. **Testing.** Most patients with physiologic gynecomastia can be readily identified and no further evaluation is required. If pathology is suspected, additional testing may be needed.
   A. **Clinical laboratory testing.** Liver, kidney, and thyroid function should be assessed, if clinically indicated.
   B. **Diagnostic imaging.** Neither mammography nor ultrasound of the breast is usually helpful.
   C. **Special tests.** If an underlying endocrine disorder is suspected, serum HCG, testosterone, estradiol, and luteinizing hormone (LH) levels should be checked. Fine needle aspiration of a mass may be considered to diagnose breast cancer.

V. **Diagnostic assessment.** The medical history and PE may be sufficient for diagnostic assessment. The directed PE should focus on detecting breast cancer, testicular tumors, and endocrine disease. Further evaluation is indicated if these conditions are suspected. In cases of gynecomastia that do not resolve, progressive or rapid onset of gynecomastia, or history and PE suggestive of a possible endocrine disorder, measure the levels of serum LH, estradiol, testosterone, and HCG, which constitutes a reasonable screening evaluation for underlying endocrinopathies.

A. **Benign gynecomastia.** If true gynecomastia appears in one of the expected age ranges and neither the history nor PE suggests an underlying medical or endocrine disorder, then only reassurance and observation are required. Gynecomastia will resolve in 1 to 2 years in most patients; however, those cases that progress or fail to resolve may require further evaluation.

B. **Medications.** Drugs that cause gynecomastia should be discontinued, if possible, and the patient followed for the resolution of gynecomastia.

C. **Testicular insufficiency** results in an elevated LH serum level and a normal to low testosterone serum level.

D. **Klinefelter's syndrome.** This abnormality is associated with small, firm testes, behavioral abnormalities or mental retardation, an elevated estradiol level, and a diagnostic chromosome analysis.

E. **Androgen resistance.** Elevated LH and testosterone levels suggest this syndrome.

F. **Neoplasia.** High HCG levels may indicate a HCG-secreting tumor of the lung, stomach, liver, or kidney, or a testicular or extragonadal germ cell tumor. An elevated HCG should prompt a search for one of these cancers with a detailed PE, a radiograph of the chest, and a computed tomographic scan of the abdomen.

References

1. Braunstein GD. Gynecomastia. *N Engl J Med* 1993;328:490–495.
2. Frantz AG, Wilson JD. Disorders of breasts in men. In: Wilson JD, Foster DW, eds. *Williams textbook of endocrinology*, 9th ed. Philadelphia: WB Saunders; 1998:885–900.

14.3 Hirsutism

Richard D. Blondell

The growth of terminal hair (long, coarse hair) in areas other than the scalp and eyebrows is dependent on androgens. Different hair follicles have varying degrees of sensitivity to androgens. Axillary and pubic hair follicles are relatively sensitive to androgens and respond to the androgens produced by the adrenal glands of girls during puberty. Women develop some terminal hair on their forearms and lower legs. Some will get hair on the chest and abdomen, but few will grow facial hair. Men grow more terminal hair than women because of testicular androgens.

I. **Approach.** The goal is to distinguish hirsutism from other patterns of hair growth and determine its cause.

A. **Patterns of hair growth.** *Hirsutism* in women is characterized by the development of a male pattern of terminal hair growth, which occurs on the upper lip, chin, chest, back, linea alba, upper portions of the limbs, and within the superior pubic triangle. Some hirsute women with excessive androgen levels will also develop male-pattern baldness. *Hypertrichosis* is the excessive growth of non–androgen-dependent villus hair (short, fine hair) over all areas of the body, which can be caused by neoplasms, hypothyroidism, or anorexia nervosa.

B. **Causes of hirsutism.** Many causes are found for hirsutism (Table 14.1). Some causes are functional and are thought to result from an increased sensitivity of the hair follicle to normal female levels of androgens, whereas others result from pathologic hyperandrogenism (1).

Table 14.1 Causes of hirsutism

IDIOPATHIC
Very common ($\approx$1 of 30 women), often familial

CONSTITUTIONAL
Pregnancy, obesity, normal menopause

MEDICATIONS
Oral contraceptives (high androgen), phenytoin, danazol, cyclosporin

POLYCYSTIC OVARIAN DISEASE
Common

CUSHING'S SYNDROME
Iatrogenic and pathologic causes

ANDROGEN-SECRETING TUMOR
Ovarian, adrenal, lung, choriocarcinoma

PITUITARY DISEASE
Hyperprolactinemia, adenoma

CONGENITAL ADRENAL HYPERPLASIA
Late-onset type

II. History

A. **Onset.** It is useful to determine the age of the onset of the hirsutism, its rate of progression, and the timing of any exacerbation of hair growth. The patient's menstrual history, pregnancy history, or general medical history can yield important clues about an underlying endocrinopathy or another medical disorder.

B. **Medications.** A detailed medication history is important. Some medications cause hirsutism directly (e.g., androgenic oral contraceptives, anabolic steroids in body-builders) and can produce an increased libido. Others cause hirsutism indirectly by causing hyperprolactinemia (e.g., phenothiazines, tricyclic antidepressants), which can be associated with galactorrhea and menstrual abnormalities.

C. **Family history.** A familial pattern can be associated with idiopathic hirsutism, polycystic ovarian disease, and late-onset congenital adrenal hyperplasia.

III. Physical examination

A. **Hair growth.** The exact distribution of terminal hair growth should be noted. A male type escutcheon (hair filling the superior pubic triangle) is a presumptive sign of hyperandrogenism. Some patients will have had unwanted hair removed, altering the clinical presentation.

B. **Secondary sexual characteristics.** Pathologic androgen excess is suggested by acne, oily skin, and signs of *virilization* (frontal balding, deepening of the voice, increase in muscle mass, and clitoromegaly). This is especially true if *defeminization* (loss of breast tissue, vaginal atrophy) is also present.

C. **Other findings.** A bimanual pelvic examination may reveal ovarian enlargement. Obesity with *acanthosis nigricans* (dark, velvety hyperpigmentation of the axilla, groin, neck, umbilicus) is suggestive of the insulin-resistant form of polycystic ovarian disease. Corticosteroid excess can produce the signs of Cushing's syndrome.

IV. Testing.
Diagnostic testing is directed at confirming the cause of hirsutism suggested by the medical history and the physical examination (2).

A. **Clinical laboratory tests.** It is useful to measure the serum concentrations of testosterone and dehydroepiandrosterone sulfate (DHEAS) if an androgen-secreting neoplasm is suspected. If pituitary abnormalities, polycystic ovarian disease, or premature menopause are possibilities, then determine the

serum levels of luteinizing hormone (LH), follicle-stimulating hormone (FSH), and prolactin, as indicated by the clinical impression.
   B. **Diagnostic imaging.** Ultrasonography can be used to detect ovarian cysts, but other imaging studies may be indicated if a neoplasm of the adrenals or ovaries is suspected.
   V. **Diagnostic assessment.** The vast majority of patients with hirsutism will have either an idiopathic cause or polycystic ovarian disease. Studying other hirsute women can become a major diagnostic exercise that is best left to a physician with experience in these unusual cases. A patient can be considered to have idiopathic hirsutism if she has mild hirsutism that began shortly after the onset of puberty and progressed slowly, has regular menses, has an otherwise normal physical examination, does not have galactorrhea or virilization, and is not taking any medication associated with hirsutism. No further diagnostic assessment is needed for these women. Polycystic ovarian disease is seen in women between the ages of 15 and 25 years and is associated with a mildly elevated serum level of testosterone and DHEAS, a LH:FSH ratio of 2 or more, and cystic ovaries on ultrasonography. Among women with hirsutism, an adrenal tumor is unlikely if the serum levels of testosterone and DHEAS are normal (3). A dexamethasone suppression test is indicated for women with elevated values of testosterone or DHEAS to exclude a sinister cause of hirsutism. Treatment is cosmetic in women with idiopathic hirsutism, otherwise the underlying cause is targeted (4).

References
1. Toscano V. Hirsutism: pilosebaceous unit dysregulation. Role of peripheral and glandular factors. *J Endocrinol Invest* 1991;14:153–170.
2. Kalve E, Klein JF. Evaluation of women with hirsutism. *Am Fam Physician* 1996;54: 117–124.
3. Derksen J, Nagessar SK, Meinders AE, Haak HR, van de Velde CJH. Identification of virilizing adrenal tumors in hirsute women. *N Engl J Med* 1994;331:968–973.
4. Knochenhauer ES, Azziz R. Advances in the diagnosis and treatment of the hirsute patients. *Curr Opin Obstet Gynecol* 1995;7:344–350.

14.4 Hypothyroidism

Stephen F. Wheeler and David E. Bybee

Hypothyroidism is the clinical syndrome resulting from deficient thyroid hormone action. Overt hypothyroidism is found in 2% of women aged more than 70 years and in 0.5% of women aged 40 to 60 years. Hypothyroidism is present in 0.8% of men older than 60 years and is rare in women younger than 40 years and men younger than 60 years (1).

   I. **Approach.** Mild to moderate hypothyroidism often exhibits subtle, nonspecific signs and symptoms of insidious onset. Severe disease tends to have more characteristic findings. The key diagnostic tasks are to suspect and confirm the presence of hypothyroidism and consider the level of disease.
      A. **Hypothalamic-pituitary-thyroid axis.** Thyrotropin-releasing hormone, secreted by the hypothalamus, stimulates the anterior pituitary to produce thyroid-stimulating hormone (TSH). The major hormone produced by the pituitary in response to TSH is thyroxine (T_4). The most sensitive indicator of thyroid status is the level of TSH, which is controlled in classic negative-feedback fashion by the concentration of active thyroid hormones.
      B. **Level of disease.** *Primary hypothyroidism*, by far the most common type, is the result of thyroid gland failure. Hypothyroidism caused by pituitary or hypothalamic disease is termed *secondary* or *tertiary*, respectively.
      C. **Special concerns.** *Myxedema* refers to the hypothyroidism-associated, nonpitting edema caused by glycosaminoglycan accumulation in the skin, subcutaneous tissues, and other organs. *Subclinical hypothyroidism* is dis-

tinguished by an elevated sensitive test for thyroid-stimulating hormone (sTSH), normal thyroid hormone levels, and few, if any, symptoms. Transient hypothyroidism can follow the initial thyrotoxic phase of subacute or postpartum thyroiditis.

II. **History.** Symptoms generally correspond directly to the duration and severity of disease.

    A. **Present illness**

        1. The probability of thyroid disease is directly related to the number of typical symptoms manifested by the patient (2), including weakness, lethargy, skin changes (dry, coarse, cold, yellow), coarseness or loss of hair, cold intolerance, weight gain, constipation, memory or concentration impairment, depression, hoarseness, goiter, menstrual abnormalities (most commonly menorrhagia), and fluid infiltration of tissues (eyelids, face, peripheral) (3).

        2. Loss of axillary or pubic hair, headaches, visual field defects, amenorrhea, galactorrhea, and symptoms of postural hypotension are suggestive of secondary or tertiary hypothyroidism.

    B. **Past and family history**

        1. Chronic autoimmune thyroiditis (Hashimoto's disease), previous radioactive iodine therapy, and prior thyroid surgery are the most common causes of primary hypothyroidism. Other groups with an increased risk for this type include women 4 to 8 weeks postpartum; women aged more than 50 years; patients with immunologically mediated diseases such as diabetes mellitus type 1, pernicious anemia, vitiligo, Addison's disease, and rheumatoid arthritis; and persons with a family history of thyroid disease. Screening these patients for hypothyroidism using sTSH may be appropriate (1).

        2. A pituitary tumor is the most common cause of secondary hypothyroidism. Other historical diagnoses that increase the likelihood of secondary or tertiary disease include pituitary surgery, cranial radiation therapy, postpartum hemorrhage (Sheehan's syndrome), head trauma, granulomatous diseases, metastatic disease (breast, lung, colon, prostate, others), and infectious diseases (tuberculosis, others) (4).

III. **Physical examination (PE).** The features frequently found in hypothyroidism should be sought.

    A. **Observation.** A welcoming handshake may reveal cold skin and further observations uncover altered affect, hoarseness, facial or eyelid edema, hair loss (scalp, eyebrows), and physical or mental slowing.

    B. **General examination.** Vital sign abnormalities commonly include weight gain, diastolic hypertension, and bradycardia. All major organ systems are affected by thyroid hormone deficiency. The heart may be enlarged, because of both dilation and pericardial effusion, which is indicated by a cardiac rub or distant heart sounds. Adynamic ileus, rarely, can result in megacolon or intestinal obstruction. Tissue glycosaminoglycan accumulation and reduced lymphatic clearance of interstitial proteins can produce carpal tunnel syndrome. The relaxation phase of deep tendon reflexes is prolonged, creating the characteristic "hung-up reflex." Orthostatic hypotension suggests secondary or tertiary disease, as do visual field defects and galactorrhea.

    C. **Thyroid examination.** Inspect the neck below the thyroid cartilage from the front and side. During palpation, approach the patient from the front or from behind and palpate using the fingers or thumbs. Having the patient swallow during both inspection and palpation causes the thyroid to move and aids in developing a three-dimensional impression of the gland. The size, consistency, and tenderness of the gland should be noted, as should the presence and characteristics of any nodules.

IV. **Testing**

    A. **Laboratory tests.** The most useful test is a sTSH, which is elevated (>10 µU/ml) in the vast majority of patients with hypothyroidism (1). Primary hypothyroidism is confirmed by a low free thyroxine index (FTI) or

free T_4 (fT_4) measured directly (5). Antithyroid antibodies are not usually necessary in the evaluation of patients with hypothyroidism.
    B. **Diagnostic imaging.** Radionuclide scans are not commonly helpful in the evaluation of patients with hypothyroidism. Radioactive iodine uptake is typically low in hypothyroidism of any cause. Notable exceptions are the rare cases of iodine deficiency or an intrathyroidal block in thyroid hormone production or release. The underlying pathology determines the distribution of the isotope in the gland.
V. **Diagnostic assessment**
    A. **Pitfalls of sTSH.** The sTSH is characteristically elevated in primary hypothyroidism. Starvation, corticosteroid administration, and use of dopamine can lower sTSH, even in hypothyroid patients, making the diagnosis more difficult. In patients with severe nonthyroidal illness, low peripheral thyroid hormone levels may suggest hypothyroidism. However, the sTSH is usually normal unless affected by starvation or therapies.
    B. **Primary hypothyroidism.** Most patients have primary disease. Typical findings on history and PE, coupled with an elevated sTSH and low FTI or fT_4, are sufficient for the diagnosis. Hypothyroid patients should be treated with T_4, and replacement therapy monitored using sTSH (5). Retest annually or at least 6 to 8 weeks after changes in therapy.
    C. **Secondary or tertiary hypothyroidism.** In a patient with overt hypothyroidism, a sTSH that is low, normal, or only mildly elevated suggests secondary or tertiary hypothyroidism. The historical and clinical features previously discussed support the diagnosis, and evaluation of the pituitary is necessary (4). Multiple endocrine end-organ failure caused by the autoimmune destruction of endocrine glands (Schmidt's syndrome) is a special case of primary hypothyroidism that mimics secondary level disease.
    D. **Severity.** Most patients will have only mild or moderate disease at the time of diagnosis. Profound hypothyroidism with hypothermia and stupor (*myxedema coma*) is life threatening and requires hospitalization. Factors that predispose to myxedema coma include infection, trauma, cold exposure, and central nervous system depressants.
    E. **Subclinical hypothyroidism.** In patients with subclinical hypothyroidism not treated with thyroid hormone replacement, monitor clinical and biochemical markers for evidence of progressive thyroid dysfunction. An appropriate follow-up interval has not been firmly established, but every 2 to 5 years may be adequate (1).

References
1. Helfand M, Redfern CC. Screening for thyroid disease. *Ann Intern Med* 1998;129: 144–158.
2. White GH, Walmsley RN. Can the clinical assessment of thyroid function be improved? *Lancet* 1978;2(8096):933–935.
3. Thyroid Guidelines Task Force of the American Association of Clinical Endocrinologists and the American College of Endocrinology. ACCE Clinical Practice Guidelines for the Evaluation and Treatment of Hyperthyroidism and Hypothyroidism. *Endocrine Prac* 1995;1:54–62.
4. Vance ML. Medical progress: hypopituitarism. *N Engl J Med* 1994;330:1651–1662.
5. Lindsay RS, Toft AD. Hypothyroidism. *Lancet* 1997;349:413–417.

14.5 Polydipsia

Soraya Nasraty

Polydipsia is a symptom that can be attributed to medical or psychogenic causes and has a prevalence of 3% to 39% among chronic psychiatric inpatients (1). It is a common symptom in patients with diabetes mellitus (DM) (Chapter 14.1) and prominent in patients with diabetes insipidus (DI). Polydipsia is usually seen with polyuria.

I. **Approach.** Initially try to classify and identify the cause of polydipsia.
   A. **Poorly resorbed solutes.** DM should be suspected in any patient with polydipsia and polyuria of recent onset that is caused by the osmotic diuresis from glucose (Chapter 14.1). Mannitol, sorbitol, or urea can also cause polyuria.
   B. **Primary polydipsia.** Increased fluid intake of up to 20 L/day may be seen in patients with psychogenic polydipsia. This can be caused by hyperactivity of hypothalamic thirst centers or by the anticholinergic effects of neuroleptic medications which cause dry mouth. Other patients may have delusions leading to increased fluid intake (1).
   C. **Diabetes insipidus** can result from either a central (neurogenic DI) or renal cause (nephrogenic DI).
      1. Central (complete or partial) DI is caused by a defect in the secretion of antidiuretic hormone (ADH) by the pituitary gland. Neurogenic DI can be idiopathic or be caused by an intracranial event such as a brain tumor, head trauma, neurosurgery, toxic brain injury, or metastatic cancer. Rare forms include granulomatous disease (tuberculosis, sarcoidosis) and an inherited autosomally dominant form. Vasopressin-induced DI occurs in the last trimester of pregnancy and is often associated with preeclampsia.
      2. Nephrogenic DI is caused by the nephrons not responding to ADH, which could be congenital or acquired. It can be secondary to medications (lithium, methoxyflurane, demeclocycline) or result from systemic hypokalemia and hypercalcemia.
   D. **Iatrogenic polydipsia** can occur because a patient misinterprets the physician's instructions to drink plenty of water (2).
II. **History.** Thirst, which is the chief complaint of patients with DM, DI, and psychogenic polydipsia, is associated with polyuria. Nocturia occurs more frequently with DM and DI than with psychogenic polydipsia. Polydipsia usually starts abruptly in central DI and patients often have a preference for ice cold water (3). In eliciting the history, take note of neurologic symptoms (problems with visual fields, headaches, numbness), a prior history of cancer (particularly metastatic brain cancer), a history of trauma, neurosurgery, and infections (e.g., encephalitis). The patient's psychiatric history may also be relevant.
III. **Physical examination.** A thorough general physical examination, including vital signs, is helpful in making the diagnosis, but the emphasis is on the neurologic examination (i.e., visual fields, cranial nerve deficits, oculomotor palsies, and reflexes). Signs of recent weight loss or presence of peripheral neuropathy is helpful in making the diagnosis of DM (Chapters 2.13 and 4.6).
IV. **Testing**
   A. **Clinical laboratory tests.** A urinalysis needs to be performed to look for glucosuria of DM or the low specific gravity associated with DI. A chemistry panel is helpful in checking for elevated serum glucose levels of DM or an elevated creatinine seen with renal disease or nephrogenic DI. A calcium level could be useful if hypercalcemia is suspected (Chapter 17.4). Serum and urine osmolality are useful in differentiating between DI, which presents with increased serum osmolality and in an appropriately low urine osmolality (specific gravity < 1.005), and excessive water intake, which presents with low or normal serum osmolality and an appropriately low urine osmolality. Normal serum values are between 285 and 295 mOsm/L.
   B. **Diagnostic imaging.** Magnetic resonance imaging (MRI) of the head may be indicated to exclude pituitary or hypothalamic tumors. In neurogenic DI, MRI is quite specific because the normal bright spot of a functioning pituitary gland will be absent (3).
   C. **Water deprivation test.** This indirect test may be useful in making the diagnosis of DI and to differentiate between neurogenic and nephrogenic DI

by determining the effects of water deprivation (mild dehydration) on ADH secretion by measuring serum, urine osmolality, urine-specific gravity, and serum sodium in a controlled environment (3). This test needs to be carefully supervised by someone able to treat severe hypertonic dehydration if necessary. Patients with mild polydipsia are placed on fluid restriction starting at midnight prior to testing, but fluids are restricted in those with severe polydipsia during the day only. Baseline body weight, plasma osmolarity, serum sodium, and urine osmolarity are determined. Urine osmolarity and weight are assessed on an hourly basis. Adequate dehydration is noted by a decrease in body weight by 5% and serum osmolarity by more than 275 mOsm/L. A normal response would show normal plasma osmolarity and sodium concentration with decreased urine output and increasing urine osmolarity to more than 800 mOsm/L (i.e., two to four times greater than the plasma). In contrast to healthy patients, patients with DI cannot concentrate their urine in response to dehydration. Patients with central DI respond to desmopressin (a synthetic analog of vasopressin) administered intranasally, whereas patients with nephrogenic DI do not (4). Sometimes patients do not fall into definite categories (e.g., partial central DI). The direct form of testing where ADH levels are measured after infusing hypertonic saline is rarely performed.

V. **Diagnostic assessment.** Often important clues about the cause of polydipsia can be obtained with a directed clinical history with particular attention paid to the onset of symptoms, the presence of nocturia, and the medication history. The value of the physical examination is limited unless signs are evident of defects caused by a pituitary tumor (e.g., progressive headaches, visual field defects) or endocrinologic symptoms (e.g., amenorrhea, galactorrhea, acromegaly, Cushing's disease). Often the diagnosis is made with routine laboratory tests. Sometimes a water deprivation test needs to be performed to make the diagnosis, but this test should be done in a hospital setting with the patient monitored closely for dehydration.

References
1. Greendyke RM, Bernhardt AJ, Tasbas HE. Polydipsia in chronic psychiatric patients. *Neuropsychopharmacology* 1998;18:272–281.
2. Olpade-Olaopa EO, Morley RN, Ahiaku ER, Bramble FJ. Iatrogenic polydipsia: a rare cause of water intoxication in urology. *Br J Urol* 1997;7:488.
3. Adam P. Evaluation and management of diabetes insipidus. *Am Fam Physician* 1997;55:2146–2153.
4. Blevins LS Jr, Wand GS. Diabetes insipidus. *Crit Care Med* 1992;20:69–79.

14.6 Thyroid Enlargement/Goiter

Stephen F. Wheeler and David E. Bybee

Goiter, an enlarged thyroid gland, is the most common thyroid abnormality. Goiter is termed *endemic* if it occurs in more than 10% of a population. Endemic goiter most commonly results from dietary iodine deficiency and is extremely rare in the United States. *Sporadic* goiter arises in nonendemic areas and from various causes (1). Mean thyroid gland weight in iodine-sufficient populations is 10 g, with 20 g representing the upper limit of normal (2).

I. **Approach**
    A. **Goiter types.** *Simple* goiter, also referred to as *diffuse*, is present in approximately 5% of the population. Its incidence increases with age and it is three to five times more common in women than men. Simple goiter is usually accompanied by a normal metabolic state, although functional status can change with time. A palpable goiter may represent a solitary nodule or mul-

tiple nodules (*multinodular goiter*) (Chapter 14.7). The functional status of a goiter can be hypothyroid (Chapter 14.4), normal, or hyperthyroid [also referred to as *toxic* (Chapter 14.8)].

  B. **Etiology.** Any process that impedes thyroid hormone synthesis or release can cause simple goiter. Inherited defects of thyroid-stimulating hormone (TSH) receptors and virtually all biochemical steps in thyroid hormone synthesis and release have been identified as causes of goiter. The resulting thyroid hyperplasia is initially dependent on elevated levels of TSH from the pituitary; however, because of increased thyroxine production by the enlarged gland, serum TSH levels in patients with established goiter are usually normal (3). Goitrogens, substances that interfere with thyroid hormone production and action, can cause sporadic goiter. This category includes certain drugs (thioamide derivatives, lithium, iodides, amiodarone and others) and foods (rutabagas, cabbage, turnips, soybeans, kelp and others) (1).

 II. **History.** In simple goiter, patients are asymptomatic or, if the gland is sufficiently enlarged, they present with symptoms caused by mechanical pressure. Substernal goiters are frequently responsible for tracheal pressure symptoms, including dyspnea and inspiratory stridor. They can also obstruct the large cervical veins at the thoracic inlet, causing suffusion of the face, giddiness, and syncope (Pemberton's sign). Esophageal compression can lead to dysphagia (Chapter 9.5). Hoarseness caused by compression of or traction on the recurrent laryngeal nerve is rare in simple goiter and suggests a malignancy (Chapter 6.3). Generalized thyroid pain suggests subacute thyroiditis, whereas sudden localized pain and swelling are consistent with hemorrhage into a nodule. Although simple goiters are usually euthyroid, typical symptoms of hypothyroidism or thyrotoxicosis should be sought. A family history of goiter and a personal history of residing in an endemic goiter area or ingesting goitrogens may be significant (1).

III. **Physical examination**

  A. **General examination.** Look for typical vital and physical signs consistent with hypothyroidism or thyrotoxicosis. Pemberton's sign can be induced by having the patient raise both arms above the head.

  B. **Thyroid examination.** Inspect the neck below the thyroid cartilage from the front, using cross-lighting to accentuate shadows and masses. Full extension of the neck enhances visibility of the gland. Inspection from the side with measurement of any prominence of the normally smooth and straight contour between the cricoid cartilage and the suprasternal notch is useful. Palpitation is done using the technique with which the examiner is most experienced and skilled. Approach the patient from either the front or behind and palpate using the fingers or thumbs. If felt between the cricoid cartilage and the suprasternal notch, the thyroid isthmus can be used to help locate the gland. Palpation of the lobes can be improved by relaxation of the sternocleidomastoid; for example, the left lobe can be defined better by having the patient slightly flex and rotate the neck to the left. Other useful maneuvers include measuring the circumference of the neck or the dimensions of each lobe. Note the location, size, consistency, mobility, and tenderness of any nodules. Having the patient swallow during both inspection and palpation causes the thyroid to move and aids in developing a three-dimensional impression of gland shape and size. This maneuver can also make a low-placed gland accessible. Categorize thyroid size as "normal" or "goiter," and subcategorize "goiter" as "small" (two or less times normal) or "large" (more than two times normal) (2).

 IV. **Testing**

  A. **Laboratory testing.** The sensitive TSH (sTSH) assay is the single best test to evaluate thyroid status. Elevated sTSH is highly suggestive of hypothyroidism (Chapter 14.4). If sTSH is suppressed, an elevated free thyroxine index (FTI) or free thyroxine (fT_4) measured directly, confirms thyrotoxicosis (Chapter 14.8). In a patient with a suppressed sTSH and a normal FTI or fT_4, serum triiodothyronine (T_3) should be measured to assess for possible T_3 thyrotoxicosis.

B. **Diagnostic imaging.** Nuclear scans and ultrasound studies are not warranted in the routine evaluation of simple or multinodular goiter (4). Ultrasonography may be helpful in patients with equivocal findings on palpation. Symptoms suggestive of substernal mechanical pressure require evaluation, usually by computed tomography (CT) or magnetic resonance imaging (MRI).

C. **Other tests.** Fine needle aspiration biopsy (FNAB) should be performed in cases of a solitary or dominant nodule found by palpation. Pulmonary function tests are warranted with evidence of inspiratory impairment. Barium swallow is indicated to evaluate goiter-associated dysphagia.

V. **Diagnostic assessment.** The evaluation of goiter focuses on the history, thyroid palpation, and functional status of the gland. An asymptomatic patient with a simple or multinodular goiter associated with a normal metabolic state does not necessarily require further diagnostic studies or treatment. Periodic assessment, at least annually, to evaluate growth, function, and symptoms is warranted. A palpable solitary nodule or dominant nodule in a multinodular gland should be evaluated by FNAB or excisional biopsy (Chapter 14.7). Goiter with compressive symptoms requires CT or MRI evaluation and referral for probable surgery. Further assess a goiter associated with an abnormal metabolic state as outlined for hypothyroidism (Chapter 14.4) or thyrotoxicosis (Chapter 14.8). Thyroid hormone suppression of any goiter type is controversial, and the risks associated with subclinical hyperthyroidism must be included in the risk-to-benefit analysis (5).

References

1. Petrone LR. A primary care approach to the adult patient with nodular thyroid disease. *Arch Fam Med* 1996;5:92–100.
2. Siminoski K. Does this patient have a goiter? *JAMA* 1995;273:813–817.
3. Peter HJ, Burgi U, Gerber H. Pathogenesis of nontoxic diffuse and nodular goiter. In: Braverman LE, Utiger RD, eds. *Werner and Ingbar's the thyroid*, 7th ed. Philadelphia: JB Lippincott, 1996:890–895.
4. Tan GH, Gharib H. Thyroid nodular disease: diagnostic evaluation and management [Letter]. *Arch Intern Med* 1997;157:575.
5. Gharib H, Mazzaferri EL. Thyroxine suppressive therapy in patients with nodular thyroid disease. *Ann Intern Med* 1998;128:386–394.

14.7 Thyroid Nodule

Stephen F. Wheeler and David E. Bybee

Palpable nodules are present in 4% to 7% of adults. Prevalence is four to nine times greater in women than men. Approximately 5% of all solitary nodules are carcinomas.

I. **Approach.** The evaluation of nodular thyroid disease focuses on the functional status of the gland and detection of clinically significant cancer.

A. **Functional status.** Thyroid function is evaluated through history, physical examination, and appropriate testing (Chapters 14.4 and 14.8).

B. **Cancer risk.** Prior radiation exposure increases the rate of development of both benign and malignant new nodules by approximately 2% per year. Peak incidence is 15 to 25 years after exposure. Because similar frequencies of cancer have been found in glands having solitary or multiple nodules on palpation, consider dominant nodules in multinodular thyroids for diagnostic evaluation (1). Age less than 20 or more than 60 years and male gender are also commonly cited risk factors for thyroid cancer.

II. **History.** Although history is neither sensitive nor specific for diagnosing thyroid cancer, an appropriately focused history can significantly alter the clinical likelihood of malignancy (2).

A. **Family history.** Approximately 3% of cases of papillary cancer are familial and a high incidence has been reported in patients with adenomatous polyposis coli (Gardner's syndrome). Medullary cancer often occurs in a hereditary pattern.

B. **Personal history.** Recent increase in size of a nodule, hoarseness, dysphagia, stridor, or dyspnea can indicate growth or invasiveness and increase the suspicion of cancer. Recurrence of cystic nodules after aspiration is also suggestive of cancer.

   1. External beam irradiation before the age of 15 to 20 years, which has been done for conditions such as acne and thymic or tonsillar enlargement, or exposure to ionizing radiation from a nuclear accident, increases the risk of thyroid carcinoma. The risk increases for 15 to 25 years after exposure, remains maximal and stable for 20 years, and then slowly declines.

   2. Sudden onset of localized swelling, pain, or tenderness suggests hemorrhage into a preexisting nodule or cyst. Subacute thyroiditis is suggested by fever, a preceding viral illness, and a gradual onset of swelling, pain, and tenderness. Typical symptoms of hypothyroidism suggests Hashimoto's thyroiditis, whereas thyrotoxicosis suggests toxic adenoma or toxic multinodular goiter (3).

III. **Physical examination.** As with the history, physical examination is neither sensitive nor specific for malignancy.

   A. **General examination.** Look for typical vital and physical signs consistent with hypothyroidism or thyrotoxicosis.

   B. **Thyroid examination.** Inspect the neck below the thyroid cartilage from the front and side, using cross-lighting to accentuate shadows and masses. Full extension of the neck enhances visibility of the gland. During palpation, approach the patient from either the front or behind and palpate using the fingers or thumbs. Having the patient swallow during both inspection and palpation causes the thyroid to move and aids in developing a three-dimensional impression of the gland. Note the location, size, consistency, mobility, and tenderness of all nodules. Findings suggestive of cancer include a nodule that is hard, irregular, nontender, greater than 4 cm in size, fixed to surrounding structures or associated with local lymphadenopathy.

IV. **Testing**

   A. **Laboratory testing.** Serum thyroid-stimulating hormone, performed by a sensitive method (sTSH), should be assessed in every patient. It is the best screen for both hypothyroidism (elevated sTSH—Chapter 14.4) and thyrotoxicosis (suppressed sTSH—Chapter 14.8). A family history of medullary thyroid cancer or multiple endocrine neoplasia, type II, warrants a basal serum calcitonin (4).

   B. **Diagnostic imaging.** Because diagnostic imaging cannot reliably differentiate benign from malignant nodules, it is not part of the routine assessment of thyroid nodules. Diagnostic imaging, however, may be helpful in certain circumstances. Ultrasonography can be useful when findings on palpation are inconclusive regarding the presence of a single nodule or a dominant nodule in a multinodular gland (5). Some clinicians also apply ultrasonography when an abnormality has been detected fortuitously by other imaging procedures or in patients with a history of head and neck irradiation (1). A radionuclide scan, usually done with ^{123}I, can also be helpful when thyroid palpation is inconclusive or to differentiate the functional status of nodules in a multinodular gland. A nodule identified as hyperfunctioning by radionuclide scan is almost invariably benign, but such lesions constitute less than 10% of all nodules.

   C. **Fine-needle aspiration biopsy (FNAB),** performed and interpreted by experienced individuals, is the most important test in the evaluation of thyroid nodules. In various studies, FNAB has demonstrated a sensitivity of 68% to 98% (mean, 83%) and specificity of 72% to 100% (mean, 92%). Use of FNAB has allowed many centers to increase the yield of thyroid cancer in excised nodules from 15% to 45% (2).

V. Diagnostic assessment. When the initial examination is suggestive of cancer, an immediate surgical consultation is appropriate. In all other patients, FNAB is the cornerstone in the evaluation of solitary or dominant thyroid nodules.

  A. Management strategy. The cytopathologic interpretation of the FNAB dictates management. If the specimen is insufficient for diagnosis, repeat FNAB is necessary. Even in experienced hands, approximately 10% of biopsies are nondiagnostic (1). If the biopsy is clearly benign, periodic follow-up is necessary. If the biopsy is malignant, suspicious, or indeterminate, surgical consultation is warranted.

  B. Follow-up. During follow-up of nodules not surgically explored, the significant historical and physical elements previously discussed should be reexamined. Although the intervals of follow-up will vary, based on patient and nodule characteristics, a standard protocol is to reexamine patients at intervals of 1.5, 3, 6, and 12 months, and then annually if the nodule is stable. Consider the judicious use of laboratory testing, diagnostic imaging, and repeat FNAB, again based on patient and nodule characteristics. Thyroid hormone suppression is commonly used in both the diagnosis and treatment of thyroid nodules. Recent controlled trials have raised questions about this practice. If suppressive therapy is considered, the risks associated with subclinical hyperthyroidism must be included in the risk-to-benefit analysis (2).

References

1. Singer PA, Cooper DS, Daniels GH, et al. Treatment guidelines for patients with thyroid nodules and well-differentiated thyroid cancer. *Arch Intern Med* 1996;156: 2165–2172.
2. Thyroid Nodule Task Force of the American Association of Clinical Endocrinologists and the American College of Endocrinology. AACE Clinical Practice Guidelines for the Diagnosis and Management of Thyroid Nodules. *Endocrine Prac* 1996;2:78–84.
3. Petrone LR. A primary care approach to the adult patient with nodular thyroid disease. *Arch Fam Med* 1996;5:92–100.
4. Mazzaferri EL. Management of a solitary thyroid nodule. *N Engl J Med* 1993;328: 553–559.
5. Tan GH, Gharib H. Solitary thyroid nodule: comparison between palpation and ultrasonography. *Arch Intern Med* 1995;155:2418–2423.

14.8 Thyrotoxicosis/Hyperthyroidism

Stephen F. Wheeler and David E. Bybee

Thyrotoxicosis affects 1.9% of women and 0.16% of men. Approximately 15% of cases occur in persons aged more than 60 years. Graves' disease is more common in younger patients, whereas toxic nodular goiter is more common in older patients. Although routine screening for thyrotoxicosis is controversial and may not be cost-effective, mild disease is often overlooked and atypical presentations of overt disease, more common in older patients, can delay diagnosis (1).

  I. Approach. Accurate diagnosis requires distinguishing between disorders that result from primary thyroid hyperactivity and those in which such hyperactivity is absent. Etiologic diagnosis is important because it influences both prognosis and therapy.

  A. Thyrotoxicosis is the clinical syndrome of increased metabolism caused by elevations of thyroid hormone, regardless of cause. In the absence of hyperthyroidism, thyrotoxicosis is usually secondary to thyroiditis or exogenous thyroid hormone.

B. **Hyperthyroidism** refers to a sustained increase in the production and secretion of thyroid hormone by the thyroid gland (2). Common causes of hyperthyroidism are Graves' disease, which accounts for up to 90% of cases, and toxic nodular goiter.

II. History

A. **Clinical features.** Severity can vary with duration of illness, magnitude of hormone excess, age of the patient, and presence of disease in other organs, such as the heart. Typical patient complaints include thyroid enlargement (depending on cause), dyspnea on exertion, fatigue, proximal muscle weakness (often manifested by difficulty with stair climbing), palpitations, heat intolerance, excessive sweating, tremor, weight loss, nervousness or emotional lability (more common in younger patients), decreased menstrual flow, alterations in appetite, frequent bowel movements, and sleep disturbances (3). A recent viral illness can be an antecedent for subacute thyroiditis.

B. **Effect of age.** Older patients present with fewer clinical features than younger patients. Tachycardia, fatigue, and weight loss are the only clinical features found in more than 50% of patients aged more than 70 years (4).

III. Physical examination (PE)

A. **Observation.** Clothing may be loose because of weight loss. Clothing choices may suggest inappropriate heat intolerance, whereas the welcoming handshake may present warm moist hands with a fine tremor. Other possible observations include nervousness or restlessness, a characteristic stare with widened palpebral fissures, lid lag and infrequent blinking, and silky fine hair.

B. **General examination.** Vital sign abnormalities commonly include weight loss, sinus tachycardia, arrhythmias, and systolic hypertension with a widened pulse pressure. Systolic murmurs, cardiac enlargement, and, occasionally, overt heart failure may be found on cardiovascular examination (Chapters 7.4, 7.5 and 7.7). Besides the classic stare noted above, Graves' disease can also present with proptosis (which may be asymmetric), ophthalmoplegia (with impaired conjugate eye movement and strabismus), orbital congestion (with periorbital edema and potential compression of the optic nerve), and inflammation of the conjunctiva and cornea. Pretibial myxedema, an unusual but pathognomonic finding in Graves' disease, is a painless raised thickening of the subcutaneous tissue, most often found in the anterior lower leg or dorsal foot. It produces a *peau d'orange* texture, which can be pruritic and hyperpigmented. Clubbing of the fingers and toes is also found in Graves' disease, but is very rare. An ovarian mass, usually unilateral, may indicate struma ovarii. Thyrotoxicosis (but not hyperthyroidism) can result from this teratoma, which infrequently produces thyroid hormone.

C. **Thyroid examination.** Inspect the neck below the thyroid cartilage from the front and side. During palpation, approach the patient from the front or from behind and palpate using the fingers or thumbs. Having the patient swallow during both inspection and palpation causes the thyroid to move and aids in developing a three-dimensional impression of the gland. The size, consistency, and tenderness of the gland are important, as are the presence and characteristics of any nodules. Auscultation of a bruit over the gland correlates with increased vascularity, usually indicative of Graves' disease.

IV. Testing

A. **Laboratory testing.** A sensitive assay for thyroid-stimulating hormone (sTSH) is the best test for detecting thyrotoxicosis. Thyrotoxicosis from any cause, except the extremely rare instance of excess TSH production, results in a suppressed sTSH. Thyrotoxicosis is confirmed by an elevated free thyroxine index (FTI) or an elevated free thyroxine (fT$_4$), measured directly. If the FTI or fT$_4$ is normal, T$_3$ should be measured to evaluate for T$_3$ toxicosis. Assays for thyroid autoantibodies, including TSH receptor antibodies, are usually not required. However, they can be helpful in selected cases (e.g., pregnancy, where levels correlate with risk to the fetus).

B. **Diagnostic imaging.** Radioactive iodine uptake (RAIU) can help clarify the cause of thyrotoxicosis. A diffuse increase in RAIU is consistent with Graves' disease, whereas nodular concentration is consistent with toxic adenoma (a single increased area) or multinodular goiter (multiple areas of increased uptake) (3). A decrease in RAIU is consistent with exogenous (iatrogenic or factitious) thyrotoxicosis, thyroiditis, iodine-induced thyrotoxicosis, or struma ovarii.

V. **Diagnostic assessment.** Accurate diagnosis depends on the appropriate combination and interpretation of history, PE, and testing.

A. **Graves' disease.** If ophthalmopathy is present, the diagnosis of Graves' disease is usually obvious. Typically, the thyroid gland is increased in size, smooth, and nontender. A bruit is present in 50% of patients. The RAIU is homogeneously increased and pretibial myxedema may be present.

B. **Toxic nodular goiter** is the most common cause of thyrotoxicosis in those aged more than 40 years. The thyroid gland is typically increased in size, nontender, but with multiple nodules. The RAIU is increased in a heterogeneous pattern. A single toxic nodule is more common in younger people and has the RAIU concentrated in one spot, with suppression of the remaining gland.

C. **Exogenous (iatrogenic or factitious) thyrotoxicosis** is associated with a gland that is small or normal sized and a low or absent RAIU. A psychiatric evaluation should be considered in factitious thyrotoxicosis.

D. **Thyroiditis.** Thyrotoxicosis can be produced as hormone leaks from an inflamed gland. Typically, the symptoms of the diverse thyroiditis entities are of recent onset and have escalated rapidly. The gland is enlarged and either tender (*subacute thyroiditis*) or nontender (*painless thyroiditis* or *postpartum thyroiditis*). RAIU is very low or absent. Transient hypothyroidism often follows as the intrathyroidal stores of hormone are depleted. *Acute suppurative thyroiditis* is a rare infectious disorder, usually caused by pyogenic organisms (5).

E. **Other diagnoses.** Thyrotoxicosis with hyperthyroidism and an inappropriately elevated sTSH suggests a TSH-secreting pituitary tumor. Thyrotoxicosis without hyperthyroidism and an increased RAIU over the pelvis suggests struma ovarii. A low sTSH with normal T_3 and FTI or fT_4 indicates subclinical hyperthyroidism or TSH suppression by nonthyroidal factors (e.g., corticosteroid administration or starvation).

References

1. Helfand M, Redfern CC. Screening for thyroid disease: an update. *Ann Intern Med* 1998;129:144–158.
2. Hennessey JV. Diagnosis and management of thyrotoxicosis. *Am Fam Physician* 1996;54:1315–1324.
3. Thyroid Guidelines Task Force of the American Association of Clinical Endocrinologists and the American College of Endocrinology. AACE Clinical Practice Guidelines for the Evaluation and Treatment of Hyperthyroidism and Hypothyroidism. *Endocrine Prac* 1995;1:54–62.
4. Trivalle C, Doucet J, Chassagne P, et al. Differences in the signs and symptoms of hyperthyroidism in older and younger patients. *J Am Geriatr Soc* 1996;44:50–53.
5. Sakiyama R. Thyroiditis: a clinical review. *Am Fam Physician* 1993;48:615–621.

15. VASCULAR AND LYMPHATIC SYSTEM PROBLEMS

PAUL M. PAULMAN

15.1 Lymphadenopathy, Generalized

Jeffrey D. Harrison

Lymph nodes of abnormal size, consistency, or number define lymphadenopathy. Generalized lymphadenopathy refers to these abnormal nodes when they are found in two or more noncontiguous sites. Generalized lymphadenopathy should prompt further investigation by the physician.

I. **Approach**
   A. **Epidemiology.** Few reliable studies exist regarding the incidence of unexplained lymphadenopathy; however, one large Dutch study places the incidence at 0.6% annually (1). Generalized lymphadenopathy comprises approximately 25% of these cases (3). No gender differences occur in regard to incidence (2). Nonspecific lymphadenopathy is found more frequently in those aged less than 40 years.
   B. **Causes.** Infectious, autoimmune, granulomatous, or malignant diseases can cause generalized lymphadenopathy. Studies have shown a 4% cancer risk in those patients older than 40 years and a 0.4% cancer risk in those less than 40 years who present with generalized lymphadenopathy (1). Lymphadenopathy present for more than a year is usually from a nonspecific cause, whereas that present less than 2 weeks usually has an infectious cause.
II. **History** should focus on those common causes of generalized lymphadenopathy.
   A. **History of present illness** should focus on the duration, location, quality, and context of the lymphadenopathy. Note associated signs and symptoms such as rash, fever, sore throat, and cough (4) (Chapters 2.6, 8.1, and 13.6). The goal is to ascertain if the adenopathy is attributable to a specific cause.
   B. **Past medical history** should focus on known illness, medication usage, and allergies. Serum sickness from antibiotic use as well as diphenylhydantoin for seizure prevention can cause generalized lymphadenopathy. Common chronic illnesses (e.g., lupus erythematosus and rheumatoid arthritis) can also cause generalized lymphadenopathy.
   C. **Social history** should focus on the patient's occupation, sexual history, and alcohol use. Hepatitis B, secondary syphilis, and early human immunodeficiency virus (HIV) can all present with generalized lymphadenopathy. Patients with Hodgkin's disease can develop painful adenopathy with alcohol use.
   D. **Family history.** Inquire about family illness with a genetic predisposition as well as any exposures to household contacts with infectious diseases (e.g., tuberculosis, infectious mononucleosis, or hepatitis B).
   E. **Review of systems** should focus on constitutional symptoms such as weight loss, fatigue, night sweats, malaise, arthralgias, nausea, and vomiting (1).
III. **Physical examination**
   A. **General.** A comprehensive physical examination should be performed on all patients with generalized lymphadenopathy. Focus on those findings consistent with the most frequent causes of generalized lymphadenopathy. Note the patient's temperature and weight, because fever and weight loss are frequent findings. Examine the skin, mucous membranes, abdominal organs, and joints; specifically, the presence of rash, mucocutaneous ulceration, organomegaly, and arthritis can be a guide to possible causes of the adenopathy. The presence of splenomegaly in a patient with adenopathy implies a systemic illness (e.g., infectious mononucleosis, lymphoma, leukemia, lupus, sarcoidosis, toxoplasmosis, or cat scratch disease) (Chapter 15.4). Additionally, search for other abnormal lymph nodes. Studies have shown that clinicians identified only 17% of those cases of generalized lymphadenopathy when it was present (1).

  B. **Nodal examination.** The abnormal lymph node groups should be specifically examined.
    1. **Size.** Lymph nodes enlarged up to 1 cm in diameter can be considered normal in size. These have a low malignancy risk and can usually be observed. Lymph nodes greater than 1.5 cm × 1.5 cm in area have been shown to have a 38% risk of cancer involvement and merit further workup (2).
    2. **Location.** Anterior cervical, submandibular, and inguinal nodes are normally palpable. The presence of supraclavicular adenopathy is always abnormal and carries a 90% cancer risk in those aged more than 40 years. Postocciptal nodes are associated with infectious mononucleosis, scalp lesions, toxoplasmosis, and non-Hodgkin's lymphoma. Axillary nodes are associated with upper extremity infections, breast cancer, cat scratch disease, and lymphomas. Epitrochlear nodes are associated with pyogenic infections, sarcoidosis, tularemia, and syphilis. Inguinal nodes are associated with lower extremity infections and sexually transmitted diseases.
    3. **Pain.** The presence or absence of pain is not a reliable indicator of the cause of adenopathy. Capsular swelling from acute infections can cause pain as can necrotic hemorrhage from a malignant lymph node.
    4. **Consistency.** Rock hard nodes are consistent with metastatic disease (2). Firm rubbery nodes are found with lymphomas. Soft nodes tend to occur with infectious causes; however, this should not be considered diagnostic.
IV. **Testing**
  A. **Primary laboratory test.** Initial laboratory testing should include a complete blood count (CBC) and a slide test for infectious mononucleosis (IM) (1). Atypical lymphocytes are suggestive of IM, cytomegalovirus, or toxoplasmosis. Neutropenia is found with viral illness, lupus, brucellosis, and bone marrow replacement. Severe anemia can be seen with malignancy and autoimmune processes. If the initial mononucleosis spot is negative, the test should be repeated at intervals of 1, 2, and 3 weeks, if atypical lymphocytes are present in the CBC.
  B. **Secondary testing.** If the initial laboratory results are nondiagnostic, order a purified protein derivative (PPD), antinuclear antibody, hepatitis B surface antigen, HIV, rapid plasma reagin, cytomegalovirus serology, and chest X-ray (CXR) study. Although the CXR is seldom positive, it can be helpful in finding tuberculosis (TB), histoplasmosis, lymphoma, or sarcoidosis. Although a PPD will not be diagnostic of TB, it can be helpful in differentiating sarcoid from TB on a node biopsy (2).
  C. **Lymph node biopsy.** If the aforementioned laboratory testing is nondiagnostic, then lymph node biopsy may be indicated. The largest and most pathologic node should be removed. Axillary and inguinal nodes should be avoided as they often reveal only reactive hyperplasia. Biopsy should be avoided in cases of suspected IM and drug reaction because the histologic picture is easily confused with malignant lymphoma (2). Experienced hematologists or hematopathologists should handle all specimens. The value of fine needle aspiration is controversial, with reasonable arguments both for and against (4).
V. **Diagnostic assessment.** Generalized lymphadenopathy merits evaluation beyond mere observation, as a specific systemic illness will be the likely cause. The history and examination should focus on infectious, autoimmune, granulomatous, and malignant causes. If a specific entity is suspected based on the history and physical examination, then that entity should be specifically evaluated. In the event the cause is unclear, first order a CBC and mononucleosis spot. If these are negative, then serologic testing and a CXR are warranted. Consider lymph node biopsy in those cases where the node is rock hard or larger than 1.5 cm × 1.5 cm in size (1). Biopsy should be avoided in those cases where viral causes are clinically suggested.

References
1. Ferrer R. Lymphadenopathy: differential diagnosis and evaluation. *Am Fam Physician* 1998;58:1313–1320.
2. Pangalis GA, Vassilalopoulos TP, Boussiotis VA, Fessas P. Clinical approach to lymphadenopathy. *Semin Oncol* 1993;20:570–582.
3. Williamson HA. Lymphadenopathy in a family practice. *J Fam Pract* 1985;20: 449–452.
4. Henry P, Longo D. Enlargement of lymph nodes and spleen. *Harrison's on line* 1999;61. www.harrisonsonline.com/

15.2 Lymphadenopathy, Localized

Laeth S. Nasir

I. **Approach.** In clinical practice, the enlargement of a single lymph node or multiple contiguous lymph nodes is observed most commonly as a reaction to a well-defined process (e.g., impetigo or cellulitis) and requires no attention beyond treatment of the primary condition. However, lymphadenopathy as a primary complaint is often seen, and it requires further evaluation. Knowledge of the lymphatic drainage patterns of various regions of the body and the pathologic conditions most likely to affect these areas is critical in evaluating localized lymphadenopathy. The context in which lymphadenopathy is seen is very important. The age of the patient, the past medical history, and the presence of associated symptoms are all factors that need to be taken to account when planning a diagnostic assessment (1).

The lymphatic tissue of children is prominent when compared with that of adults. In fact, the absence of palpable lymph nodes in a child is sometimes the first clinical manifestation of an underlying immune deficiency. Viral or minor bacterial infections can lead to reactive lymphadenopathy, which is sometimes dramatic. The likelihood that lymphadenopathy is secondary to a benign process falls with increasing age. Patients aged less than 30 years are found to have a benign process causing their lymphadenopathy 80% of the time. However, 60% of individuals aged more than 50 years without a clear cause for localized lymphadenopathy will be found to have a malignancy on further evaluation (2).

II. **History.** A comprehensive history is critical in evaluating lymphadenopathy. It is important to elicit as accurately as possible the time course of the process. Progressive enlargement of a lymph node over several weeks or months suggests an underlying malignancy or granulomatous inflammation (e.g., tuberculosis or sarcoidosis). However, reactive lymphadenopathy can also persist for months. The presence of localizing or systemic signs (e.g., weight loss, night sweats, rash, or fever) suggests a particular pathologic process. Epidemiologic clues such as exposure to cats may suggest cat scratch disease. A history of contact with a new sexual partner raises the possibility of a sexually transmitted disease. Manifestations of regional lymphadenopathy within the thorax or abdomen can present as cough, shortness of breath, abdominal pain, urinary frequency, or intestinal obstruction. Rarely, pain in an area of lymphadenopathy following alcohol ingestion is the presenting symptom of Hodgkin's disease.

III. **Physical examination.** On physical examination, the first question that needs to be answered is whether the structure being palpated is truly a lymph node. Parotid enlargement, thyroid masses, sternocleidomastoid tumors, dermoid cysts, hemangiomas, or other tumors occasionally mimic lymphadenopathy. Thoroughly examine the anatomic region or regions drained by the affected nodes. Carefully note the characteristics of the lymph nodes and surrounding tissues. Tender lymph nodes that are mobile often represent lymphadenitis or acute inflammation. Matted, hard lymph nodes that are fixed to surrounding tissue imply an underlying metastatic carcinoma. Rubbery, nontender nodes may be seen in lymphoma.

In otherwise healthy children, lymph nodes up to 2.5 cm in diameter, particularly in the inguinal, suboccipital, and cervical regions, may be seen (3). In adults, lymph nodes larger than 1 cm in diameter should arouse suspicion, and nodes larger than 3 cm are highly suggestive of a malignant process (2). In both children and adults, supraclavicular lymph nodes larger than 1 or 2 cm in diameter should be investigated aggressively.

IV. Testing. Testing is often done to uncover pathology involving the region of the body drained by the affected lymph nodes. For example, cultures for venereal disease may be obtained in inguinal adenopathy, or sinus films in cervical adenopathy if clinically indicated. Consider radiographic techniques such as ultrasound or computerized tomographic scanning of the thorax or abdomen if lymphadenopathy is suspected in these locations. In some cases, watchful waiting may be diagnostically useful. In cases where a serious condition is suspected or cannot be ruled out, the test of choice is an excisional biopsy of the node or nodes involved. The lymph node chosen for biopsy is important. In general, it is preferable to obtain a biopsy from large nodes that have recently enlarged. Mediastinal nodes can be biopsied via bronchoscopy, mediastinoscopy, or thoracotomy. Intraabdominal adenopathy can be evaluated by fluoroscopically guided needle biopsy or exploratory laparotomy. The biopsy material obtained by any of these methods can be submitted for both pathologic study and bacteriologic testing. In lymph nodes that are fluctuant, consider needle aspiration or biopsy. Carefully follow up patients who are diagnosed as having nonspecific changes or reactive hyperplasia, because a proportion of these will ultimately be diagnosed as having a lymphoma. Patients who are human immunodeficiency virus-positive or have a history of a previous malignancy have a higher likelihood of serious pathology, and the threshold for aggressive investigation should be low (4).

V. Diagnostic assessment. The cause of localized lymphadenopathy can be conveniently classified based on the location of the enlarged nodes. Enlarged occipital nodes, which are common in children, most often are caused by scalp infections such as tinea capitis. Seborrheic dermatitis, rubella, and roseola are other common causes. In both children and adults, enlarged preauricular nodes caused by conjunctival infections or cat scratch disease may be seen. Cervical adenopathy can be caused by infections of the sinuses, pharynx, or soft tissues of the face. In children, Kawasaki's disease can result in cervical adenopathy, which may be unilateral. Acute leukemias, rhabdomyosarcoma, or neuroblastoma can also present in this way (5). Hodgkin's disease or non-Hodgkin's lymphoma can present with cervical adenopathy. Squamous cell carcinoma from the nasopharynx or laryngeal area is a common occurrence in older individuals.

Supraclavicular lymphadenopathy is a particularly worrisome finding in both children and adults, as this pattern of nodal enlargement is frequently associated with granulomatous conditions and malignancies. Classically, the right supraclavicular area is described as receiving drainage from the intrathoracic organs, whereas the left supraclavicular lymph nodes drain the abdomen. The supraclavicular lymph nodes also receive lymphatic drainage from the breasts. Enlarged axillary nodes may be seen secondary to inflammatory or malignant disease of the upper extremity, or breast, as a reaction to immunizations in the ipsilateral arm, and occasionally in autoimmune disorders such as juvenile rheumatoid arthritis. Isolated epitrochlear or popliteal lymphadenopathy is most commonly caused by local infection; however, local melanoma should be carefully excluded. Enlarged inguinal nodes are most commonly caused by local infection. In children, this includes diaper dermatitis and infections of the lower extremities. In adults, lymphogranuloma venereum or syphilis commonly presents with unilateral inguinal adenopathy. Common causes of mediastinal adenopathy include bronchogenic carcinoma, lymphoma, tuberculosis or sarcoidosis, histoplasmosis or coccidioidomycosis, and Hodgkin's disease. Intraabdominal adenopathy is often caused by Hodgkin's and non-Hodgkin's lymphoma or tuberculosis.

References
1. Slap GB, Connor JL, Wigton RS, Schwartz JS. Validation of a model to identify young patients for lymph node biopsy. *JAMA* 1986;225:2768–2773.
2. Simon HB. Evaluation of lymphadenopathy. In: Goroll AH, May LA, Mulley AG. *Primary care medicine: office evaluation and management of the adult patient*, 3rd ed. Philadelphia: JB Lippincott, 1995:54–58.
3. Bedros AA, Mann JP. Lymphadenopathy in children. *Adv Pediatr* 1981;28:341–376.
4. Ferrer R. Lymphadenopathy: differential diagnosis and evaluation. *Am Fam Physician* 1998;58:1313–1320.
5. Marcy SM. Cervical adenitis. *Pediatr Infect Dis J* 1985;4:S23–S26.

15.3 Petechiae and Purpura

John L. Smith

Purpura are the visible extravasation of blood into the skin or mucous membranes. Petechiae are purpura less than 2 mm in diameter and ecchymoses are greater than 1 cm in diameter.

I. **Approach.** Purpura are a sign of another illness or pathologic process. After initially ruling out emergent or life-threatening disorders, which are the norm in newborns and occasionally with infectious causes, a specific cause is sought. Purpuric rashes are secondary to a quantitative or qualitative platelet abnormality, coagulation disorder, or congenital or acquired vascular disorder.

II. **History**

   A. **Have there been any recent illnesses?** Henoch-Schönlein purpura is associated with a preceding upper respiratory infection in 60% to 75% of cases (1). *Streptococcus pneumoniae* is the most commonly cited organism. Various other infections may be responsible for thrombocytopenias and vasculitis.

   B. **Has there been any recent medication usage?** Quinidine, quinine, sulfa, aspirin, and many other medications have been associated with purpuric lesions.

   C. **Are there any additional symptoms, such as abdominal or joint pain, or gastrointestinal symptoms including changes in stool characteristics?** Henoch-Schönlein purpura is associated with all of these; abdominal pain is noted in 40% to 80% of patients (1).

   D. **Is there a history of heavy menses or mucous membrane bleeding?** Coagulation abnormalities such as von Willebrand's disease (present in 0.5% to 1% of the population) or platelet abnormalities are most likely (3) (Chapter 11.5).

   E. **Is there a history of prior transfusions or heavy bleeding with previous operations?**

   F. **Are there risk factors for a history of liver disease?** There may be impaired synthesis of coagulation factors.

   G. **Has there been a similar rash in the past?** A long history of purpura may be present in idiopathic thrombocytopenic purpura (ITP) as it tends to be a chronic course with an insidious onset in adults.

   H. **If the patient is a newborn, was there maternal illness, drug exposure, maternal ITP, or was vitamin K given?** Hemorrhagic disease of the newborn develops on the second or third day of life. The most common causes of *purpura fulminans* in the neonatal period are congenital deficiencies of proteins C and S (1).

III. **Physical examination**

   A. **General and vital signs.** Does the patient appear toxic or unstable? Considerations would include meningococcemia, Rocky Mountain spotted fever,

disseminated intravascular coagulation (DIC), sepsis from *Staphylococcus aureus*, or thrombotic thrombocytopenic purpura.
- **B. Skin.** Purpura should not blanch or only partially blanch with pressure. Petechiae are generally indicative of a quantitative or qualitative platelet abnormality. These nonpalpable petechiae may be caused by thrombocytopenia, which is either congenital or acquired (Chapter 16.7). The acquired thrombocytopenia can be caused by decreased platelet production as seen with viral infections, B_{12} or folate deficiency, iron deficiency, or a drug reaction. It is also seen with evidence of platelet destruction as present in ITP, connective tissue disease, leukemia, drugs, DIC, and thrombotic thrombocytopenic purpura. Abnormal platelet function is seen with aspirin ingestion, kidney and liver dysfunction, and in the thrombocytosis seen with myeloproliferative disorders. Significant straining with the Valsalva maneuver can cause petechiae. Lastly, the chronic pigmented purpura are the brown-orange spots occasionally seen on the lower extremities of adults. Schamberg's disease is the most frequently seen and well known of the group. In these disorders, petechia are often intermixed with the pigmentation.

  Ecchymoses are usually associated with coagulation disorders (e.g., in hemophilia, von Willebrand's disease, anticoagulant usage, DIC, and vitamin K deficiency). Also responsible for ecchymoses are weakened connective tissue with less protection for vessels, as in senile purpura; glucocorticoid excess; vitamin C deficiency; and congenital disorders, such as Ehlers–Danlos syndrome.

  Palpable purpura are usually secondary to a vasculitis. The causes are many and include hypersensitivity vasculitis to drugs; infections, including viral, rickettsial, and bacterial illnesses; cryoglobulinemias, such as Waldenström's; and granulomatous causes, such as Wegener's granulomatosis.
- **IV. Testing**
  - **A. Test selection.** Initial laboratory: Complete blood count (CBC), platelet count, peripheral smear, prothrombin time (PT), activated partial thromboplastin time (APTT), and possibly a bleeding time (3). If the lesions appear vasculitic, consider a sedimentation rate and C-reactive protein determination. Serum creatinine and urinalysis can be ordered to screen for renal involvement. In vasculitis, the laboratory findings are often nonspecific and a skin biopsy for histology is employed (2).
  - **B. Significance of test results**
    1. Isolated thrombocytopenia: most often ITP in nonpregnant women. Without atypical features, no follow-up laboratory study is recommended (4).
    2. Isolated, increased APTT: low levels of factors VIII, IX, XI. Follow-up studies: factor VIII level and von Willebrand's factor assay and activity.
       A slightly increased APTT and slightly decreased factor VIII are consistent with von Willebrand's disease. A very prolonged APTT and very low factor VIII is consistent with an acquired factor VIII inhibitor (3).
    3. Thrombocytopenia with increased PT, APTT: consider DIC and liver failure. Follow-up study: d-dimer, fibrinogen, fibrin degradation products.
       In newborns with purpura, evaluation for sepsis, serologies for the TORCH syndrome (acronym for Toxoplasmosis, Other infections, Rubella, Cytomegalovirus infection, and Herpes simplex), and coagulation factors are also recommended. Proteins C and S activities are also indicated in purpura fulminans (diffuse ecchymoses that become bullous and necrotic); neutropenia or abnormal neutrophils may indicate leukemia. Other laboratory tests when evaluating vasculitis can include complement levels, antinuclear antibody, and cryoglobulins.
- **V. Diagnostic assessment (4).** With petechiae resulting from lone thrombocytopenia, ITP may be difficult to differentiate from pregnancy-induced thrombocytopenia (which tends to be milder), viral infection, or drugs. ITP is designated if no other clinically obvious cause is noted.

  Thrombotic-thrombocytopenic purpura (TTP) and hemolytic uremic syndrome (HUS) are seen in many clinical situations, including pregnancy, cancer, infections, chemotherapy, and so on. Signs include the pentad of fever, thrombocytopenia, microangioipathic hemolytic anemia, hemorrhage (including purpura), and neurologic abnormalities. Because of serious consequences, the diagnosis should be considered if thrombocytopenia and fragmented red blood cells are seen on the peripheral smear. TTP-HUS has a normal PT, APTT, and d-dimer as opposed to DIC.

In regard to coagulation factor abnormalities, hemophilia A and B can cause increased bruising and ecchymoses but not nearly as frequently as von Willebrand's disease. Children being investigated for nonaccidental bruising should be evaluated for coagulation disorders with a CBC, platelet count, PT, APTT, and a bleeding time. With the sudden onset of large ecchymoses and hematomas in an adult with normal platelets, an acquired factor VIII deficiency (autoantibody) should be investigated in cases of a prolonged PT, APTT.

In newborns, a blueberry muffin baby (from extramedullary hematopoiesis) may appear purpuric, and this condition must be differentiated from purpura fulminans secondary to protein C or S deficiency, or sepsis.

Vasculitis causing palpable purpura in children is most common with Henoch–Schönlein purpura. In connective tissue diseases, purpuric lesions are usually a secondary finding.

The causes of purpuric lesions are many. A thorough history and physical examination, along with some basic laboratory studies and an occasional skin biopsy, are all that is needed to establish a likely diagnosis.

References

1. Baselga E, Drolet BA, Esterly NB. Purpura in infants and children. *J Am Acad Dermatol* 1997;37:673–705.
2. Cuttica RJ. Vasculitis in children: a diagnostic challenge. *Curr Probl Pediatr* 1997 27:309–317.
3. Loserh JM. Screening and diagnosis of coagulation disorders. *Am J Obstet Gynecol* 1996;175:778–783.
4. Diagnosis and treatment of idiopathic thrombocytopenic purpura: Recommendations of the American Society of Hematology. The American Society of Hematology ITP Practice Guideline Panel. *Ann Intern Med* 1997;126:319–326.

15.4 Splenomegaly

Audrey Paulman

The spleen is an encapsulated reticuloendothelial organ in the left upper quadrant of the abdomen with two basic functions: (a) the white pulp makes humoral antibodies, B and T lymphocytes, and plasma cells; and (b) the red pulp scavenges unneeded matter from the blood, including such items as Howell-Jolly bodies, bacteria, and aging blood cells.

I. **Approach.** Most cases of splenomegaly are caused by familial or acquired needs for increased scavenger activity, disease process infiltrating the spleen, abnormal blood flow, or infectious disease.

II. **History**

  A. **Presentation.** The most common symptom of splenomegaly is a heaviness in the left upper quadrant of the abdomen. The patient may have pain believed to be caused by stretching of the splenic capsule. However, splenomegaly can be entirely asymptomatic. Even rupture of the spleen by trauma or disease process can be without pain.

  A history of fevers, night sweats, pain, and fatigue might lead to an infectious cause, whereas alcohol abuse and a history of liver or heart failure would be important in splenomegaly caused by abnormal blood flow.

  B. **Family history** may give clues to inherited red blood cell disorders and inherited disorders of metabolism.

III. Physical examination. The diagnosis of splenomegaly is made by palpation of a mass in the left upper quadrant. *Harrison's Textbook of Medicine* cites that a spleen is palpable in 3% of normal college freshmen, whereas in tropical countries, the incidence of splenomegaly may reach 60% (1). Percussion is also used to delineate the size of the spleen. Percussion is only approximately 60% accurate in most studies, with palpation about 50% accurate. To palpate the spleen, the patient is in the supine position with the knees flexed to decrease abdominal muscle tone. Begin the examination by palpating the right lower quadrant and move upward across the abdomen as the patient breathes in deeply. Beginning the examination low in the abdomen, allows the lower edge of a markedly enlarged spleen to be detected.

IV. Testing

  A. Diagnostic imaging. The most accurate methods of determining spleen size include nuclear scans, computed tomography (CT) scan, and ultrasound. Ultrasound offers the most sensitivity and specificity, with the widest availability at the lowest cost. Magnetic resonance imaging has an advantage over CT scan in that it allows for delineating the blood flow patterns that cause congestion in the spleen. None of the methods are reliable in determining the underlying cause of splenomegaly.

  B. Clinical laboratory tests. Most of the laboratory tests used in splenomegaly are those used to delineate other systemic disease processes (2–4). A complete blood count with peripheral smear will identify many of the hematologic diseases that cause splenomegaly. These include elevated white blood cell levels associated with leukemias, spherocytes in spherocytosis, and anemias. A bone marrow biopsy may show increased production of those cells that are low in the peripheral blood, leading to the diagnosis of hypersplenism. Also, the biopsy may show lymphocyte infiltration, increased myeloid elements, blast cells, fibrosis, abnormal staining in disease processes (e.g., amyloidosis), and macrophages in storage-related diseases (2).

  Studies such as ^{51}CR-labeled red blood cell count, platelet survival, and splenic survival studies help to determine if the spleen is sequestering an abnormal number of cells.

V. Diagnostic assessment

  A. The diseases that are associated with splenomegaly include:

  1. Infectious diseases. Infectious mononucleosis, bacterial endocarditis, tuberculosis, sarcoidosis, acquired immune deficiency syndrome, cytomegalovirus infection, hepatitis, splenic abscess, histoplasmosis, and tropical diseases.

  2. Inflammatory diseases. Connective tissue disease, Felty's syndrome, and serum sickness.

  3. Abnormal blood flow. Cirrhosis; hepatic, splenic, or portal vein obstruction; and portal hypertension.

  4. Storage diseases. Gaucher's disease, Nieman–Pick disease, and Hand-Schuller-Christian disease.

  5. Infiltrative disease. Leukemia, lymphoma, and Hodgkin's disease.

  6. Chronic anemia. Spherocytosis, sickle cell disease, and thalassemia.

  B. Hypersplenism occurs when the size and activity of the spleen interfere with normal cells in the peripheral blood and increased bone marrow production of these cells. The treatment of hypersplenism is reversal of the underlying cause or splenectomy. Splenectomy can be performed by a laparoscopic technique. Preoperative pneumococcal vaccine should be considered for patients undergoing splenectomy.

References

1. Fauci A, Braunwald E, Isselbacher K, et al., eds. *Harrison's principles of internal medicine*, 14th ed. New York: McGraw-Hill, 1998:347–350.
2. Nelson W, Behrman R, Kliegman R, Arvin A, eds. *Nelson textbook of pediatrics*, 15th ed. Philadelphia: WB Saunders, 1996:1439.
3. Rakel R. *Saunders manual of medical practice*. Philadelphia: WB Saunders, 1996:610.
4. Ferrer R. Lymphadenopathy: differential diagnosis and evaluation. *Am Fam Physician* 1998;58(6):1313–1320.

16. LABORATORY ABNORMALITIES: HEMATOLOGY AND URINE DETERMINATIONS

LARS C. LARSEN

16.1 Anemia

S. Shekar Chakravarthi

Anemia is defined as a reduction of more than 10% below mean values in the quantity or quality of the concentration of red blood cells (RBC) or circulating hemoglobin. In 1972, the World Health Organization standardized the normal hemoglobin values for men and women as 13 g/dl and 12 g/dl, respectively. Variations for age include children aged 6 months to 2 years, 10.5 g/dl; 2 to 12 years, 11.5 g/dl; in men aged more than 65 years, a 1 to 2 g/dl decline may be seen, probably because of decreased androgen production (1).

I. **Approach**
   A. **Classification.** Anemia can be categorized based on the size of the RBCs (mean corpuscular volume, MCV) or the cause of the anemia:
      1. Size. Microcytic (MCV < 80 FL); normocytic (MCV 80 to 100 FL); macrocytic (MCV > 100 FL).
      2. Etiology.
         a. Hypoproliferative or caused by decreased red cell production from:
            i. Reduced iron supply (e.g., blood loss, chronic inflammation, or malnutrition)
            ii. Decreased stimulus (e.g., renal disease or hypothyroidism)
            iii. Marrow defect (e.g., drugs, fibrosis, or tumors)
         b. Hemolytic or caused by red cell destruction (e.g., decreased red cell survival time)
            i. Immunologic: idiopathic or secondary to drugs
            ii. Extrinsic: mechanical or caused by a lytic substance
         c. Ineffective hematopoiesis
            i. Megaloblastic anemias (abnormality in nuclear maturation)
            ii. Thalassemia and sideroblastic anemia (abnormality at cytoplasmic maturation).
      3. Worldwide, the most common type of anemia results from iron deficiency. Among hospitalized patients, the most common form is anemia of chronic disease.
   B. **Screening for anemia.** Patients at risk, where screening may prove useful, include those who are institutionalized, of African descent, have poor nutritional status, and those who have had a gastrectomy (2).
II. **History.** The severity of symptoms is directly related to the rapidity of anemia development. Fatigue and a decreased level of activity may be noticed with mild anemia. In those with cardiovascular disease, angina, palpitations, or dyspnea on exertion, headaches or dizziness may be the presenting symptom. In the elderly, the symptoms may be more subtle and vague. Other relevant history includes the use of prescription and over-the-counter medications, exposure to toxic agents or chemicals (e.g., lead), alcohol use, history of cancer, history of surgery, type of diet, and a family history of anemia. In younger women, menstrual and reproductive histories will be helpful.
III. **Physical examination.** The patient may appear pale, tachycardia may be present unless blocked by a drug, and the patient may have orthostatic hypotension. A systolic murmur may be heard. Dark stool that is hematoccult positive suggests gastrointestinal bleeding. Jaundice can indicate increased red cell destruction. Bone tenderness, lymphadenopathy, splenomegaly, or neurologic signs can suggest diagnoses such as multiple myeloma and other malignancies, hypersplenism, or vitamin B_{12} deficiency.
IV. **Testing.** Complete blood count with red cell indices, reticulocyte count, and peripheral blood smear examination is the initial step, and subsequent workup will depend on these results. The red cell indices along with the red cell distribution width (RDW) (normal, = 13 ± 1.5) will help to differentiate anemias (Table 16.1).

Table 16.1 Red blood cell indices and red cell distribution width (RDW) in the diagnosis of anemia

	Increased RDW	Normal RDW
Low MCV	Iron deficiency, thalassemias	Anemia of chronic disease, thalassemia traits
Normal MCV	Early iron deficiency, uremia, liver disease, myelofibrosis, sideroblastic anemia	Anemia of chronic disease, hemorrhage, hypothyroidism, chronic lymphocytic leukemia, chronic myelocytic leukemia
High MCV	Vitamin B_{12} deficiency, folate deficiency, and immune hemolytic anemias	Aplastic anemia, preleukemia, alcohol and other drugs

MCV, mean corpuscular volume.
Reticulocyte index = observed reticular count × packed cell volume (PCV)% / normal PCV.
If the reticulocyte count is less than 2%, the anemia is due to inadequate production of red cells.
If the index is greater than 2%, the anemia is due to increased loss from bleeding or destruction.
Reticulocyte count should be corrected for the degree of anemia.

V. **Diagnostic assessment**. In iron deficiency anemia, the serum iron and ferritin level will be low with an elevated total iron binding capacity (TIBC). In some cases, ferritin can be falsely elevated as an acute phase reactant. Also, with adequate iron replacement therapy, a rise of 2 g/dl in hemoglobin can be expected in 3 weeks (3).

In contrast, in anemia of chronic disease the TIBC is not elevated, ferritin is normal, serum iron may be low or normal, and the hemoglobin is usually more than 8 g/dl. Subacute or chronic inflammation can cause sideropenic anemia; nonsideropenic anemias can result from kidney, liver, thyroid, or adrenal failure.

Depending on the history, a lead level may be indicated, especially in children (4). Hemoglobin electrophoresis is performed when sickle cell traits or thalassemias are suspected. Decreased plasma haptoglobin, elevated serum lactate dehydrogenase, and hemoglobinuria can indicate increased intravascular hemolysis; a positive Coombs' test indicates immune-mediated red cell destruction. Premature destruction can occur from prosthetic valves, G-6-PD or pyruvate deficiency, or it can be drug induced or caused by cold or warm antibodies.

In macrocytic anemias a serum Vitamin B_{12}, folate, and thyroid stimulating hormone may be checked. Other causes include leukemias, hemolytic anemia, alcohol, or drugs.

Indications for a bone marrow aspiration include pancytopenia, presence of immature cells in the peripheral blood, or an unexplained normocytic anemia (5). Marrow biopsy is considered if aspiration is unsuccessful or if myelofibrosis or metastatic cancer is suspected.

References

1. Welborn JL, Meyers FJ. A three point approach to anemia. *Postgrad Med* 1991;89(2): 179–183, 186.
2. Farley PC, Foland J. Iron deficiency anemia: how to diagnose and correct. *Postgrad Med* 1990;87(2):89–93, 96, 101.
3. Massey AC. Microcytic anemia: differential diagnosis and management of iron deficiency anemia. *Med Clin North Am* 1992;76(3):549–566.
4. Kline NE. A practical approach to the child with anemia. *J Pediatr Health Care* 1996;10(3):99–105.
5. Colon-Otero G, Menke D, Hook CC. A practical approach to the differential diagnosis and evaluation of the adult patient with anemia. *Med Clin North Am* 1992; 76(3):581–597.

16.2 Eosinophilia

Samuel B. Adkins, III

Eosinophilia is an elevation of the peripheral eosinophil count above the normal value of 350 to 500 cells/mm^3. It is most commonly associated with allergic disease (United States) or parasitic disease (worldwide) (1).

  I. **Approach.** Eosinophilia occurs in many different conditions. A detailed history and physical examination will guide the testing and lead to a diagnosis.
 II. **History**
   A. **Allergic disease.** Included in this category are allergic rhinitis, asthma, atopic dermatitis, angioneurotic edema, and urticaria.
     1. Allergic rhinitis can cause rhinitis, itchy eyes, pharyngitis, or cough.
     2. Patients with asthma may complain of cough, chest pain, shortness of breath, or wheezing (Chapter 8.9).
     3. Atopic dermatitis, angioneurotic edema, and urticaria all produce itchy rashes (Chapter 13.5).
     4. Angioneurotic edema produces swelling of the oropharynx.
     5. Urticaria produces a wheal and a flare-type rash (Chapter 13.7).
   B. **Parasitic disease.** Strongyloidiasis, trichinosis, echinococcosis, cysticercosis, schistosomiasis, filariasis, and toxocariasis can all be associated with eosinophilia.
     1. Abdominal pain and a change in bowel habits are common in gastrointestinal parasitic infection.
     2. Consumption of infected meat can cause trichinosis and result in muscle soreness, malaise, and fever.
     3. A history of travel to an area endemic for parasitic infections suggests parasitic infection as the cause of eosinophilia.
   C. **Neoplastic disease.** Malignancies associated with eosinophilia include bronchogenic, cervical, liver, pancreatic, kidney, and breast carcinomas; Hodgkin's lymphoma; and T-cell and eosinophilic leukemia (2).
     1. Unexplained weight loss, night sweats, skeletal pain, change in bowel habits with or without bleeding, painless jaundice, and fatigue can indicate the presence of one of these malignancies.
     2. A family history of one of these types of malignancies may be found.
   D. **Medications (prescription and over-the-counter).** The list of medications that can produce eosinophilia includes phenytoin, sulfonamides, aspirin, allopurinol, and, in the past, contaminated L-tryptophan (eosinophilia myalgia syndrome) (3).
   E. **Collagen vascular disease.** Systemic lupus erythematosus, polyarteritis nodosa, scleroderma, and the rare Churg–Strauss syndrome (hypereosinophilia, systemic vaculitis, and asthma) can have associated eosinophilia.
   F. **Adrenal insufficiency.** Primary or secondary adrenal insufficiency can produce eosinophilia. Possible symptoms include fatigue, anorexia, nausea, hypotension, abdominal pain, and increased skin pigmentation.
   G. **Human immunodeficiency virus.** Sexual promiscuity or sex with an infected partner, blood transfusion, and intravenous drug use are risk factors for human immunodeficiency virus (HIV).
   H. **Other eosinophilic syndromes.** Eosinophilia is also seen in idiopathic hypereosinophic syndrome, Löffler's syndrome (pulmonary symptoms with *Ascaris* infection), Will's syndrome (pruritic rash), and Shulman's syndrome (muscle pain and weakness).
III. **Physical examination**
   A. All patients should have measurements of vital signs, as well as examination of the skin, lymph nodes, thyroid gland, breasts, heart, lungs, and abdomen. Adults should have pelvic and rectal examination.

  B. Muscle and joint examinations should be done in symptomatic patients.

  C. Neurologic examination should be done for patients suspected of having the idiopathic hypereosinophilic syndrome.

IV. Testing

  A. Examination of the peripheral blood smear may reveal microcytic anemia, suggesting blood loss (parasitic disease or malignancy).

  B. Urinalysis should be done looking for white blood cells and proteinuria.

  C. Three stool specimens should be examined for ova and parasites.

  D. The patient's age, symptoms, and family history should direct cancer screening (colonoscopy, mammography, chest radiographs, and so on).

  E. The patient's history and physical examination should direct other testing (HIV, liver function tests, corticotropin stimulation test, chest radiographs, and so forth).

V. Diagnostic assessment. Determining the cause of eosinophilia requires knowledge of the possible causes and some detective work. Because of their frequency, allergic disease and parasitic infections must always be considered. Those patients who either lack symptoms or have nonspecific symptoms (e.g., weight loss, malaise, or fatigue), require a thorough history looking for increased risk of neoplastic, collagen vascular, immunodefiency or adrenal disease, which is then followed by appropriate laboratory testing. Several drugs (noted above) are known to cause eosinophilia. Others, which are not yet associated with eosinophilia, may also lead to this condition. These include prescription as well as over-the-counter products.

References

1. Rothenberg ME. Eosinophilia. *N Engl J Med* 1998;338:1592–1599.
2. Grathwohl K, LeBrun C, Tenglin R. Eosinophilia of the blood. *Postgrad Med* 1995;97:169–172.
3. Blackburn WD. Eosinophilia myalgia syndrome. *Semin Arthritis Rheum* 1997;26: 788–793.

16.3 Erythrocyte Sedimentation Rate, Elevated

Joseph P. Garry

 I. Approach. The erythrocyte sedimentation rate (ESR) is an acute phase reactant, which is sensitive but nonspecific. The two main determinants of the ESR are the degree of red blood cell aggregation and the packed cell volume. As such, the ESR is influenced by erythrocyte membrane characteristics, hematocrit levels, and levels of plasma proteins, such as fibrinogen, α_2-macroglobulin, immunoglobulins, and albumin (Table 16.2) (1–4).

 II. History. The ESR has been considered a measure of the presence and intensity of inflammation or tissue destruction within the body. The Westergren method is currently recommended for use in the clinical setting by the International Committee for Standardization in Hematology (4).

III. Physical examination

  A. The ESR is a test to be used in conjunction with a thorough physical examination. An ESR alone should serve only as a guide and not a screen, and only in symptomatic patients.

  B. Age, gender, race, and pregnancy have each been demonstrated to alter the ESR, with higher rates found in the elderly, females, African-Americans, and pregnant women (1–2,4–5).

IV. Testing

  A. The ESR is both a rapid and inexpensive test.

Table 16.2 Factors known to alter the sedimentation rate (1–5)

Increase	Decrease
Anemia	Microcytosis
Macrocytosis	Anisocytosis
Hypercholesterolemia	Spherocytosis
African-American race	Polycythemia
Female sex	Marked leukocytosis
Pregnancy (oral contraceptives)	Sickle cell disease
Elderly	Congestive heart failure
Inflammation or infection	
Heparin	
ESR > 100 mm/h	**ESR < 10 mm/h**
Abscess	Polycythemia vera
Subacute bacterial endocarditis	Macroglobulinemia
Osteomyelitis	Hypofibrinogenemia
Temporal arteritis	Disseminated intravascular coagulation
Collagen vascular disease	Massive hepatic necrosis
Multiple myeloma	Cachexia
Leukemia or lymphoma	Chronic fatigue syndrome
Neoplasm	Trichinosis
Drug hypersensitivity reactions	

ESR, erythrocyte sedimentation rate.

B. The modified Westergren method uses anticoagulated venous blood (in EDTA), which is placed in a 200-mm glass tube with a 2.5-mm internal diameter. At the end of 1 hour, the distance from the meniscus to the top of the column of erythrocytes is recorded as the ESR and expressed in millimeters per hour.

C. The range of "normal values" is generally determined by each laboratory performing the test. Although age, gender, and race are known to affect the ESR, the choice of an upper limit of normal is somewhat arbitrary. An empirical formula for the derivation of the value of the ESR, which includes 98% of healthy persons aged 20 to 65 years, is for men, age in years divided by two; for women, age in years plus ten, divided by two (5).

V. **Diagnostic assessment**

A. **The ESR should never be used as a screening test in asymptomatic patients.** An isolated finding of a very low ESR in this group has little clinical significance (<6% of patients with an ESR <1 mm/h are diagnosed with a disease associated with a low ESR) (1,3). An elevated ESR in an asymptomatic patient is best evaluated by a period of watchful waiting and retesting at a later date, as 60% or more of such findings will revert to normal (2).

B. **The ESR is most helpful when extreme elevations are observed** (>100 mm/h) because of the very low false–positive rate for serious underlying disease. It is less helpful, diagnostically, when elevations in the range of 25 to 50 mm/h are observed because these suggest a wide variety of illnesses (Table 16.2). Clinical conditions in which the ESR *may* be helpful are collagen vascular diseases, autoimmune diseases, multiple myeloma, paraproteinemias, sickle cell disease, ischemic stroke (as an early predictor of severity), infectious diseases [e.g., acute otitis media, osteomyelitis, pelvic inflammatory disease, subacute bacterial endocarditis, human immunodeficiency virus (HIV) infection], and neoplastic diseases. The ESR cannot differentiate between types of malignancy or infectious processes. For patients with sickle cell disease, a low ESR is so common that even slight elevations should raise the suspicion for a comorbid condition, such as infection (1,4).

C. **The ESR is used most frequently in disease diagnosis and monitoring, and as a marker for underlying disease in the symptomatic patient (2).**

1. **Diagnosis.** An elevated ESR is diagnostic in two conditions: temporal arteritis and polymyalgia rheumatica, but normal values do not preclude these conditions (2). Remember, the ESR has, at best, a limited role in the diagnosis of inflammatory arthritis (e.g., rheumatoid arthritis, systemic lupus erythymatosus).

2. **Disease monitoring.** Measurement of the ESR can aid in assessing response to treatment or determining the course of disease relapse. This type of monitoring has been best described in temporal arteritis, polymyalgia rheumatica, rheumatoid arthritis, and Hodgkin's disease (2,5). *Note: high dose salicylate therapy and corticosteroids can act to lower the ESR independently* (1). The elevated ESR may be an indicator of metastatic disease in patients with a known tumor, whereas a normal or decreased sedimentation rate significantly reduces the likelihood of metastases in cancer patients (5).

3. **Initial screening in symptomatic patients.** Although the ESR should not be used to screen for occult malignancy, a small proportion of patients with an elevated ESR will be found to harbor a malignancy (3,5). An elevated sedimentation rate can aid in raising the suspicion of autoimmune, rheumatologic, or neoplastic conditions; however, additional diagnostic testing is necessary to confirm these conditions. Certain infectious disease processes are also aided by the finding of an elevated ESR. Pelvic inflammatory disease can be differentiated from an unruptured appendicitis (3). Osteomyelitis and septic arthritis can be differentiated from more benign conditions, such as synovitis (3) (Chapter 12.6). Elevation of the ESR also aids in the diagnosis of subacute bacterial endocarditis with sensitivities approaching 95% (3). Newer applications of the ESR involve its use in the diagnosis of bacterial otitis media in afebrile children, with elevations indicating a higher risk for recurrence (4); the prediction of ischemic stroke severity, with higher initial values associated with a poorer prognosis (4); prediction of progression to acquired immunodeficiency syndrome in a HIV-positive patient with a CD4 count less than $500 \times 10^6/\mu L$ and an elevated β_2-macroglobulin (4); and the association of an elevated ESR with disease progression and death in prostate cancer (2,4).

References

1. Bedell SE, Bush BT. Erythrocyte sedimentation rate, from folklore to facts. *Am J Med* 1985;78:1001–1009.
2. Brigden M. The erythrocyte sedimentation rate. *Postgrad Med* 1998;103:257–274.
3. Olshaker JS. The erythrocyte sedimentation rate. *J Emerg Med* 1997;15:869–874.
4. Saadeh C. The erythrocyte sedimentation rate: old and new clinical applications. *South Med J* 1998;91:220–225.
5. Sox HC, Liang MH. The erythrocyte sedimentation rate: guidelines for rational use. *Ann Intern Med* 1986;104:515–523.

16.4 Neutropenia

Julie A. Reeves

Neutropenia is not simply a low white blood count (WBC) value. It is defined by the absolute neutrophil count (ANC). The ANC can be calculated as follows: ANC = WBC × (% bands + % neutrophils) × 0.01.

I. **Approach.** The many causes of neutropenia can be divided into acute and chronic (1–3).
  A. **Acute** causes occur more frequently and produce some external effect on the body, so as to alter a normally functioning bone marrow.
     1. **Drug-induced.** Two mechanisms have been identified—immune-mediated and direct toxicity to the bone marrow. Although theoretically recognized, the exact mechanisms are not clearly understood. Examples include antibiotics (penicillin, cephalosporins, trimethoprim-sulfamethoxazole, chloramphenicol), antithyroidals (propylthiouracil), antipsychotics (thioridazine, clozapine), angiotensin-converting enzyme inhibitors (captopril), antirheumatics (nonsteroidal antiinflammatories, gold, penicillamine), antidepressants (desipramine, imipramine), anticonvulsants (phenytoin, phenobarbital, carbamazepine), and antiarrhythmic drugs (procainamide).
     2. **Infection.** Three mechanisms of infection-induced neutropenia are identified—increased margination of neutrophils, bone marrow suppression, and neutrophil destruction. Bacterial types include gram-positive organisms (*Staphylococcus, Streptococcus, Enterococcus, Corynebacterium*), gram-negative organisms (*Escherichia coli, Klebsiella, Pseudomonas*), and anaerobes. Tuberculosis and brucellosis are further examples. Viral sources are seen particularly in children. Respiratory syncytial virus, varicella, influenza A and B, measles, and rubella are implicated. Infection with human immunodeficiency virus (HIV), mononucleosis, or hepatitis can produce severe, protracted neutropenia. In addition, protozoal, fungal, and rickettsial infections may be culprits.
     3. **Others.** Other less common acute or extrinsic factors include bone marrow replacement (leukemia and lymphoma), chemotherapy, radiation, and autoimmune disorders (4).
  B. **Chronic** causes of neutropenia involve impairment of the bone marrow. Such intrinsic factors are usually genetic and, therefore, present in early childhood.
     1. **Chronic benign neutropenia of childhood** can be either congenital or acquired (e.g., viral), and presents in patients aged less than 4 years. Antineutrophil antibodies have been linked to 80% of cases. The ANC is less than 500/mm^3, seemingly placing the child in a high risk category. However, as implied in the disease name, children actually have a decreased risk of infection. Although neutrophil production can be impaired, other immunologic defense systems (e.g., lymphocytes) are functioning normally and are adequate to fight off viral invaders. Management is conservative; routinely, it consists of observation and antibiotics only with confirmed infection. The median duration is 20 months, so that by age 4, the disease has regressed (1).
     2. **Congenital agranulocytosis** is a much more worrisome disease with the onset of life-threatening infections in the first year of life. An intrinsic stem cell defect has been implicated. The ANC is less than 500/mm^3.
     3. **Cyclic neutropenia.** The hallmark is non–life-threatening infections occurring every 21 days. The repetitive nature of this disease results from oscillations in neutrophil counts. This phenomenon can be confirmed by obtaining a complete blood count (CBC) two to three times a week for 2 months (or two cycles). There appears to be some abnormal regulation of early neutrophil precursor cells. The disease is usually benign, but unfortunately can be life-long.
II. **History.** The initial workup of neutropenic disease includes an extended history regarding recent or remote drug use, chemotherapy, radiation, or recent infection (5,6). With children, inquire into unexplained childhood deaths in the family. Next, thoroughly examine the skin, mouth, liver, lymph nodes, and perianal regions.
III. **Physical examination.** The clinical manifestations of neutropenic disease, regardless of cause, are generally the same. That is, they represent signs and

symptoms of infection—fever, erythema, pain, tenderness, and increased warmth of localized tissues. All initially involve the skin and mucous membranes. The location of physical features and severity of infection are determined by the ANC. If the ANC is between 500 and 1,000/mm³, oropharyngeal problems (stomatitis, gingivitis, otitis media) and cellulitis are present. Perirectal abscess, pneumonia, and sepsis are seen with an ANC less than 500/mm³.

IV. **Testing.** Laboratory data should include serial CBC to check for pattern (cyclic vs. random) and evolution (transient vs. chronic). Liver function tests, electrolytes, blood urea nitrogen, creatinine, pan-cultures (blood, stool, urine, lesion), and chest x-ray study are all routine. Optional laboratory studies are a serum immunoglobulin, serum antinuclear antibody, and a bone marrow biopsy (7).

V. **Diagnostic assessment.** ANC values are classified as mild (1,000–1,500/mm³), moderate (500–1,000/mm³), or severe (<500/mm³). This classification helps to distinguish those patients at low or high risk for infection.

Normal values for the circulating neutrophil count are listed in many texts. In the first day of life, the neutrophil count is approximately 8,000/mm³. Thereafter, counts drop off. Between 6 and 12 months of age, neutrophil counts reach an expected nadir of 1,000/mm³ (1). Beyond 1 year to adult, values of 1,500/mm³ to 10,000/mm³ are considered normal. Interestingly, African-Americans tend to have lower values than the white population.

References

1. Bernini JC. Diagnosis and management of chronic neutropenia during childhood. *Pediatr Clin North Am* 1996;43:773–792.
2. Boxer LA, Blackwood RA. Leukocyte disorders: quantitative and qualitative disorders of the neutrophil, part 1. *Pediatr Rev* 1996;17:19–28.
3. Drug-induced agranulocytosis. *Drug Ther Bull* 1997;35:49–52.
4. Hathorn JW, Lyke K. Empirical treatment of febrile neutropenia: evolution of current therapeutic approaches. *Clin Infect Dis* 1997;24(Suppl 2):S256–S265.
5. Hughes WT, Armstrong D, Bodey GP, et al. 1997 Guidelines for the use of antimicrobial agents in neutropenic patients with unexplained fever. *Clin Infect Dis* 1997;25:551–573.
6. Kim SK, Demetri GD. Chemotherapy and neutropenia. *Hematol Oncol Clin North Am* 1996;10:377–395.
7. Welte K, Dale D. Pathophysiology and treatment of severe chronic neutropenia. *Ann Hematol* 1996;72:158–165.

16.5 Polycythemia

Gary I. Levine

Polycythemia [from the Greek *poly* (many) and *kytos* (cells)] is used to describe the state of having an increased number of red blood cells. The term erythrocytosis, often used synonymously with polycythemia, indicates an elevated hematocrit (packed red cell volume)—more than 51% in males and more than 48% in females (1,2). Polycythemia vera (PV) has an estimated annual incidence of 0.5 to 2.0/100,000, a peak incidence between ages 50 and 70 years, and no significant gender predominance. Relative polycythemia (Gaisbock's disease, stress polycythemia) primarily occurs in obese, hypertensive men, aged 45 to 55 years, with a prevalence of 0.5 to 0.7% of men in the United States (3).

I. **Approach**

A. **Etiology.** An increased hematocrit can result from a decrease in plasma volume (relative polycythemia) or from an increase in red cell mass (absolute polycythemia). An increased red cell mass (RCM) can result from enhanced renal erythropoietin synthesis because of tissue hypoxemia or aberrant erythropoietin release from various renal and hepatic disorders (secondary polycythemia), or a myeloproliferative disorder associated with hyperplasia of erythroid, myeloid, and platelet elements (polycythemia vera) (2). Treatment is targeted at both the elevated hematocrit and the underlying pathologic process, making it essential that a thorough diagnostic evaluation be undertaken for all individuals with polycythemia.

B. Differential diagnosis of polycythemia or erythrocytosis (2)
    1. Relative polycythemia (Gaisbock's, spurious, stress, apparent)
    2. Absolute polycythemia
        a. Secondary polycythemia caused by tissue hypoxemia
            (1) High altitude erythrocytosis (Monge)
            (2) Cor pulmonale
            (3) Congenital heart disease with right-left shunt
            (4) Hypoventilation (Pickwickian), sleep apnea, or both
            (5) High affinity hemoglobinopathy
        b. Secondary polycythemia caused by aberrant erythropoietin production
            (1) Hypernephroma
            (2) Hepatocellular carcinoma
            (3) Cerebellar hemangioma
        c. Polycythemia vera (polycythemia rubra vera)
        d. Idiopathic primary polycythemia

II. History. Individuals with an elevated hematocrit, regardless of cause, often exhibit symptoms related to increased blood viscosity. These include headache, dizziness, fatigue, tinnitus, decreased mental acuity, and a bleeding tendency (4). Pruritus after a hot shower or bath (aquagenic pruritus) is pathognomonic for PV (3). Between 30% and 50% of patients with PV initially present with symptoms of venous thrombosis or arterial microvascular occlusion. History or current symptoms of pulmonary, congenital cardiovascular, or renal disease suggests secondary polycythemia. A history of dyspnea, snoring, hypersomnolence, weight loss, and smoking should be sought. A family history of polycythemia at a young age suggests a hemoglobinopathy. The combination of obesity, hypertension, diuretic use, and smoking is suggestive of relative polycythemia (5).

III. Physical examination. Most patients with an increased hematocrit exhibit a characteristic ruddy cyanosis (2) (Chapter 8.2). The presence of splenomegaly and, to a lesser degree, hepatomegaly, is highly suggestive of PV (Chapter 15.4). Fingers and toes may be erythematous and tender despite the presence of normal peripheral pulses. Hypoventilation, rales, systolic murmur, augmented second heart sound (P_2), and digital clubbing are findings suggestive of secondary polycythemia.

IV. Testing
    A. Blood tests. Individuals who present with an elevated hematocrit should have repeat testing done on a specimen obtained without venous occlusion. A measurement of red cell mass should be done early in the investigation of all polycythemic patients. This measurement is obtained by labeling a small sample of a patient's blood with radioactive chromium-51, re-injecting this known quantity, and obtaining a second sample at least 90 minutes later (3). Values above 32 ml/kg (men) and 28 ml/kg (women) are elevated (1). Plasma volume is measured in a similar manner using ^{125}I-labeled albumin. Although it appears intuitive that measuring erythropoietin levels would be the key to differentiating primary from secondary polycythemia, this has not proved to be the case (2). Hemoglobin electrophoresis with measurement of the P50 (oxygen pressure at which hemoglobin is half saturated) is valuable in patients with a family history of polycythemia. A complete blood count (CBC) may reveal a white blood cell count of more than 15,000/mm^3 and platelet count more than 400,000/mm^3 in patients with PV. Elevated vitamin B_{12}, B_{12} binding capacity, uric acid, and leukocyte alkaline phosphatase levels are also seen in PV.
    B. Other tests. Measurement of supine arterial oxygen saturation by pulse oximeter is a key diagnostic study. An O_2 saturation less than 92% is

suggestive of tissue hypoxemia, and should be confirmed by formal arterial blood gas analysis (5). Bone marrow aspiration and biopsy evaluation, not required for the diagnosis of PV, typically shows erythroid, granulocytic, and megakaryocytic hyperplasia. Chromosomal analysis of the marrow may be abnormal in 10% to 15% of patients with PV (3). Diagnostic imaging studies of value include chest x-ray, echocardiography in suspected congenital and acquired heart disease with right-left shunts, ultrasound or computed tomography (CT) of the abdomen to assess splenic size and identify renal or hepatic tumors, and magnetic resonance imaging (MRI) to screen for cerebellar hemangioma (4).

V. **Diagnostic assessment.** Obtain RCM and plasma volume. If RCM is normal and plasma volume is decreased—*relative polycythemia.* If RCM is elevated—*absolute polycythemia*—obtain O_2 saturation. If O_2 saturation is less than 92%—*secondary polycythemia caused by hypoxemia.* If O_2 saturation is normal, obtain CBC, B_{12}, B_{12} binding capacity, and leukocyte alkaline phosphatase (LAP). If the WBC count is more than 12,000/mm³, platelets more than 400,000/mm³, elevated B_{12}/B_{12} binding capacity or LAP, and splenomegaly—*polycythemia vera*—consider bone marrow to confirm. If CBC is normal, obtain abdominal CT, head MRI, and hemoglobin (Hb) electrophoresis and erythropoietin level. Abnormal findings on diagnostic imaging and elevated erythropoietin level—*secondary polycythemia caused by aberrant erythropoietin.* If Hb electrophoresis is abnormal—*high affinity hemoglobin.* A normal CBC and other diagnostic studies—*idiopathic (primary) polycythemia.*

References

1. Prchal JT. Primary polycythemias. *Curr Opin Hematol* 1995;2(2):146–152.
2. Means RT. Polycythemia: erythrocytosis. In: Lee GR, ed. *Wintrobe's clinical hematology*, 10th ed. Baltimore: Williams & Wilkins, 1999:1538–1554.
3. Broudy VC. The polycythemias. *Sci Am Med* 1996;5 Hema V:1–10.
4. Fauci AS, ed. *Harrison's principles of internal medicine*, 14th ed. New York: McGraw-Hill, 1998:206–207.
5. Pearson TC, Messinezy M. Investigation of patients with polycythemia. *Postgrad Med* 1996;72(851):519–524.

16.6 Proteinuria

Irene M. Hamrick

The prevalence of proteinuria in the general population is 3%, and 5% in healthy adolescents (1). Heavy and persistent proteinuria is associated with the development of end-stage renal disease in patients with glomerular pathology. For example, 40% to 50% of patients with type I diabetes and 8% to 20% of patients with type II diabetes (2) develop end-stage kidney disease, usually preceded by proteinuria in excess of 3.5 g/day.

I. **Approach.** Normal urine protein is less than 150 mg/d/1.73 m² and consists of approximately 40% albumin, and 40% Tamm-Horsfall protein, synthesized by the kidney tubule, and the rest is small globulins and immunoglobulins, including IgA and light chains. Proteinuria that is persistent should be quantitated. Nephrotic range proteinuria is more than 3.5 g/d/1.73 m² and is the hallmark of increased permeability to serum proteins and, in turn, the development of progressive renal failure.

II. **History.** Presentation is usually by abnormal urinalysis or urine dipstick, most often found during routine sports, insurance, or employment physical examinations. Proteinuria causes the urine to foam or form bubbles in the commode but patients generally do not have subjective complaints, so that underlying illnesses have to be asked about.

A. **Medical history.** Urologic or renal problems may have been evaluated in the past by urinalysis or radiology, revealing infections or stones. Chronic illnesses such as hypertension, diabetes or autoimmune diseases can cause proteinuria. Recent history of infectious illness (e.g., strep throat, impetigo, endocarditis) may indicate a causative factor.

B. **Medications.** Ask for prior intake of medications that can cause proteinuria [e.g., penicillamine, gold, nonsteroidal antiinflammatory drugs, angiotensin-converting enzyme inhibitor (ACE inhibitor), or an aminoglycoside].

C. **Family history.** A family history of renal disease or renal abnormalities (e.g., polycystic kidneys), hypertension, diabetes, or autoimmune diseases can point to a diagnosis.

D. **Review of systems.** Ask for symptoms in the musculoskeletal, dermatologic, infectious, immune, and cardiovascular systems (4).

III. **Physical examination** includes vital signs (notably blood pressure), funduscopic eye examination (looking for diabetic retinopathy or vascular changes), and abdominal examination for masses (polycystic kidney). The cardiovascular examination is important for evaluation of murmur and renal artery bruits, and the extremities for edema or rheumatologic joint changes.

IV. **Testing**

A. **Clinical laboratory tests.** Urine dipstick is more specific for albumin and may not react to Bence Jones or other proteins. A dipstick test for microalbuminuria identifies urine protein in the range of 30 to 300 mg/d (2). Initial evaluation includes urinalysis with microscopy to identify casts, cells, and hematuria. Red cells and red cell casts indicate acute nephritic syndrome and leukocytes indicate acute infection or inflammation, including interstitial nephritis. Oval fat bodies are present in nephrotic syndrome (1). The next step is to evaluate creatinine clearance and to quantify proteinuria as nephrotic range or nonnephrotic. This is best done by 24-hour urine collection. If this is not feasible, or if the result is questionable, the creatinine clearance (CCL) can be calculated using the Cockcroft-Gault formula, using lean body weight:

CCL males = (140-age) × weight in kg/serum creatinine × 72

For females = CCL males × 0.85

Similarly, a spot urine protein:creatinine ratio can give a fairly accurate estimate of the quantity of protein excreted per day:

Urine protein (mg/dl)/Urine creatinine (mg/dl)

(>0.2 is abnormal and >3.5 is nephrotic range)

In addition to quantification of proteinuria, the type of protein can be assessed by serum or urine protein electrophoresis. Complete blood count, sedimentation rate, serum levels of electrolytes, parathyroid hormone, uric acid, complement (C3, C4), IgA, rheumatoid factor, antistreptolysin-O, antiglomerular basement membrane, anticentromere, and antinuclear antibodies can be helpful in further characterizing glomerular pathology.

B. **Other studies.** Imaging studies may include ultrasound of kidneys (e.g., polycystic kidneys) and Doppler studies of renal arteries (e.g., hypertension). Depending on history and physical examination results, rectal biopsy (for amyloid) or renal biopsy may be indicated, particularly when protein excretion exceeds 3.5 g/day.

V. **Diagnostic assessment**

A. **Diagnosis of proteinuria.** If the history and physical examination do not reveal a causative factor, the key to diagnosis is to differentiate transient from persistent proteinuria. Transient (also called benign or functional proteinuria) proteinuria is caused by hemodynamic changes, whereas persistent proteinuria, present in three or more specimens, indicates a pathologic process (2), particularly when proteinuria exceeds 1.0 g/day. Causes of transient proteinuria include orthostasis, exercise, emotional stress, exposure to cold, fever, prolonged lordotic posture, norepinephrine excess, albumin infusion, pericardial effusion, pulmonary edema, congestive heart failure, head injury, and cerebrovascular accident (1). Long-term follow-up of these patients shows a benign course (2). Persistent proteinuria, especially in the nephrotic range requires nephrology evaluation and renal biopsy. A renal biopsy is usually not necessary when the history and physical examination reveal a causative factor (e.g., Bence Jones proteinuria), collagen vascular screens for systemic lupus erythematosus or a history (10–15 year) of diabetes, especially with diabetic retinopathy (4).

B. **Significance of proteinuria in specific diseases.** Early detection of proteinuria by microalbumin testing can identify patients who would benefit from the renal-protective effects of ACE inhibitors. Although the most common cause of proteinuria is glomerulosclerosis resulting from diabetes, ACE inhibitors will decrease proteinuria and improve prognosis in patients with glomerular pathology of various causes.

Extrarenal manifestations of nephrotic syndrome include alterations in cellular immunity leading to increased infections, hyperlipidemia, changes in calcium and bone metabolism, and hypercoagulable state. Those patients with membranous glomerulonephritis, especially, should be counseled about the risk of deep vein thrombosis (e.g., long periods of immobilization).

References

1. Hurst JW. *Medicine for the practicing physician*, 4th ed. Stamford, CT: Appleton & Lange, 1996.
2. Hassan A. Proteinuria. *Postgrad Med* 1997;101(4):173–180.
3. Glassock RJ. Proteinuria. In: Massry SG, Glassock RJ, eds. *Textbook of nephrology*, 3rd ed. Baltimore: Williams & Wilkins, 1995.
4. Barker LR, Burton JR, Zieve PD. *Principles of ambulatory medicine*, 4th ed. Baltimore: Williams & Wilkins, 1995.

16.7 Thrombocytopenia

Mark D. Darrow

A low platelet count is usually brought to the attention of the practitioner as the result of an automated complete blood count in an asymptomatic patient (1).

I. **Approach.** In working through the differential diagnosis of thrombocytopenia, it is helpful to categorize it by cause and severity of clinical presentation.

A. **Causes.** Platelet counts fall secondary to a decrease in production, increased consumption, destruction, sequestration or dilution, and from physiologic causes. Errors in measurement and specimen collection also contribute to the causes of thrombocytopenia (Table 16.3).

B. **Common concerns.** When does bleeding become a problem? Susceptibility to bleeding is specific to the individual; however, bleeding is rare above a platelet count of 100,000/mm^3 (100 × 10^9/L). With platelet counts between 20,000 mm^3 to 50,000/mm^3 (20 – 50 × 10^9/L), bleeding from trauma or surgery can occur. At this level, bleeding in the form of petechiae can occur in the mouth, on legs, along brassiere straps and undergarments, and in the genital area. Spontaneous bleeding occurs with counts less than 20,000/mm^3 (20 × 10^9/L) from or within many body organs. Life-threatening hemorrhage from the gastrointestinal tract or the central nervous system usually occurs at extremely low platelet counts, 5000/mm^3 (5 × 10^9/L) or less (2) (Chapter 9.7).

Table 16.3 Causes of a low platelet count

DECREASED PRODUCTION
Congenital megakaryocyte disorders, chemical agents, drugs, aplastic anemia,
    myelophthisic and myelodysplastic disorders, vitamin deficiencies (B_{12}, folate)

INCREASED CONSUMPTION OR DESTRUCTION/LOSS
Immunologic (autoantibodies, allergies, incompatibility), disseminated intravascular
    coagulation disorders, microangiopathic processes (heart valves, thrombotic thrombo-
    cytopenic purpura) infections, large volume transfusions

POOLING, DILUTION, AND PHYSIOLOGIC SEQUESTRATION
Hypersplenism, posttransfusion, pregnancy, hypothermia

MISCELLANEOUS CAUSES
Laboratory error (in collection from clumping, in reporting)

II. History

A. **Pertinent recent and past history**. Has there been any indication of a
    low platelet count? Easy bruisability, nose bleeds, petechiae, for example.
    Does the patient have any acute or chronic medical conditions such as preg-
    nancy, infections, connective tissue diseases, alcohol abuse, medication use
    (quinidine, heparin), or liver disease?

B. **Family history**. Are there any relatives with a history suggestive of con-
    genital thrombocytopenic or platelet function disorders?

C. **Surgical history.** Has the patient had a cardiac valve or other device im-
    planted in the past? Does the patient have an implanted artificial joint that
    can serve as a source of infection? Is there is history of a splenectomy?

D. **Medications.** Heparin, quinidine, and gold therapy are well known to be
    associated with drug-related, immune-mediated thrombocytopenia. Recre-
    ational use of cocaine can also cause this condition. Many other drugs can
    lower platelet counts through various other mechanisms (antiinflammatory
    agents, β-lactamase–resistant antibiotics) (2,3).

III. Physical examination.
The physical examination should be directed at finding
evidence of bruising or bleeding. Look for petechiae on the skin or mucosa, particularly in dependent areas and in areas of pressure, as well as in the mouth and
perianal and vulvar areas. Stool guaiac evaluations are also important (2–4)
(Chapters 9.11 and 15.3).

Evidence of lymphadenopathy, hepatosplenomegaly, jaundice, fever, and neurologic abnormalities suggests the presence of systemic illnesses that can be
associated with and be the cause of the patient's thrombocytopenia (4,5).

IV. Testing

A. **Blood tests.** The first step in the laboratory evaluation is to repeat the platelet
    count. Clumping or laboratory error may have occurred during the first read-
    ing. A complete blood count and an evaluation of the peripheral blood smear
    help narrow the differential diagnosis based on the presence and number of
    certain cell types and forms. The remainder of the laboratory evaluation—liver
    function tests, renal function tests, vitamin B_{12} and folate levels, and antibody
    screening—should be guided by historical and physical findings. A bone mar-
    row evaluation may be appropriate if the peripheral smear suggests bone
    marrow-based pathology (hypoplasia, malignancy, and fibrosis) (2,4,5).

B. **Diagnostic imaging.** Imaging studies (e.g., an ultrasound of the abdomen
    for evaluation of liver and spleen size) are appropriate in some situations
    where the physical examination of these organs was not adequate. Comput-
    erized tomographic (CT) images of the brain should be considered when neu-
    rologic findings exist. CT images of the chest, abdomen, and pelvis will help
    evaluate adenopathy if present peripherally and its extent in the thoracic
    and abdominal cavities (4,5).

V. Diagnostic assessment. To determine the cause of thrombocytopenia, give equal consideration to the history, physical examination, and laboratory findings. Some causes may be obvious; others may consume time and require some further evaluation. For example, the thrombocytopenic patient recently started on quinidine for a cardiac dysrhythmia should have this medication discontinued and the platelet count followed for return to the normal range. A second patient with multiple sexual partners, a history of systemic lupus erythematosus, pain medication abuse, and newly diagnosed adenopathy may require a more extensive evaluation.

Whatever the cause, urgency in the workup of the thrombocytopenia is often driven by the clinical presentation and any clinically significant bleeding that may be present.

References

1. George JN, el-Haroke MA, Raskob GE. Chronic idiopathic thrombocytopenia purpura. *N Engl J Med* 1994;331:1207–1211.
2. Goldstein KH, Abramson N. Efficient diagnosis of thrombocytopenia. *Am Fam Physician* 1996;53(3):915–920.
3. Rithell T. *Wintrobe's clinical hematology*, 9th ed. Philadelphia: Lea and Febiger, 1993:1325–1373.
4. Schrier SL, Leung LLK. Disorders of hematosis and coagulation. In: Dale DC, Federman DD. *Scientific American Medicine*. Scientific American, Inc., 1997:11–39.
5. Shuman M. Hemorrhagic disorders: abnormalities of platelet and vascular function. In: Wyngaarden JB, Smith LH, Bennett JC, eds. *Cecil textbook of medicine*, 19th ed. Philadelphia: WB Saunders, 1992:987–999.

17. LABORATORY ABNORMALITIES: BLOOD CHEMISTRY AND IMMUNOLOGY

JUDITH A. FISHER

17.1 Alkaline Phosphatase, Elevated

Judith A. Fisher and M. Gina Glazier

Alkaline phosphatase (ALP) is an enzyme expressed on the plasma membrane of many cells. It has two primary sources: the liver (specifically, the biliary tree) and bones (it marks new bone formation) (1). In adults, approximately half of the circulating ALP comes from the liver and the other half from bone. Small amounts are produced by the intestines and vascular endothelium. In pregnancy, significant amounts are produced by the placenta.

The range of normal serum ALP levels varies throughout life. Normal ranges are:

Infant: 50–165 U/L
Child: 20–150 U/L
Adult: 20–70 U/L
Adult aged more than 60 years: 30–75 U/L

I. **Approach.** A serum ALP should be ordered only if suspecting bone or liver disease. No role is seen for a "screening" or "routine" ALP. If the ALP level is found to be elevated, normal physiologic elevation owing to age or pregnancy should be excluded, along with spurious elevation caused by a recent albumin infusion (2), the use of an anticoagulant tube for the blood collection, or leaving the serum sample standing at room temperature for prolonged periods (increases the level by 30%). Recently, an ALP has been described that is produced by malignant tumors ("the Regan isoenzyme"), which closely resembles placental ALP.

Although a reasonable attempt can usually be made at estimating the source of elevated ALP, occasionally, it may be necessary to identify the isoenzymes biochemically. Heat inactivation and l-phenylalanine inhibition have been used. Placental and tumor ALP tend to be heat stable, whereas bone is heat labile. These tests are technically difficult and expensive and are rarely used. However, monoclonal antibodies are now being developed for this purpose and show promise (3).

Further testing should be done, based on the results of a careful history and physical examination, and be targeted to specific clinical suspicions (Table 17.1).

Table 17.1 The alkaline phosphatase levels, elevated

II. History	III. Physical examination	IV. Further testing	V. Diagnostic assessment
A. Bone Disorders			
Asymptomatic or bone pain	Frontal bossing	24-hour urine hydroxyproline	Paget's disease
Male	Dilated superficial vessels	Serum osteocalcin	
Hearing/vision problems	Saber tibia	Serum calcium— normal	
Headaches	Deafness	X-ray involved bone(s)	
Pain increased with walking (tibia involved)	Congestive heart failure	Visual fields	
		Audiometry	
Female	Neck mass (rare)	Parathyroid hormone	Hyperparathyroidism
>60 years	Muscle weakness	Serum calcium	
Diffuse aches and pains	Height loss (osteoporosis)	Urinary blood/ calcium	

Table 17.1 *Continued*

II. History	III. Physical examination	IV. Further testing	V. Diagnostic assessment
Vague abdominal pain Depressive symptoms Renal calculi Gastric ulcers		Serum phosphate Serum chloride	
>50 years Unexplained weight loss Smoker Cough Hemoptysis Shortness of breath	Decreased air entry (wheeze) Pleural effusion Dull to percussion Horner's syndrome Clubbing	CXR Chest CT scan Bone scan Serum calcium	Lung cancer ± Metastatic disease
Female >50 years Family history Breast mass	Breast mass Axillary or supra-clavicular nodes Liver enlargement	Mammogram Bone scan Serum calcium	Breast cancer ± metastatic disease
Female >45 years Family history Abdominal bloating Unexplained weight loss	Ovarian mass Ascites	Pelvic ultrasound Pelvic CT scan CA125 CT scan Serum calcium	Ovarian cancer ± metastatic disease
Male >50 years Hematuria Flank/abdominal pain	Unilateral flank mass Conjunctival pallor	Urinalysis CT scan abdomen Serum calcium	Renal cell carcinoma
Male >50 years Voiding symptoms (rare) Family history	Prostate mass on rectal examination Diffusely enlarged hard prostate	Rectal ultrasound with prostate biopsy Bone scan—blastic lesions Prostate-specific antigen Serum calcium	Prostate cancer
10–30 years			Osteosarcoma
Male Pain near joint Very high ALP	Mass near joint Tender over mass	X-ray area (mixed sclerotic or lytic lesion of bone) MRI Bone scan CXR/CT scan—metastases Biopsy	

Table 17.1 *Continued*

II. History	III. Physical examination	IV. Further testing	V. Diagnostic assessment
Recent trauma	Bone pain in area	X-ray—callus formation	Healing fracture
B. Biliary or Liver Disease			
ALP 2 times normal	Spider nevi	Serum AST/ALT levels—	Cirrhosis
Alcohol use or abuse—chronic	Leukonychia	– ↑ in early disease,	Hepatitis
Family history of liver disease	Dupuytren's contracture	– ↓↔ late disease	Fatty liver
Risky sexual practices	Tender RUQ	Bilirubin elevated	
Blood transfusions	Liver may be enlarged	Hepatitis screen (A,B,C)	
Intravenous drug use	Jaundice	Coagulation screen	
Obesity		Liver biopsy	
Fatigue			
Weight loss			
Female	RUQ tenderness + Murphy's sign (only in acute chole-cystitis)	AST/ALT may be ↑	Gallstones
>40 years		Ultrasound of gallbladder	Biliary colic
Obese		Bilirubin elevated	Acute chole-cystitis
Family history of gallstones	Jaundice		
Pain after meals/episodic			
Bloating or gas			
ALP 5 times normal	Fever	Monospot test	Infectious mononucleosis
10–25 years	Tender RUQ	AST/ALT	Toxoplasmosis
Fever	Splenomegaly	CBC	Cytomegalovirus infection
Sore throat or fatigue	Lymphadenopa-thy (mainly cervical)	Toxoplasma titers	
History of contact with infected friend or relative			
ALP 10 times normal	Palpable gallbladder	CT scan abdomen	Pancreatic carcinoma
Weight loss	Cachectic	Elevated bilirubin	Gallbladder carcinoma
Anorexia	Epigastric mass	CT or ultra-sound-guided biopsy	
Back or RUQ pain	Jaundice		
Jaundice			
ALP 10–20 times normal	Frequently normal	AST/ALT	Drug-induced elevation of ALP
Chlorpropamide use	RUQ tenderness	Liver biopsy if problem per-sists	
Antineoplastic agents	Excoriations		
Immune modulators	Jaundice		

continued

Table 17.1 *Continued*

II. History	III. Physical examination	IV. Further testing	V. Diagnostic assessment
ALP 5–20 times normal	Skin pigmen- tation	Antimitochon- drial antibodies	Primary biliary cirrhosis
Female	RUQ tenderness	Liver biopsy	
35–60 years (90%)	Xanthelasma	Elevated biliru- bin (late)	
Frequently asymptomatic	Liver or spleen enlarged	Elevated liver enzymes (late)	
Itching (palms, soles first)		Cholesterol ele- vated	
Fatigue			
Bone pain			
Steatorrhea			
Jaundice			
ALP > 5–20 times normal	RUQ tenderness	ERCP	Sclerosing cholangitis (primary or secondary)
Male	Jaundice		
30–60 years			
RUQ pain			
Jaundice			
Pruritus			
Inflammatory bowel disease			
Fatigue			

CT, computed tomography; CXR, chest x-ray (study); MRI, magnetic resonance imaging; AST/ALT, aspartate/alanine aminotransferase; RUQ, right upper quadrant; CBC, complete blood cell (count); ERCP, endoscopic retrograde cholangio-pancreatography.

Other rarer causes of elevation include hyperthyroidism, vitamin D deficiency (particularly in the elderly and debilitated), hepatic infiltration (caused by lymphoproliferative disorders, granulomatous disease, or primary and secondary malignancies of the liver), and intestinal conditions such as bowel obstruction, and infarction. Because of the presence of ALP in the vascular system, infarction of any solid organ can cause ALP elevation.

References

1. Taylor AK, Lueken SA, Libanati C, Baylink DJ. Biochemical markers of bone turnover for the clinical assessment of bone metabolism. *Clin Rheum Dis* 1994;20:589–607.
2. Bark CJ. Albumin-induced elevation in alkaline phosphatase. *JAMA* 1971;216: 518–520.
3. Broyles DL, Nielsen RG, Bussett EM, Lu WD, Mizrahi IA, Nunnelly PA, et al. Analytical and clinical performance characteristics of Tandem-MP Ostase, a new immunoassay for serum bone alkaline phosphatase. *Clin Chem* 1998;44:2139–2147.

17.2 Aminotransferase Levels, Elevated

Douglas J. Ivins and Judith A. Fisher

I. **Approach.** Serum aspartate aminotransferase (AST or SGOT) or alanine aminotransferase (ALT or SGPT) can be elevated in a wide variety of liver diseases. A normal AST is 8 to 26 U/L. A normal ALT is 4 to 46 U/L. When evaluating elevated ALT or AST levels, it is important to know the reason behind ordering the test (1–4) (Table 17.2).

Table 17.2 Evaluation of the patient with elevated aminotransferase levels

II. History	III. Physical examination	IV. Further testing	V. Diagnostic assessment
ALT/AST often elevated to >10 × normal Patient often asymptomatic or experiences transient flulike illness Antecedent illness of several days to weeks with nausea, vomiting, anorexia, malaise, diarrhea, arthralgias, or low-grade fever 5% to 10% of patients have a serum sicknesslike presentation Recent shellfish ingestion Risky sexual practices Past or present intravenous drug use Past or present blood transfusion	Jaundice Clay-colored stools Dark urine Hepatic tenderness Hepatomegaly Urticaria Maculopapular skin eruptions Isolated joint swelling, redness, or tenderness Edema	CBC ALP and LDH Serum bilirubin Hepatitis A IgM Hepatitis B antigen and IgM anti-hepatitis B core antibody Hepatitis C RNA Epstein-Barr virus or cytomegalovirus titers	Acute viral hepatitis
Excessive somnolence Obtundation History of rectal or upper GI bleeding Rapidly progressive course in 65% to 95% of patients Symptoms of severe sepsis Prior hepatitis History of aspirin ingestion in children < 17 years with influenza or chicken pox	Diminution in liver size Ascites Refractory hypotension Petechia Bleeding from mucous membranes	Prothrombin time (profoundly prolonged) Low blood glucose Low total serum protein and serum albumin CBC Serum ammonia (may be severely elevated)	Fulminant hepatitis Acute hepatic failure associated with Reye's syndrome 1% of the elderly or immunocompromised patients with hepatitis
ALT/AST values of 500–1000 IU/L ALT:AST >2:1 Chronic or acute alcohol ingestion Younger age drinker Past or present pancreatitis or erosive gastritis	Jaundice ± fever Weight loss Hepatomegaly with mild tenderness Spider angiomas Ascites in 25%	Gamma-glutamyl transferase CBC (possible anemia) Vitamin B_{12}, folic acid Upper endoscopy	Alcoholic hepatitis

continued

Table 17.2 *Continued*

II. History	III. Physical examination	IV. Further testing	V. Diagnostic assessment
Cirrhotic liver disease Anorexia Nausea Vomiting Abdominal pain	Palmar erythema Caput medusae		
ALT/AST are variably elevated Often asymptomatic Previous episode of hepatitis Coagulopathy	May be no findings Thin Jaundiced Small liver	Albumin (often low) Prothrombin time (may be elevated) Liver biopsy	Chronic hepatitis
Right upper quadrant pain Gallstones Middle-aged Overweight Female	Jaundice Intermittent fever Rigors Right upper quadrant tenderness ± rebound	Alkaline phosphatase elevated more than the ALT or AST Bilirubin CBC Abdominal ultrasound ERCP	Biliary tract obstruction with or without an infection
Cirrhosis Abdominal pain Weakness Anorexia Hepatitis B infection Males aged 50–60 Known malignancy	Weight loss Ascitis	ALP, LDH Magnetic resonance imaging Serum α-fetoprotein Liver biopsy	Malignancy (primary or metastatic)
Child or young adult Hepatitis Dysarthria Dysphagia	Kayser–Fleischer rings in cornea Tremors	Liver function tests often non-specific Ceruloplasmin (possibly reduced)	Wilson's disease
Use of isoniazid, phenothiazines, erythromycin, progesterone, halothane, opiates, indomethacin, corticosteroids	Often none	Repeat ALT and AST after discontinuation of the medication	Medication effect

ALT/AST, alanine aminotransferase/aspartate aminotransferase, CBC, complete blood cell (count); ALP, alkaline phosphatase; LDH, lactate dehydrogenase; GI, gastrointestinal; ERCP, endoscopic retrograde cholangiopancreatography.

Elevated ALT and AST levels can also be seen in myocardial infarctions, hemolytic anemia, after trauma, and intramuscular injections.

References
1. Jacobs D. *Laboratory test handbook*, 3rd ed. Hudson, OH: Lexi-Comp, Inc., 1994: 100–101, 135–137.

2. Mezey E. Diseases of the liver. In: Barker RL, ed. *Principles of ambulatory medicine*, 4th ed. Baltimore, MD: Williams & Wilkins, 1995:507–517.
3. Pincus M, Schaffner J. Assessment of liver function. In: Henry J, ed. *Clinical diagnosis and management by laboratory methods*, 4th ed. Philadelphia: WB Saunders, 1996:253–267.
4. Wallach J. *Interpretation of diagnostic tests*, 6th ed. Boston: Little, Brown and Company, 1996:57–59.

17.3 Antinuclear Antibody Titer, Elevated

Judith A. Fisher and Douglas J. Ivins

In the practice of cost-effective medicine, no value is seen to routine laboratory testing. An antinuclear antibody titer (ANA) should only be ordered in cases of a clinical suspicion of a rheumatologic disease (also known as connective tissue disorder) (1–2).

I. **Approach.** The patient may present with vague complaints of malaise, aches, or skin rash. On the other hand, the complaint may be of a red, hot, or swollen joint or joints. If a rheumatologic disease is suspected, an ANA can be ordered. It is important to remember that the specificity of a positive ANA titer for all rheumatic diseases is only 50% (3). With that in mind, ANA titers of more than 1/160 may be significant (1). The characteristic staining patterns associated with ANAs can be helpful. Homogeneous (diffuse) and speckled patterns are relatively nonspecific.

Peripheral patterns are often seen in systemic lupus erythematosus. Nucleolar patterns are more typical for scleroderma. A mildly elevated ANA and no disease process (falsely positive ANA) is found in 5% of young adults and in 18% of individuals aged more than 65 years (1).

The history and physical examination will help to place the patient into one of several diagnostic categories (Table 17.3).

Table 17.3 Evaluation of the patient with an elevated antinuclear antibody titer

II. History	III. Physical examination	IV. Further testing	V. Diagnostic assessment
A. Connective Tissue Disorders			
Pain, redness or heat in two or more joints	Malar rash (presents in one-third to one-half of patients)	Urinalysis (look for persistent proteinuria or casts)	SLE (ANA positive in 95% of patients with SLE (3)
Photosensitivity reaction			Anti-Smith Ab+ and double-stranded DNA + titers are diagnostic for SLE)
Pericarditis or pleural effusion	Discoid rash	VDRL (may be falsely positive)	
Seizures or psychosis	Recurrent oral ulcers		
Hemolytic anemia, leukopenia, lymphopenia, thrombocytopenia, immunologic disorder	Focal neurologic deficits (15% of patients)	CBC (look for evidence of anemia)	
More common in females and African-Americans		Specialized nuclear antigen tests: ribonucleo-protein, anti-	

continued

Table 17.3 *Continued*

II. History	III. Physical examination	IV. Further testing	V. Diagnostic assessment
		bodies to anti-Smith, anti-SS-A/Ro, anti-SS-B/La (SLE patients may produce different auto-antibodies) Creatinine (look for occult renal disease)	
Chronic, symmetric joint, complaints	± Red, hot, swollen joint(s) and subcuta-neous nodules are evidence of vasculitis	± Elevated rheumatoid factor CBC (look for an anemia of chronic disease)	Rheumatoid arthritis
Excessive dryness of eyes and/or mouth Recurrent oral ulcers	Dry tongue Decreased salivation Decreased tearing	Biopsy of salivary glands or lip to demonstrate lymphocytic infiltration CBC (looking for anemia of chronic disease) Cryoglobulins (if positive should screen for hepatitis C) Immunoglobulin electrophoresis (to demon-strate a mono-clonal spike) Complement lev-els (low levels may suggest vasculitis)	Sjögren's syndrome
Generalized weakness Muscle tenderness Muscle weakness is usually symmetric, gradual in onset, greater loss in lower limbs	Muscle strength may be diminished Skin rashes: heliotrope rash on eyelids or erythematous	Serum creatine kinase is typi-cally elevated Normal electro-lytes and renal function	Idiopathic inflammatory myopathy (e.g., dermato-myositis) Mixed connective tissue disorder

Table 17.3 *Continued*

II. History	III. Physical examination	IV. Further testing	V. Diagnostic assessment
Skin rash Arthralgia May have a history of malignancy	papules over joints (proximal interphalangeal, elbow, or knee)	Muscle biopsy can be definitive for a diagnosis	
B. Drugs Patient is taking: Procainamide (10% will develop lupus, 50% will get elevated ANAs) (2), isoniazid, hydralazine, carbamazepine, methyldopa, beta-blockers, anticonvulsants	Physical examination as per SLE	ANA is often negative Erythrocyte sedimentation rate is often elevated	Drug-induced lupus
And has any of complaints listed in the block on SLE plus fever; weight loss; arthralgas are common			
These patients are generally older and male			
Patient is taking: carbamazepine, chlorpromazine, phenytoin, ethosuximide, isoniazid, griseofulvin, penicillin, phenylbutazone, procainamide, propylthiouracil	None	None	Medication effect (false-positive test secondary to patient's medication)
C. Systemic Illness Weight loss Fatigue Malaise Cigarette smoking Family history of cancer	Physical findings are dependent on the type of malignancy suspected	Laboratory testing is dependent on type of malignancy suspected	Malignancy
Exposure to inorganic dusts, asbestos, or free silica Occupational history of mining, ceramics, or foundry work Exposure to the above often occurs for 5–20 years ±	± Barrel chest ± Adventitial lung sounds ± Finger clubbing	± Decreased forced vital capacity and/or total lung capacity on pulmonary function testing ± CXR with discrete nodular	Pneumoconiosis

continued

Table 17.3 *Continued*

II. History	III. Physical examination	IV. Further testing	V. Diagnostic assessment
Exertional dyspnea		infiltrates suggest silicosis	
		± Linear, irregular opacities in lower half of lung field (suggest asbestos exposure)	
Episodic visual changes Intermittent paresthesias or gait disturbance Trigeminal neuralgia Focal neurologic changes lasting days to weeks	± Abnormal neurologic examination Decreased visual acuity Internuclear ophthalmoplegia Limb or trunk ataxia	MRI-weighted T_2 images often show demyelination. Cerebrospinal fluid samples (elevated IgG in ≈ 80% of patients)	Multiple sclerosis
Fever (in 50% to 80%) Malaise Weight loss Night sweats Cough (nonproductive in early stages, may eventually be productive of sputum/heme) Pleuritic pain Dyspnea Extrapulmonary involvement (15% of cases)	± Adventitial lung sounds ± Lymph adenitis	Tuberculin skin test CXR if positive skin test Acid-fast staining and culture for mycobacteria if positive CXR Possibly bronchoscopy	Tuberculosis
History compatible with heat or chemical injury	Erythema of the skin with or without blistering ± Loss of sensation to the area	Typically, a transient rise in ANA	First, second, or third degree burns
Fatigue Chills Nonspecific sore throat Headache Sleep disturbances	Often normal May have nonspecific fever, lymphadenopathy or joint swelling	ANA rise is often transient Other laboratory abnormalities are unusual, but can be specific to the particular viral agent suspected	Chronic viral infections (e.g., Epstein-Barr)

Table 17.3 *Continued*

II. History	III. Physical examination	IV. Further testing	V. Diagnostic assessment

Female
Abdominal pain
Fever
Amenorrhea
Diarrhea
Pleuritic pain/
  polyarthritis
	Jaundice
	  (common)
	Hepatomegaly
	  (> 50% of
	  patients)
	Splenomegaly
	Spider angiomas
		Serum
		  immunoglo-
		  bulins (often
		  associated with
		  elevated
		  gamma globu-
		  lin level)
		CBC (checking
		  for anemia/
		  thrombo-
		  cytopenia)
		Liver function
		  tests (variable
		  elevations)
		Liver biopsy
		  (cirrhotic
		  changes)
			Chronic auto-
			  immune
			  hepatitis

CBC, complete blood cell (count); SLE, systemic lupus erythematosus; ANA, antinuclear antibody; CXR, chest x-ray (study); MRI, magnetic resonance imaging.

It is important to remember to order an ANA only with a clinical suspicion of a disease process in which the ANA value plays a significant role.

References

1. Jacobs D. *Laboratory test handbook*, 3rd ed. Hudson, OH: Lexi-Comp, Inc., 1994: 638–640.
2. Nakamura R. *Clinical diagnosis and management by laboratory methods*, 4th ed. Philadelphia: WB Saunders, 1996:1013–1023.
3. Wallach J. *Interpretation of diagnostic tests*, 6th ed. Boston: Little, Brown, and Company, 1996:817–820.

17.4 Hypercalcemia

M. Gina Glazier and Judith A. Fisher

The normal concentration of calcium in the extracellular fluid is 8.5 to 10.5 mg/dl. Symptoms usually occur when the calcium level rises to 12.5 mg/dl or above. Serum calcium levels between 10.5 and 12 mg/dl are usually asymptomatic.

I. Approach

    A. Manifestations. Although most patients with hypercalcemia are asymptomatic (1), patients with symptomatic hypercalcemia can have a variety of vague complaints: generalized muscle weakness, muscle aches or pains, incoordination, change in level of consciousness, headache, loss of appetite, nausea, vomiting, constipation, increased salivation, dysphagia, severe abdominal pain, abdominal distension, or itching. These patients may present with a renal calculus or a history of a renal calculus. Physical examination may reveal mental confusion, poor memory, slurred speech, acute psychotic behavior, lethargy or coma, ataxia, poor over-all muscle strength, hypotonia, hyperextensible joints, increased deep tendon reflexes, positive Babinski's sign, incoordination, loss of pain or vibration sense, calcium deposits on the conjunctiva near the palpebral fissure or on the cornea around the iris, an acute abdomen, or an ileus. Patients with hypercalcemia can also present with another diagnosis such as malignancy. In malignancy, hypercalcemia is often a sequitor. A calcium level should be ordered only if hypercalcemia is suspected after the history and physical examination.

It is important to note that calcium levels are frequently ordered to investigate nonspecific symptoms and mild, asymptomatic hypercalcemia is a frequent incidental finding. In dehydration with hemoconcentration, serum calcium can be falsely elevated. If this is the case, a second blood sample should be drawn after the hemoconcentration has resolved.

B. **Common causes.** Of the cases of hypercalcemia in adults, 90% are caused by hyperparathyroidism or malignancy. Hyperparathyroidism is the most common outpatient cause of hypercalcemia. In primary hyperparathyroidism, the serum calcium is less than 14.5 mg/dl, with serum chloride more than 102 mEq/L in the setting of a normal alkaline phosphatase, increased parathyroid hormone level (PTH), and no clinical evidence of malignancy.

Malignancy is the most common cause of hypercalcemia in hospitalized patients (2–3). Hypercalcemia secondary to malignancy occurs through metastatic involvement of bone, or the tumor itself may secrete a parathyroid hormone-related-protein that causes bone resorption. In multiple myeloma, hypercalcemia is caused primarily by impairment of glomerular filtration and subsequent renal failure. Patients with malignancy and hypercalcemia have higher calcium levels that are less amenable to treatment. Most of these patients will die within 3 to 6 months. In hypercalcemia associated with malignancy, the serum calcium is 14 mg/dl or higher, with a serum chloride less than 100 in the setting of anemia, a serum alkaline phosphatase of more than two times the upper limit of normal, and a normal or less than twice the upper limit of normal PTH.

The less common causes of hypercalcemia (e.g., renal failure and hyperthyroidism) can be ruled out with normal renal and thyroid functions (Chapters 10.5 and 14.8). Sarcoidosis can be ruled out with a normal chest x-ray study.

C. **Special concerns.** Symptomatic hypercalcemia with levels above 12.5 mg/dl can be a life-threatening metabolic emergency. It is important to order an electrocardiogram and begin treatment immediately, as cardiac arrest, convulsions, or coma can occur. Further testing can be done while the serum calcium is being lowered (Table 17.4).

Table 17.4 Evaluation of the patient with hypercalcemia

II. History	III. Physical examination	IV. Further testing	V. Diagnostic assessment
A. Spurious Elevation			
Laboratory studies ordered for another reason	Normal	Repeat calcium (may be normal) Serum albumin	High serum albumin Tight tourniquet at time of blood draw
Excessive thirst Vomiting or diarrhea with poor oral intake	Dry mucous membranes	Repeat calcium after re-hydration	Dehydration

Table 17.4 *Continued*

II. History	III. Physical examination	IV. Further testing	V. Diagnostic assessment
	Decreased skin turgor		
	Confusion/lethargy		
B. Hormonal Abnormalities			
Female	Neck mass (unlikely)	Serum calcium <14.5 mg/dl	Hyperparathyroidism (primary or secondary)
>60 years	No clinical evidence of malignancy	Parathyroid hormone—elevated	
Aches and pains		Serum chloride >102 mg/dl	
Vague abdominal pain		Alkaline phosphatase—normal	
Depressive symptoms		Serum phosphate	
Renal calculi		Bicarbonate	
		X-ray hands and clavicles	
Headaches	Hypertension (labile, resistant to treatment)	Urinary 24-hour excretion of vanillylmandelic acid, metanephrines, and free catecholamines	Pheochromocytoma
Nosebleeds			
Palpitations			
Profuse sweating	Pallor/flushing (during an attack)		
Apprehension		Computed tomography (CT) scan of abdomen to define lesion	
Nausea/vomiting	Weight loss		
	Sweating		
Anxiety/tremor	Thin	Thyroid function tests	Thyrotoxicosis
Weight loss	Exophthalmos		
Family history	Eyelid tremor		
Intolerance of heat	Tachycardia		
Eye problems	Sweating		
	Hyperreflexia		
Fatigue	Hypotension	Potassium (elevated)	Addison's disease
Weight loss	Lethargy	Sodium (decreased)	
Family history	Increased mucosal/skin pigmentation	Blood sugar (low)	
Nausea/vomiting		Adrenal cortical hormone (ACTH) stimulation test	

continued

Table 17.4 *Continued*

II. History	III. Physical examination	IV. Further testing	V. Diagnostic assessment
C. Malignancy			
>50 years Weight loss Smoker Family history Other symptoms specific to particular tumor site	Weight loss Signs specific to particular tumor site	Serum calcium >14 mg/dl Serum chloride <100 mg/dl Alkaline phosphatase >2 × normal Parathyroid hormone <2 × normal CBC—anemia frequent Further workup according to the site where primary tumor most likely to be found Bone scan	Malignancy with or without metastasis Lung cancer Renal cell carcinoma Squamous cell carcinoma
>50 years Female	Weight loss Signs specific to particular tumor site	Further workup according to the site where primary tumor most likely to be found Alkaline phosphatase Bone scan	Breast cancer Ovarian cancer (± metastatic disease)
>50 years Male Urinary complaints of hesitancy, postvoid dripping, or split stream Family history	Prostate mass on rectal examination or a diffusely enlarged hard prostate	Rectal ultrasound with prostate biopsy Bone scan Prostatic-specific antigen (PSA) Alkaline phosphatase	Prostate cancer
>60 years Bone pain (mainly back pain) Weight loss Fatigue	Pallor Hepatomegaly Splenomegaly Tenderness over bones	CBC—anemia Serum protein electrophoresis BUN Creatinine Erythrocyte sedimentation rate	Multiple myeloma
D. Medications/Vitamins			
Lithium Furosemide Thiazide diuretics Aminophylline	Physical examination—normal or shows signs of hypercalcemia	Repeat serum calcium elevated Other serum electrolyte	Medication use

Table 17.4 *Continued*

II. History	III. Physical examination	IV. Further testing	V. Diagnostic assessment
		values may be abnormal	
Use of calcium-based antacids	Normal or shows signs of hyper-calcemia	Phosphate BUN Creatinine Bicarbonate	Milk-alkali syndrome
Vitamin pill use Bone pain Headaches	Normal physical examination or tenderness over bones Papilledema	Repeat serum Ca^{2+} Serum phosphate and chloride levels For suspected vitamin A overuse, a computed tomography scan of the head	Vitamin D over-dose Vitamin A over-dose
E. Other Prolonged bed or chair rest	Physical examination—normal or shows signs of hypercalcemia	Consider dexa-scan for osteoporosis	Immobilization
History of acute renal failure	Physical examination—normal or shows signs of hypercalcemia	BUN Creatinine Urinalysis	Chronic or diuretic phase of acute renal failure
Fever Fatigue Malaise Anorexia Cough Dyspnea Retrosternal chest discomfort	Findings dependent on sites involved Erythema nodosum Uveitis Lymphadeno-pathy	CBC (lympho-cytopenia) Chest x-ray study Pulmonary function testing Transbronchial biopsy	Sarcoidosis or other granulo-matous disease
Polyarthritis			
Family history of hypercalcemia	May be normal or show signs of hypercalcemia		Familial hypo-calciuric hypercalcemia

CBC, complete blood cell (count); BUN, blood urea nitrogen.

References
1. Bushinsky DA, Monk RD. Calcium. *Lancet* 1998;352:306–311.
2. Al Zahrani A, Levine MA. Primary hyperparathyroidism. *Lancet* 1997;349:1233–1238.
3. Mundy GR, Guise TA. Hypercalcemia of malignancy. *Am J Med* 1997;103:134–145.

17.5 Hyperkalemia

Kent D.W. Bream and Judith A. Fisher

Hyperkalemia is probably the most serious electrolyte abnormality. Normal serum potassium is 3.5 to 5.0 mEq/L. Severe hyperkalemia, however, is patient specific and not simply defined by a cut-off of 5.0. A serum potassium (K^+) of 6.0, for example, in one patient may lead to a fatal cardiac arrhythmia, whereas it is asymptomatic and without morbidity in another.

I. **Approach.** Hyperkalemia is usually not sustained without a disorder of the normal potassium regulatory system. In an otherwise healthy individual, routine screening of potassium is not indicated. Potassium, however, should be monitored in patients on certain medications, or with acid-base disorders, abnormalities in renal function, and disorders of aldosterone secretion. These patients are at risk for potentially fatal hyperkalemia (1–4).

A. **Special concerns.** In diagnosing hyperkalemia, the most important characteristic to rule out is cardiac electrical abnormality on the electrocardiogram (ECG). Hyperkalemia can remain asymptomatic until its effects on cardiac conduction lead to cardiac arrest. This potential consequence requires that hyperkalemia be diagnosed and treated promptly. ECG changes include flattening of the P wave, widening of the QRS complex, and peaking of the T wave. When the QRS and T waves merge, a sine wave pattern develops which represents the severest form of cardiac abnormality.

Depending on the K^+ level, some patients will require emergent evaluation for hyperkalemia. Patients with a K^+ greater than 7.0 in any circumstance should have immediate cardiac evaluation. When the potassium is below 7.0, numerous factors determine the urgency of evaluation including the historical cause, the possible duration of hyperkalemia, and the probability that the level will continue to increase without treatment. These three factors, and the absolute value of serum K^+, suggest the timing of cardiac evaluation.

B. **Causes of hyperkalemia.** Four causes of hyperkalemia are seen: spurious causes, redistribution abnormalities, renal disorders, and hormone deficiencies. Spurious hyperkalemia is the most frequent cause of hyperkalemia in a healthy patient. The most common redistribution abnormality is acidosis. Renal causes are most frequently renal insufficiency or failure with a concomitant potassium load. Finally, uncontrolled diabetes is the major cause of hyperkalemia resulting from hormonal causes (Chapter 14.1) (Table 17.5).

Table 17.5 Evaluation of the patient with hyperkalemia

II. History	III. Physical examination	IV. Further Testing	V. Diagnostic Assessment
A. Spurious Causes			
Laboratory reading is "hemolysis" on electrolyte panel	Normal patient	Repeat serum K^+ testing; normalized in redrawn sample	Hemolysis in collection tube
Platelet count > 1 million	Normal patient, except for dis-	Repeat platelet with	Thrombocytosis (platelets

Table 17.5 *Continued*

II. History	III. Physical examination	IV. Further testing	V. Diagnostic assessment
	order causing thrombocytosis	heparinized specimen	release K⁺ during clotting)
WBC >200,000	Normal patient, except for underlying disorder causing leukocytosis	Repeat WBC with rapid processing/ spinning down specimen	Leukocytosis
K⁺ normalized in repeat draw with careful draw technique	Normal patient	Repeat serum K⁺	Tight or prolonged tourniquet or fist clenching during blood draws
B. Redistribution			
Acidosis	Often no signs specific to acidosis in otherwise ill patient	Immediate ECG Monitor cardiac rhythm ABG Sequential testing	pH <7.35
Beta-blockers Angiotensin-converting enzyme inhibitors Cardiac glycosides Neuromuscular blocking agents Salt substitutes Trimethoprim Pentamidine	No signs of hyperkalemia Physical examination may reveal underlying illness leading to medication use	Immediate ECG Cardiac rhythm should be monitored	Medication/ diet effect
Crush injury Tissue breakdown	Bruising/other signs of trauma/ necrotic wound	Immediate ECG Monitor cardiac rhythm	Cell breakdown
Rhabdomyolysis	Signs cell injury/ heat stroke/ crush injury	Urinalysis for myoglobin BUN/creatinine Immediate ECG Monitor cardiac rhythm	Cell breakdown and kidney dysfunction
Large bruise or hematoma	Hematoma	Immediate ECG Monitor cardiac rhythm	Hematoma breakdown
Muscle contraction in marathon runners	Runner		Cell breakdown and muscle release of K⁺

continued

Table 17.5 *Continued*

II. History	III. Physical examination	IV. Further testing	V. Diagnostic assessment
Cachexia	Cachetic	Immediate ECG	Tissue catabolism
Symptoms related to the cause of the cachexia	Signs related to reason for cachexia	Monitor cardiac rhythm	
Hemolytic anemia	Pallor	Immediate ECG	Hemolysis
	Petechiae	Monitor cardiac rhythm	
	Orthostatic hypotension	CBC	
	Bleeding from any orifice		
Hyperkalemic periodic paralysis	Other signs as related to the cause of hemo-lytic anemia		Transient hyper K$^+$
	Quadriplegia with sparing of the cranial nerves		
C. Renal Disorders			
Use of potassium-sparing diuretics (e.g., triamterene or spironolactone)		BUN	Diuretic use
		Creatinine	
		Cr Cl may be low	
		Low fractional excretion of potassium (FE_{K+})	
History of treatment for a *Pneumocystis carinii* infection		BUN	Trimethoprim or pentamidine effect
		Creatinine	
		Cr Cl	
Known Cr Cl<50		Cr Cl Immediate ECG, Monitor cardiac rhythm	Renal insuffi-ciency or failure with a potas-sium load
Systemic lupus erythematosus	Malar rash	ABG	Decreased GFR
	Discoid rash	Cr Cl	
	Recurrent oral ulcers	FE_{K+}	
	Focal neurologic deficits	Evaluation of underlying disease	
Sickle cell disease or trait		BUN	Decreased GFR
		Creatinine	
		Cr Cl may be low	
		Low FE_{K+}	

Table 17.5 *Continued*

II. History	III. Physical examination	IV. Further testing	V. Diagnostic assessment
		Evaluation of underlying disease	
Amyloidosis	Signs from amyloidosis	BUN	Decreased GFR
		Creatinine	
		Cr Cl may be low	
		Low FE_{K+}	
		Evaluation of underlying disease	
D. Hormone deficiency			
Diabetes mellitus	Signs DKA	Evaluate for DKA	Acidosis causing redistribution with K^+/H^+ exchange
		Check ECG/ cardiac rhythm	
		Sequential testing	
Pseudo and actual aldosterone deficiency	Hyperpigmentation	Aldosterone levels	Addison's disease
	Hypotension	Renin levels	
	Weight loss	Check ECG/ cardiac rhythm	
	Vomiting	Cosyntropin stimulation test	
Heparin use		Aldosterone levels	Aldosterone excretion low owing to heparin use
		Check ECG/ cardiac rhythm	

WBC, white blood cell (count); ECG, electrocardiogram; ABG, arterial blood gases; BUN, blood urea nitrogen; Cr Cl, creatinine clearance; GFR, glomerular filtration rate; DKA, diabetic ketoacidosis.

References
1. Evers S, Engelien A, Karsch V, Hund M. Secondary hyperkalemic paralysis. *J Neurol Neurosurg Psychiatry* 1998;64(2):249–252.
2. Halperin ML, Kamel KS. Potassium. *Lancet* 1998;352(9122):135–140.
3. Martinez-Maldonado M. Approach to the patient with hyperkalemia. In: Kelley WN, ed. *Textbook of internal medicine*. Philadelphia: Lippincott-Raven, 1997.
4. Wallach J, ed. *Interpretation of diagnostic tests*, 6th ed. Boston: Little, Brown and Company, 1996.

17.6 Hypokalemia

Judith A. Fisher and Kent D.W. Bream

Hypokalemia is a common electrolyte abnormality found on chemical assay. Through the prescribing of medication, the medical profession is responsible for many of these low potassium values. While practicing cost-effective medicine, no indication is seen for "routine blood tests." On the other hand, the patient's history often leads to an order for a serum potassium (K^+) level. The normal range for serum potassium is 3.5 to 5.0 mEq/l. In an otherwise healthy patient, dietary deficiencies rarely cause hypokalemia as the body has many compensatory mechanisms (1–4).

   I. **Approach.** The differential diagnoses for low potassium values can be sorted into iatrogenic and disease state causes. They can be further divided into the categories listed in Table 17.6 (Table 17.6).

Table 17.6 Evaluation of the patient with hypokalemia

II. History	III. Physical examination	IV. Further testing	V. Diagnostic assessment
A. Iatrogenic			
Use of loop and thiazide diurectic	Often, no signs on physical examination	Serum electrolytes	Doctor's non-vigilance
Uncontrolled diabetes with glucosuria	Generalized muscle weakness	Spot urine electrolytes if needed	
Insulin use with rapidly falling blood sugars	Constipation	Urine and serum osmolality as needed	
Albuterol, pseudo-ephedrine, terbutaline, and other β-adrenergic drugs	Cachexia	Stool electrolytes as appropriate	
Aminoglycoside antibiotics		Electrocardio-gram (looking for "U" waves) or (if rapidly replacing potassium by the intra-venous route, looking for the development of arrhythmias)	
Amphotericin B			
Chemotherapeutic agents (cisplatin)			
Mineralocorticoid administration			
Barium overuse			
Inadequate intra-venous fluid replacement			
Chloroquine			
B_{12} replacement for pernicious anemia			
Laxative or enema use causing rapid colonic transit (acute or chronic)			
Licorice use	As above	As above	Patient excesses
Chewing tobacco	May also check for evidence to support the history (e.g., low	May also check for ketones, blood sugar, serum pH, serum alcohol	
Salicylate intoxication			
Chronic laxative or enema use			
Anorexia/bulimia			

Table 17.6 *Continued*

II. History	III. Physical examination	IV. Further testing	V. Diagnostic assessment
Forced vomiting or diarrhea for any reason Neurotic spitting Excessive sweating Acute alcohol over ingestion Over-the-counter drug use of any of drugs listed above Many geophagias	weight, staining or pitting of the teeth, irritated throat or rectum, incoordination)	level, drug screen as appropriate	
B. Systemic/Illness Diarrhea from any cause Vomiting from any cause Pyloric or duodenal obstruction Pancreatic fistulas Colon adenomas	Abdominal examination for signs of peritonitis/localized pain	Serum electrolytes Evaluation for cause/site of infection, fistula, or obstruction	Gastrointestinal potassium losses
Many of the iatrogenic causes listed above lead to potassium loss through the kidneys Other renal causes: nephropathies, renal tubular acidosis, renal artery stenosis, glucosuria or any other large metabolite loss through the kidney The genetic syndromes known as Garter's, Gittleman's, and/or Liddle's syndromes Any conditions leading to high serum or body sodium. This includes disorders with aldosterone, renin, and ACTH Syndrome of inappropriate antidiuretic hormone secretion	As above May also check for signs of renal disease/adrenal corticoid excess	As above May also consider serum renin, aldosterone, ACTH, 8 AM cortisol level, thyroid function testing, and BUN/creatinine as appropriate	Renal potassium losses

continued

Table 17.6 *Continued*

II. History	III. Physical examination	IV. Further testing	V. Diagnostic assessment
Metabolic acidosis	As above	As above	Intracellular shifts of potassium
Hyponatremia		Evaluation of underlying disease	
Hypercapnea			
Rapidly falling serum glucose			
Leukemia (K⁺ is taken up by the white blood cells at room temperature)			
β-adrenergic drug use (albuterol, pseudoephedrine, terbutaline)			
Vitamin B_{12} administration			
Chloroquine use			
Cyclic generalized weakness (periodic paralysis)			
Pancreatitis	Signs from underlying disease	Evaluation for underlying disease	Third spacing of fluid
Congestive heart failure			
Toxic shock syndrome			
Pleural effusion			
Peritoneal fluid collection			
Anasarca for any reason			
Second or third degree burns			
Loss of large areas of skin surface			

ACTH, adrenocorticotropic hormone; BUN, blood urea nitrogen.

References

1. Gennari F. Current concepts: hypokalemia. *N Engl J Med* 1998;339(7):451–458.
2. Halperin ML, Kamel KS. Potassium. *Lancet* 1998;352(9122):135–140.
3. Martinez-Maldonado M. Approach to the patient with hypokalemia. In: Kelley WN, ed. *Textbook of internal medicine*. Philadelphia: Lippincott-Raven, 1997.
4. Wallach J, ed. *Interpretation of diagnostic tests*, 6th ed. Boston: Little, Brown and Company, 1996.

18. DIAGNOSTIC IMAGING ABNORMALITIES

ENRIQUE S. FERNANDEZ

18.1 Bone Cyst

Pepi Granat and Omart Robaina

The term "bone cyst" usually denotes simple or solitary bone cyst, which is a benign, smooth, lytic lesion, usually found in children in the metaphysis of long bones, especially the humerus or femur. It can also be found in adults in any location, including the jaw. Another type that is unrelated to the simple cyst, the aneurysmal bone cyst, is also benign but has vascular and blood elements within it, and can be an aggressive lesion. Bone cysts declare themselves to the physician often by spontaneous fracture, or they are found incidentally on an x-ray film.

I. **Approach**. In evaluating a lesion of bone, whether found incidentally on x-ray film or presenting as a pathologic fracture, the important tasks are deciding whether immediate consultation or referral is required and whether the working diagnosis is sufficiently secure to allow for appropriate follow-up and later referral, if indicated.
   A. **Types of bone cysts**
      1. **Simple** (also called solitary; or juvenile—a misleading term because they can be found in adults; or unicameral—also a misnomer because they often are multichambered). Because a bone cyst is picked up only by fracturing or on incidental x-ray, its true incidence is not known, but it is found in 3% of biopsied primary bone "tumors." Radiologists will often state, "They're more common than you think." Half occur at the proximal metaphysis of the humerus. They are identified in male versus female patients in a 2:1 ratio, affecting primarily children between the ages of 5 and 15 years (1).
      The cyst appears as a lytic lesion. Histologically, it is lined with fibrous cells of connective tissue origin. The fluid inside is yellow-brown in color unless previous fracture of cyst or septae formed in response to trauma, which has caused the fluid to turn bloody or dark brown. Cysts are deemed "active" when they abut onto the metaphyseal side of the epiphysial cartilage, and "inactive" when normal bone shows between the cyst and the cartilage (2).
      2. **Aneurysmal bone cyst** is considered a separate, unrelated lesion. Its origin and cause is also clouded in obscurity and controversy. A recent epidemiologic survey of incidence of aneurysmal bone cyst was believed to be the first ever done; it showed the incidence to be 0.14/100,000 population, with female to male incidence significantly greater (3).
      3. **Other lesions** which could look like bone cysts are nonossifying fibroma, enchondroma, fibrous dysplasia, Brodie abscess, chondrosarcoma, osteogenic sarcoma, and Ewing's sarcoma (very rare).
II. **History**
   A. **Pain.** Is this a new patient with sudden onset of severe pain? Is there a history of trauma, mild or severe? Is this a patient with a new bone cyst picked up incidentally on x-ray study? Or is a known bone cyst being followed? Does the patient come in complaining of pain? Or does the patient wait until asked about pain? Significant pain may indicate a traumatic or spontaneous fracture. Is there tenderness elicited over the cyst area? Usually bone cysts are painless, unless they fracture or are growing rapidly. If there is pain or tenderness associated, consider referral or further imaging to differentiate from a more serious lesion.
   B. **Disability, weakness.** Has the little-league baseball player been having trouble with his overhand throwing? Is the swimmer having difficulty with the dolphin stroke? The patient may be guarding with exercise because of pain that occurs only then. Unless the bone cyst is near the growth plate

(epiphysis), it is unlikely to produce impairment of function, but if it abuts the epiphysis, growth arrest with physis damage is likely caused by the cyst itself, not trauma (4).

C. **Distortion, growth, rate of growth.** When examining the child, do the limbs appear different lengths? Have they been measured? If near an epiphysis a bone cyst can impair growth of the limb, causing shortening. These cases need referral early.

III. **Physical examination**

A. **Focused physical examination (PE).** Bone cyst is a diagnosis that should be kept in mind during routine examinations of children, even those not suspected of harboring bone cysts. However, once it appears on x-ray, remember to examine the area on every visit. This should include careful palpation of the bone and entire limb, looking for tender areas or associated soft tissue masses. Comparative measurement should be done with the other limb in any cases of deviation from normal or any protrusion of bone or soft tissue, looking for signs of progression between visits. All these should prompt referral, because they may be signs that the cyst is actually another lesion, or that it is growing, heading for impending fracture, or impinging on the epiphysis.

B. **Additional PE.** Routine growth charts should be maintained meticulously. Measurement of leg and arm lengths to ascertain whether growth is being interfered with is especially pertinent if the bone cyst is near the epiphysial growth plate.

IV. **Testing**

A. **Clinical laboratory tests.** No special tests are necessary, apart from those usually ordered in the course of routine care.

B. **Diagnostic imaging.** The diagnosis is made by x-ray study, but further studies may be indicated to delineate the lesion better. Initial evaluation begins with routine radiography. Certain features help to determine the "biologic activity" or aggressiveness and growth rate of a lesion, which, combined with location and clinical and epidemiologic data can lead to a decision to order additional imaging studies (5).

1. **Plain radiography.** In a study of 709 cases of solitary bone lesions, 40 unicameral bone cysts (UBCs) were analyzed according to demographic, anatomic, and radiographic features (6). Of the 40, 33 (83%) were in long bones and 7 were in the pelvis or calcaneus. All 40 UBCs were geographic, medullary, and lytic. None had an associated soft-tissue mass. Pathologic fractures were present in 55% and 10% had fallen fragment signs; 98% had no cortical break and 88% had well-defined margins. In their conclusion, the authors found a quantitative sensitivity of 80% and specificity of 93% that included the radiographic features of metaphyseal, diaphyseal, or flat bone location; geographic, lytic, or medullary based; no matrix, no satellite lesions, no subarticular extension, no soft-tissue mass, and no cortical break; and a central location in long bones.

2. **Magnetic resonance imaging** has multiplanar imaging and better contrast sensitivity, allowing it to help differentiate benign lesions from malignant ones. The signal intensity on spin-density images can indicate the type of fluid and the presence of septa, and can show if the lesion is fibrous or not. T2-weighted images can show presence or absence of soft-tissue mass. The relationship to the epiphysial plate can be seen well. In addition to causing encroachment into the physis, a large cyst can cause subchondral collapse, joint incongruity, and avascular necrosis (4).

3. **Serial repeat x-ray study.** If electing to follow the cyst, serial plain x-ray studies can be done, cyst diameter measurement taken, or computer assisted densitometric image analysis of serial radiographs obtained.

V. **Diagnostic assessment.** The key to the diagnosis of bone cyst is the typical appearance on x-ray film. When a deviation from the expected image is seen, try to ascertain that the lesion is not a more serious one, either by referral or further imaging. "Active cysts," which abut the growth plate, have the potential to cause damage and should be followed carefully or treated. Fracture of the cyst is commonly the presenting sign.

References
1. Capanna R, Campanacci DA, Manfrini M. Unicameral and aneurysmal bone cysts. *Orthop Clin North Am* 1996;27:605–614.
2. Lokiec F, Wientroub S. Simple bone cyst: etiology, classification, pathology and treatment modalities. *J Pediatr Orthop* Part B 1998;7(4):262–273.
3. Leither A, Windhager R, Lang S, Hass OA, et al. Aneurysmal bone cyst: a population based epidemiological study and literature review. *Clin Orthop* 1999;363:176–179.
4. Gupta AK, Crawford AH. Solitary bone cyst with epiphyseal involvement: confirmation with magnetic resonance imaging. A case report and review of the literature. *J Bone Joint Surg Am* 1996;78:911–915.
5. Deely D, Schweitzer ME. Imaging evaluation of the patient with suspected bone tumor. In: Taveras JM, Ferrucci JT, eds. *Radiology: diagnosis-imaging-intervention*. Philadelphia: Lippincott-Raven Publishers 1998;5(74):1–6.
6. Lee JH. Reinus WR, Wilson AJ. Quantitative analysis of the plain radiographic appearance of unicameral bone cysts. *Invest Radiol* 1999;34(1):28–37.

18.2 Mediastinal Mass

Pepi Granat

Although most mediastinal masses are discovered incidentally on chest radiographs, symptoms can sometimes provide clues enabling the timely ordering of these films. The mediastinum is defined as the extrapleural space within the thorax lying between the lungs. A mass of the mediastinum, by convention, connotes a process with mass effect, whether tumorous, cystic, or vascular. Although two-thirds of all mediastinal tumors are benign and 75% of asymptomatic patients with mediastinal tumors have benign tumors, two-thirds of symptomatic patients will harbor a malignancy. A simple classification (Fraser) into anterior, middle, and posterior mediastinal compartments based on the lateral chest film is clinically useful (1). The more detailed lines and compartments divisions (Felson, Heitzman) are helpful to radiologists (2). Visualizing lung-mediastinal interfaces, where early lesions may be detected, is aided by these lines and signs in both anteroposterior and lateral roentgenograms.

I. **Approach.** Not all mediastinal masses perceived on chest radiograph require invasive investigation; although most will require surgery, histologic sampling by fine needle percutaneous biopsy, or thoracoscopy, some can be followed, depending on location and clinical clues. Some will require emergency action (thoracic aortic dissection), either spontaneous or following injury. All require further imaging usually by computerized tomography (CT). The two indications for ordering mediastinal CT are abnormal chest radiograph and clinical suspicion of mediastinal disease.
    A. **Types of mediastinal masses.** These are classified by general rather than by strict anatomic location; they can be further classified by density and behavior on contrast CT or magnetic resonance imaging (MRI). One easy mnemonic for significant mediastinal tumors is "The Terrible Ts": thymoma, teratoma (embryomal carcinoma), 'terrible' lymphoma (Hodgkin's disease), thyroid carcinoma, neurofibroma ('tingle'), renal cell carcinoma ('tinkle').
    B. Reading the plain films. First, ascertain that the mass is not from lung, pleura, or chest wall. Clues are that masses lying deep to mediastinal vessels are mediastinal in origin; those with irregular, nodular, or spiculated edges arise in the lung; and those broad-based with smooth edge arise in mediastinum or mediastinal pleura. When the rest of the pleura is normal and when no other lung tumors are present, the evidence favors a mediastinal origin. Masses coming from sternum or spine may need CT for better definition of origin. Second, consider anatomic variants such as aortic arch abnormalities, hiatal hernia, and

esophageal mass (3). In the anterioposterior projection, look for the paraspinal lines, paraesophageal line, anterior and posterior junction line, paratracheobronchial line, azygos vein, paraaortic line, and widening of the whole mediastinum. In the lateral view, look for aortic arch and tracheal wall profiles and posterior tracheal band. Masses will displace or efface these lines. Not all lines are constant and normal variations are common.

C. Anatomy and boundaries of the mediastinal compartments (varies slightly with different authors):

1. Anterior mediastinum is defined as the region posterior to the sternum, anterior to the heart and brachiocephalic vessels, extending from the thoracic inlet to the diaphragm. It contains the thymus gland, fat, and lymph nodes.

2. Middle mediastinum is defined as the space containing the heart and pericardium, including the ascending and transverse aorta, brachiocephalic vessels, vena cavae, main pulmonary arteries and veins, trachea, bronchi and lymph nodes.

3. Posterior mediastinum is defined as posterior to the heart and trachea, extending to the thoracic vertebral margin, including the paravertebral gutters. It contains the descending thoracic aorta, esophagus, azygos veins, autonomic ganglia and nerves, thoracic duct, lymph nodes, and fat.

D. Location of mediastinal masses, the most common lesions in various compartments:

1. Anterior mediastinum: aneurysm of ascending aorta, lymphoma, pericardial cyst, retrosternal thyroid, teratoid lesion, and thymic lesion.

2. Middle mediastinum: aneurysm of aortic arch, azygos vein enlargement, bronchogenic cyst, esophageal lesions, hiatal hernia, lymph node enlargement, thyroid tumor, and hilar vascular dilatation.

3. Posterior mediastinum: aneurysm or tortuosity of descending aorta, lymph node enlargement, neurogenic tumor, and paraspinal manifestations of spinal lesions.

E. Some causes of mediastinal and hilar lymph node enlargement (4): bronchogenic carcinoma; Hodgkin's disease and non-Hodgkin's lymphoma; leukemia; immunoblastic lymphadenopathy (a hyperimmune disorder of B lymphocytes); heavy-chain disease (a plasma cell dyscrasia); bronchopulmonary amyloidosis (a plasma cell dyscrasia); lymph node metastasis; Castleman's disease (giant lymph node hyperplasia); bacterial infections, including primary tuberculosis, tularemia, pertussis, anthrax, plague; viral and rickettsial diseases, including *Mycoplasma pneumoniae*, rubeola, Epstein-Barr virus, human immunodeficiency virus (HIV) and acquired immune deficiency syndrome, psittacosis, echovirus pneumonia, varicella pneumonia; fungal infections, including histoplasmosis, coccidioidomycosis, sporotrichosis, and tropical eosinophilia; sarcoidosis; silicosis; beryliosis; histiocytosis X; idopathic pulmonary hemosiderosis and Goodpasture's syndrome, cystic fibrosis, and some are drug-induced.

F. Some causes of mediastinal widening: mediastinal pseudowidening, including expiratory film, scoliosis; normal thymus (neonate); mesothelial (pericardial or pleuropericardial cysts and diverticula); diverticula of pharynx or esophagus; meningocele; tumors, including thyroid masses and tumors, thymoma, teratoma, germinal cell neoplasms, lipoma, liposarcoma, lipomatosis, fibroma, fibrosarcoma, hemangioma, hemangiosarcoma, hemangioendothelioma, lymphangioma, hygroma, leiomyoma; lymphoma (Hodgkin's or non-Hodgkin's), leukemia; metastatic lymph node enlargement; esophageal neoplasms; neurogenic neoplasms; bone and cartilage neoplasms; vascular lesions, including aortic aneurysm, dilatation or aneurysm of innominate artery (right) or subclavian artery (left); aortic arch malformation; mediastinal hemorrhage or hematoma, dilatation of superior vena cava, azygos vein, pulmonary artery; pneumomediastinum; fracture of thoracic vertebra, herniation through foramen of Morgagni, esophageal hiatal hernia, herniation through foramen of

Bochdalek, diaphragmatic eventration, diaphragmatic rupture, megaesophagus, and some occur postsurgery (reconstructions).

II. **History**

A. **Most mediastinal masses, including lymphomas, do not cause symptoms;** however, it is important to pay early attention even to vague symptoms because most symptomatic patients with a mediastinal tumor will have a malignancy. Patients may be completely asymptomatic or their complaints can relate to the underlying disease process: myasthenia gravis or anemia from red cell aplasia, with thymoma; flushing, diarrhea, or Cushing's syndrome, with thymic carcinoid; fatigue and irritability with parathyroid adenoma; fever, night sweats, and pruritus with lymphoma or Hodgkin's; cough, wheezing, dysphagia, or chest pain, with compression or invasion of mediastinal organs (5). A personal or family history of cancer or aneurysms might be significant. Be especially alert to patients with prior tumors, even if benign. Some lesions can recur after many years (thymoma).

B. **Possible symptoms** include fatigue, general weakness, cough, pruritus, chest pain, fever, night sweats, wheezing, dysphagia, stridor, voice change, hoarseness, weight loss, paresthesias, pain, proximal muscle weakness, swelling of face, and venous distention of neck (superior vena cava syndrome).

III. **Physical examination**

A. **A general examination before an x-ray study** gives clue to a mediastinal mass: vital signs, especially temperature, heart rate, and weight; check for pallor, skin lesions, lymphadenopathy, thyromegaly, splenomegaly, other abdominal or pelvic organomegaly or masses, rashes, weakness; auscultate lungs for wheezes, rales, and rhonchi.

B. **Focused reexamination after a mass is detected.** Vital signs, especially temperature, heart rate, and documentation of weight loss; check carefully for cervical adenopathy (suitable for biopsy), evidence of thyromegaly, voice quality, airway patency sitting and supine; and observe the swallowing function. Auscultate the lungs for wheezes, rales, rhonchi; the heart for pericardial rubs; recheck for adenopathy (total body), check skin for melanoma, check testes for masses, and repeat the pelvic examination for ovarian masses.

IV. **Testing**

A. Clinical laboratory tests will depend on the index of suspicion, based on the most common diagnoses in the anatomic location. These may include complete blood count, erythrocyte sedimentation rate, lactic dehydrogenase, alpha fetoprotein, beta fraction human growth hormone, serum calcium, parathormone, gamma globulins, serum antiacetylcholine receptor antibody, purified protein derivative skin test, and HIV antibody screening.

B. Imaging studies. Any patient, but especially smokers or exsmokers, with unexplained peripheral adenopathy, unexplained cough, or any of the aforementioned symptoms, should have a chest x-ray study after no more than 2 to 3 weeks of symptomatic treatment. Any mediastinal mass seen requires a CT with iodinated bolus. The indications for mediastinal MRI are suspected vascular lesion, equivocal CT findings, posterior or paravertebral masses and neurogenic tumors, and suspected tumor recurrence so that scarring can be delineated from tumor. The MRI should be ordered with T1- and T2-weighted images and gadolinium-enhanced T1 images.

V. **Diagnostic assessment.** Correlation of the clinical and imaging picture is paramount in deciding the extent of the investigation of a mediastinal mass, because of the fairly predictable location pattern of various lesions. A patient with acute, searing chest pain and mediastinal widening will need emergent attention for thoracic aortic dissection. An anterior solid mass in a patient with cough and weight loss demands a tissue diagnosis and, if operable, surgical extirpation. A posterior cystic mass in a healthy patient may allow close follow-up. However, much overlap is seen (6), and diagnostic accuracy is better based on direct clues (e.g., tissue diagnosis) and on solid clinical judgment to include surgical diagnosis or treatment or medical or oncologic methods, if inoperable.

References

1. Strollo DC, Rosado-de-Christenson ML, Jett JR. Primary mediastinal tumors. Part I: Tumors of the anterior mediastinum. *Chest* 1997;12(2):511–522.
2. Giron J, Fajadet P, Sans N, et al. Diagnostic approach to mediastinal masses. *Eur J Radiol* 1998;27(1):21–42.
3. Laurent F, Latrabe V, Lecesne R, et al. Mediastinal masses: diagnostic approach. *Eur Radiol* 1998;8(7):1148–1159.
4. Mediastinal or hilar enlargement. In: Burgener FA, Kormano M. *Differential diagnosis in conventional radiology*, 2nd revised ed. London: Thieme Medical Publishers, 1991.
5. Strollo DC, Rosado-de-Christenson ML, Jett JR. Primary mediastinal tumors. Part II. Tumors of the middle and posterior mediastinum. *Chest* 1997;112(5):1344–1357.
6. Ahn JM, Lee KS, Goo JM, Song KS, Kim SJ, Im JG. Predicting the histology of anterior mediastinal masses: comparison of chest radiography and CT. *J Thorac Imaging* 1996;11(4):265–271.

18.3 Osteopenia

Pepi Granat

Osteopenia, which means "thin bone," refers to low bone mass. It is now defined quantitatively on the basis of bone mineral density (BMD) using T scores, or the number of standard deviations (SD) below young adult reference means. A BMD of 1 to 2.5 SD below mean is osteopenia. Osteoporosis is defined as less than –2.5 T score, without fractures; established osteoporosis is less than –2.5 T score with fractures (1). The high risk of fracture makes osteoporosis a dangerous disease, leading to immobilization, atelectasis or pneumonia, morbidity, and mortality. The success of prevention and treatment makes the diagnosis of osteopenia crucial.

I. **Approach.** Whether evaluating an incidental finding of osteopenia on routine radiograph or finding low BMD on dual energy x-ray absorptiometry (DEXA, DXA) scan, consider the limitations of both tests, and possible causes of the osteopenia. Approximately 30% of the bone mineral must be lost before a decrease in BMD can be detected on plain x-ray film and the interobserver variation is wide. In women referred for BMD to help in hormone replacement therapy decisions, the frequency of osteopenia was similar to that in the low-risk population; 30% were identified at high risk of fracture. In approximately 85% of those who were referred for radiographic evidence of osteopenia, the diagnosis was confirmed by DXA scan (2). In the elderly or in those with marked degenerative joint disease, aortic calcifications, narrowed disk spaces, or osteophytes, spine BMD may be artifactually elevated; therefore, plain radiographs can help reduce errors by identifying abnormal areas to exclude from BMD analysis.

    A. **Types of osteopenia.** Two types of generalized osteopenia are seen: primary and secondary. Primary is composed of idiopathic juvenile and young adult osteoporosis, and involutional osteoporosis, type I (postmenopausal) and type II (senile). Secondary is composed of osteopenia related to medical, surgical, or medication conditions associated with bone loss, such as hyperthyroidism, hyperparathyroidism, hypogonadism, hypercortisolism, seizure disorder (anticonvulsants), malabsorption syndrome, rheumatoid arthritis, connective tissue disease, chronic neurologic disease, chronic obstructive lung disease, malignancy, inherited inborn errors of metabolism (e.g., osteogenesis imperfecta), and certain medications (e.g., glucocorticoids and heparin).

    B. **Special concerns.** The most common type of osteopenia is the postmenopausal involutional type. Both men and women lose bone mass as they age, but it is accelerated at the time of menopause. On average, women lose

8% of bone per decade after age 40, men 3% (3). Women's lower peak bone mass predisposes them to fracture rates two to three times that of men, yet the 1-year mortality rate following hip fracture in men is nearly double that of women (4). Osteopenia can be generalized or localized.

II. History

A. **Present illness.** Is the patient complaining of anything relevant to osteopenia right now? Does the patient have pain and, if so, where is the pain? Has the patient fallen? What is happening in the patient's life?

B. **Past medical history.** Carefully question your female patients about their menstrual history, even if elderly, looking for evidence of reduced peak bone mass. Ask about periods of amenorrhea, pregnancy, and lactation; anorexia or other eating disorder; steroid history (e.g., asthma therapy). Also ask about oral contraceptives and hormones, thyroid medicine, diet doctors and diet pills (in the past such pills often contained thyroid extract), and past illnesses.

C. **Family history.** A positive family history for osteopenia is associated with low BMD. Ask not just whether any family member had diagnosed osteopenia or osteoporosis, but ask whether grandma stooped over and whether grandpa broke his hip? Who in the family had broken bones?

D. **Habits.** What is the patient's diet? Does or did the patient smoke? How much? How long? How much caffeine does the patient take in? Does the patient now or ever did exercise? How far, how fast, how long, how often? Does the patient take calcium supplements? Antacids? Ask about daily calcium-containing foods. Does the patient always wear sunscreen or stay indoors? Is the patient taking Vitamin D? How much sun is in your area? In men, ask about symptoms of low testosterone. Get a detailed injury history. Ask about falling.

E. **Other information.** Get a detailed medication history. Have the patient bring in all pills in the medicine closet, not just present medication. Obtain old medical records. Ask about the home situation. For example, safety: Are throw rugs used? Are handrails installed in the bathrooms?

III. Physical examination

A. **Focused physical examination.** Vital signs, weight, gait, posture, and silhouette. Is the patient kyphotic? Palpate the patient's spine.

B. **Focal tenderness to suggest vertebral fracture.** Observe other bones. Are they deformed? Does the male patient have signs of low testosterone? How is the patient's balance? Is the patient at risk for falls?

C. **Additional physical findings.** Note signs of poor nutrition or development.

IV. Testing

A. **Clinical laboratory tests.** Specific bone-related markers and general screening tests.

1. Biochemical measurements on serum or urine measure activity of bone remodeling, formation, and breakdown (resorption). Serum markers of bone formation: osteocalcin, serum alkaline phosphatase (specific for bone), and procollagen extension peptides. Urine markers of bone resorption: pyridinoline, deoxypyridinoline, N-telopeptide of the cross-links of collagen, and C-telopeptide of the cross-links of collagen. These show rates of bone loss (or gain) and are an option most useful for diagnosing improvement during therapy. These markers can change after 3 months of treatment; it takes 2 years of therapy for BMD to show change (5).

2. A serum chemical profile helps exclude secondary causes of bone loss. A complete blood count (hematologic disorders), a C-reactive protein, or erythrocyte sedimentation rate (nonspecific inflammation or malignancy), a sensitive thyroid-stimulating hormone assay (hyperthyroidism), a blood urea nitrogen or creatinine (renal dysfunction) level, various hepatic function tests, an albumin, globulin, total protein (myeloma), or a serum protein electrophoresis are reasonable baseline measurements. A 24-hour urine for calcium, if elevated, can guide calcium dose or require separate therapy. If reduced, think of vitamin D malnutrition or malabsorption.

B. **Diagnostic imaging.** The patient at risk for osteopenia by history or physical examination can have a fairly reliable, inexpensive screening calcaneal imaging study, followed by a DXA scan if osteopenia is suggested. Newer modalities including broadband ultrasound may come into wider use. When osteopenia is identified by plain radiograph, send the patient for a DXA scan. If the patient is elderly, remember the limits of the spine DXA scan to reflect accurately the true bone density at that site; review the plain radiographs to clarify. Calcaneal imaging should not be used to follow treatment because its accuracy is not as reliable as the DXA scan. Because physicians commonly give postmenopausal women estrogen replacement, the question of routine screening for osteopenia might be appropriate in those for whom the finding of a low bone density would influence the woman's decision to take hormones.

V. **Diagnostic assessment.** The standard method of diagnosing osteopenia measures BMD using a DXA scan. Diagnosing the cause of the osteopenia is necessary for appropriate treatment and prevention of further bone loss. Radiographic evidence of osteopenia is a strong predictor of low BMD. Assess the patient's risk factors, present and past, do appropriate testing, and consider secondary causes.

References

1. Lenchik I, Sartoris DJ. Current concepts in osteoporosis. *Am J Rheum* 1997;168: 905–911.
2. Ahmed AI, Illic D, Blake GM, Rymer JM, Fogelman I. Review of 3,530 referrals of bone density measurement of spine and femur: evidence that radiographic osteopenia predicts low bone mass. *Radiology* 1998;207:619–624.
3. Burgener F. Osteopenia. In: Kormano, ed. *Differential diagnosis in conventional radiology*. London: Thieme Medical Publishers, 1991:3–12.
4. National Osteoporosis Foundation. Osteoporosis. Part II: Equipment, measurements, quality assurance and treatment. *Bull Am Coll Radiol* 1998;54:14–18.
5. Khosla S. Osteoporosis. In: Rakel R, ed. *Conn's current therapy*. Philadelphia: WB Saunders, 1998:589–593.

18.4 Solitary Pulmonary Nodule

Michael J. Dodard

The solitary pulmonary nodule (SPN) remains a challenge for the clinician despite major advances in diagnostic imaging. Expectant management carries the risk of missing a malignancy of the lung, whereas a surgical approach can be overly aggressive because most SPNs are caused by benign processes.

I. **Approach.** The SPN, which is defined as a midlateral lung density with fairly well-defined margins, surrounded by normal lung fields, measures between 1 and 5 cm. It is usually found in an asymptomatic patient and is seen in 0.1% to 0.2% of chest x-ray films (1). It is imperative to confirm that the abnormality seen on the x-ray film is really located in the lung parenchyma. Skin moles, nipple shadows, and pleural plaques can all mimic SPNs and can be correctly identified by proper radiologic techniques. The causes of SPNs are multiple: granulomatous, infectious vascular processes and immune diseases, cystic growths, and neoplasms (benign or malignant).

The probability of an SPN being malignant has been calculated to be 2% at age 30 and to increase by 10% to 15% with each succeeding decade (2). Overall, 20% to 40% of all SPNs will be found to be malignant, mostly from lung cancer.

A. **Benign causes (60% to 80%)**

　　1. 85% to 90% of benign SPNs are granulomas, caused by tuberculosis, sarcoidosis, histoplasmosis, or coccidioidomycosis. Other rare causes include pulmonary hyalinizing granulomas, *Dirofilaria immitis* ("dog heart worm") and *Mycobacterium avium intracellulare*.

  2. 5% hematomas
  3. 5% to 10% are caused by immune diseases, particularly rheumatoid arthritis, amyloidosis, pseudolymphoma, bronchogenic cysts, hydatid cysts, and arteriovenous malformations
   B. **Malignant causes (20% to 40%)**
   1. Primary lung tumor (75%)
   2. Metastatic lesions to the lungs from breast, colon, and testicular cancer (25%)
 II. **History.** Obtain a complete history, including smoking, occupational exposure, immigration, and travel. Check previous chest x-ray studies to establish prior presence of a nodule, as well as growth on an existing nodule. An absence of growth over a period of 2 years is generally accepted as a sign of the benign nature of a SPN.
III. **Physical examination** should include a search for evidence of weight loss, chronic obstructive pulmonary disease, and primary or metastatic disease of other organs.
IV. **Testing.** The key question is to determine which one of the SPNs is malignant and warrants invasive and immediate action. The following factors can help determine a course of management:
   A. **Location.** Generally, most malignant lesions are found in the upper lobes.
   B. **Appearance.** The smooth margins seen on computerized tomography (CT) scan characterize benign lesions, whereas spiculated, irregular borders are associated with malignant growths.
   C. **Size.** Small size (<2 cm) is most frequently a sign of benignity, although it can be caused by an early, isolated pulmonary metastasis from a primary cancer at another site.
   D. **Calcifications.** Peripheral, concentric patterns ("bull's eyes" in granulomas, "popcorn ball" in hematomas) (3) have been associated with benign lesions, but the presence of calcifications has not been found to be a reliable indicator in predicting malignancy, because 14% of cancerous lesions can be calcified.
   E. **Aging.** The CT scan of the chest is widely available and noninvasive. It accurately measures the nodule and defines its location and morphology.
   F. **Preliminary results** with high resolution computerized tomography with contrast indicate good accuracy in the determination of the nodule malignancy. The MRI is not a preferred imaging tool to analyze a pulmonary nodule but its superior capacity to enhance vascular structures can be useful in the differential diagnosis.
 V. **Diagnostic assessment.** Controversy exists as to the best way to manage SPN. The decision to observe or to intervene is guided by the following parameters: patient's age, smoking history, location of the nodule, availability of previous x-ray studies, and presence and type of calcifications.
   A. **Observation.** A stable (no growth in 2 years) calcified lesion in a nonsmoker, aged less than 35 years, is almost certainly benign, and can safely be managed by repeat chest x-ray study every 3 months in the first year, then every year for 2 years. The patient's cooperation and the family physician's meticulous follow-up are essential to the success of this plan.
   B. **Intervention.** An irregular, noncalcified lesion, particularly in a smoker or older patient, warrants invasive intervention to obtain a tissue diagnosis.
   1. **Fiberoptic bronchoscopy** is the procedure of choice for centrally located SPNs.
   2. For peripheral lesions, **percutaneous needle biopsy** is a quick, relatively easy procedure when done by an experienced operator. Its low rate of specificity and potential risks of pneumothorax and bleeding make it a poor choice because the goal is to reach a diagnosis with the least discomfort to the patient.
   3. **Thoracoscopic fine-needle aspiration** is becoming an alternative to percutaneous needle biopsy. In a small surgical series, it provided an accurate diagnosis in all cases and helped to define the next surgical step (4).

4. A new surgical technique, **video-assisted thoracic surgery (VATS)**, is
fast becoming the diagnostic tool of choice for suspected SPN (5). Its yield
is excellent and its capacity allows resectability of benign lesions without
thoracotomy; its very low rate of morbidity and mortality are welcome
additions to the approach to this difficult problem.

References

1. Turpin S, Maroves H, Costa P, Medeiros F, Ramos M, de Olivera JP. The solitary
   pulmonary nodule: a retrospective study of 119 cases. *Acta Med Port* 1998;11(6):
   533–538.
2. Swensen SJ, Silverstein MD, Ilstrup DM, Schleck CD, Edell ES. The probability of
   malignancy in solitary pulmonary nodules. Application to small radiologically indeterminate nodules. *Arch Intern Med* 1997;157:849–855.
3. Caskey CI, Templeton PA, Zerhouni EA. Current evaluation of the solitary pulmonary
   nodule. *Surg Clin North Am* 1990;28(3):511–520.
4. Bousahra M 2nd, Clowry L Jr. Thoracoscopic fine needle aspiration of solitary pulmonary nodules. *Ann Thorac Surg* 1997;64:1191–1193.
5. Hazelrigg SR, Magee MJ, Cetindag LB. Video assisted thoracic surgery. *Chest Surg
   Clin North Am* 1998;8:763–774, vii.

SUBJECT INDEX

Note: Page numbers in *italics* indicate figures; page numbers followed by t indicate tables.

WMD 021001